Emerging Infectious Diseases

Diseases

SOURCEBOOK

FIRST EDITION

Health Reference Series

Emerging Infectious Diseases

SOURCEBOOK

FIRST EDITION

Basic Consumer Health Information about the Immune System, Facts about the Spread of Diseases, Information on Emerging Infectious Diseases Such as Avian Influenza, Chikungunya, *Cryptococcus gattii* Infection, Ebola Virus Disease (EVD), Lassa Fever, Lyme Disease, Nipah Virus Infection (NVI), Severe Acute Respiratory Syndrome (SARS), Yellow Fever, and Zika Fever, and the Impact of Climate Change on the Outbreak of Diseases, International Travel Guidance, Diagnostic Tests, and Treatment Methods

Along with Preventing Infectious Diseases, a Glossary of Related Medical Terms, and a Directory of Sources for Further Help and Information

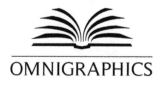

OMNIGRAPHICS

615 Griswold, Ste. 520, Detroit, MI 48226

Bibliographic Note
Because this page cannot legibly accommodate all the copyright notices, the Bibliographic
Note portion of the Preface constitutes an extension of the copyright notice.

* * *

OMNIGRAPHICS
Angela L. Williams, *Managing Editor*
* * *

Library of Congress Cataloging-in-Publication Data
Names: Omnigraphics, Inc., issuing body.

Title: Emerging infectious diseases sourcebook: basic consumer health information
about immune system, facts about the spread of diseases, information on emerging
infectious diseases such as avian influenza, chikungunya, *Crytococcus gattii* infection,
ebola virus disease (EVD), lassa fever, lyme disease, nipah virus infection (NVI),
severe acute respiratory syndrome (SARS), yellow fever, zika fever, and the impact of
climate change on the outbreak of diseases, international travel guidance, diagnostic
tests, treatment methods, and prevention and vaccination programs, along with
reports on current research initiatives, a glossary of related medical terms, and a
directory of sources for further help and information.

Description: 1st edition. | Detroit, MI: Omnigraphics, Inc., [2019] | Includes index.

Identifiers: LCCN 2019017641 (print) | LCCN 2019018249 (ebook) | ISBN
9780780817104 (ebook) | ISBN 9780780817098 (hard cover: alk. paper)

Subjects: LCSH: Communicable diseases--Popular works.

Classification: LCC RA643 (ebook) | LCC RA643.E64 2019 (print) | DDC 616.9--dc23

LC record available at https://lccn.loc.gov/2019017641

Table of Contents

Part II: Types of Emerging and Reemerging Infectious Diseases

Part III: Emerging Infectious Diseases Risk due to Climate Change

Part IV: International Travel and Infectious Diseases

Part V: Medical Diagnosis and Treatment of Infectious Diseases

Part VI: Preventing Infectious Diseases

Part VII: Additional Help and Information

Preface

About This Book

Diseases that have newly emerged within specific population groups or those with increased rate of incidence in the recent past are considered emerging infectious diseases. Ecological changes, evolution of microbial pathogens, frequent traveling, bioterrorism, etc. are some of the prime reasons for the outbreak of infectious diseases. Recent examples of such outbreaks include avian influenza, chikungunya, *Cryptococcus gattii* infection, Ebola virus disease (EVD), Lassa fever, Lyme disease, Nipah virus infection (NVI), severe acute respiratory syndrome (SARS), yellow fever, Zika fever, and more. Proper public health and vaccination programs can reduce the spread of infectious diseases to a great extent. However, the return of old communicable diseases, emergence of new ones, and evolution of antimicrobial resistance have made treatments less effective and continue to present challenges. Emerging infectious diseases remain a major public-health concern in the United States and around the world.

Emerging Infectious Diseases Sourcebook, First Edition provides information about various emerging and reemerging infectious diseases and explains how the immune system works against these infections. It describes how climatic changes impact the outbreak and spread of infectious diseases. Guidance for international travelers to protect themselves from such diseases is also provided. Types of diagnostic tests, treatment methods that are available, and preventive measures for different kinds of infectious diseases are also explained in detail. The book concludes with a glossary of related terms and a directory of additional resources.

How to Use This Book

This book is divided into parts and chapters. Parts focus on broad areas of interest. Chapters are devoted to single topics within a part.

Part I: What You Need to Know about Infectious Diseases begins with an introduction to emerging infectious diseases and explains how the diseases get transmitted. It also describes the functions of the immune system and how it works to recognize or fight against infectious diseases.

Part II: Types of Emerging and Reemerging Infectious Diseases provides facts about various diseases caused by bacteria, virus, fungi, and so on. The part discusses the mode of transmission, causes, symptoms, diagnosis, treatment, and preventive measures for specific infectious diseases.

Part III: Emerging Infectious Diseases Risk due to Climate Change explains how climatic changes influence and affect the environment around us—air, soil, water, and food—resulting in the outbreak and spread of several infectious diseases. It also discusses about the health impacts of climatic changes across different population groups in the United States and preventive measures to be taken to minimize the impact.

Part IV: International Travel and Infectious Diseases provides guidance for international travelers to stay away from infectious diseases. It also deals with aircraft and vessel management systems to prevent the spread of diseases.

Part V: Medical Diagnosis and Treatment of Infectious Diseases outlines the tests and procedures used to identify the presence of infection or infection-causing pathogens. Antibiotics, antivirals, prescription medications, and other over-the-counter (OTC) medicines available for emerging and reemerging diseases are discussed. The growing problem of antimicrobial resistance—the way microbes change to counteract the effectiveness of drug treatments—is also explained.

Part VI: Preventing Infectious Diseases offers information about a simple practice that is a key element in the fight against the spread of germs—handwashing—and also provides details on vaccines, another effective tool for halting the spread of disease. It provides vaccine recommendations for children, adolescents, and adults, and also addresses problems associated with vaccines, the vaccine adverse event reporting system, and the difficulties that can arise as a result of vaccine misinformation. It concludes by discussing quarantine and isolation for controlling contagious diseases.

Part VII: Additional Help and Information offers a glossary of important terms and a directory of government agencies and private organizations that provide help and information to patients with infectious diseases.

Bibliographic Note

This volume contains documents and excerpts from publications issued by the following U.S. government agencies: Agency for Healthcare Research and Quality (AHRQ); Centers for Disease Control and Prevention (CDC); Chemical Hazards Emergency Medical Management (CHEMM); Genetic and Rare Diseases Information Center (GARD); National Institute of Allergy and Infectious Diseases (NIAID); National Institutes of Health (NIH); Occupational Safety and Health Administration (OSHA); Office of Disease Prevention and Health Promotion (ODPHP); *Ready*, U.S. Department of Homeland Security; U.S. Department of Health and Human Services (HHS); and U.S. Global Change Research Program (USGCRP).

About the Health Reference Series

The *Health Reference Series* is designed to provide basic medical information for patients, families, caregivers, and the general public. Each volume takes a particular topic and provides comprehensive coverage. This is especially important for people who may be dealing with a newly diagnosed disease or a chronic disorder in themselves or in a family member. People looking for preventive guidance, information about disease warning signs, medical statistics, and risk factors for health problems will also find answers to their questions in the *Health Reference Series*. The *Series*, however, is not intended to serve as a tool for diagnosing illness, in prescribing treatments, or as a substitute for the physician/patient relationship. All people concerned about medical symptoms or the possibility of disease are encouraged to seek professional care from an appropriate healthcare provider.

A Note about Spelling and Style

Health Reference Series editors use *Stedman's Medical Dictionary* as an authority for questions related to the spelling of medical terms and the *Chicago Manual of Style* for questions related to grammatical structures, punctuation, and other editorial concerns. Consistent adherence is not always possible, however, because the individual volumes within the *Series* include many documents from a wide variety of different producers, and the editor's primary goal is to present material from each source as accurately as is possible. This sometimes means that information in different chapters or sections may follow other guidelines and alternate spelling authorities. For example, occasionally a copyright holder may require that eponymous terms be shown in possessive forms (Crohn's disease vs. Crohn disease) or that British spelling norms be retained (leukaemia vs. leukemia).

Medical Review

Omnigraphics contracts with a team of qualified, senior medical professionals who serve as medical consultants for the *Health Reference Series*. As necessary, medical consultants review reprinted and originally written material for currency and accuracy. Citations including the phrase "Reviewed (month, year)" indicate material reviewed by this team. Medical consultation services are provided to the *Health Reference Series* editors by:

Dr. Vijayalakshmi, MBBS, DGO, MD
Dr. Senthil Selvan, MBBS, DCH, MD
Dr. K. Sivanandham, MBBS, DCH, MS (Research), PhD

Our Advisory Board

We would like to thank the following board members for providing initial guidance on the development of this series:

- Dr. Lynda Baker, Associate Professor of Library and Information Science, Wayne State University, Detroit, MI

- Nancy Bulgarelli, William Beaumont Hospital Library, Royal Oak, MI

- Karen Imarisio, Bloomfield Township Public Library, Bloomfield Township, MI

- Karen Morgan, Mardigian Library, University of Michigan-Dearborn, Dearborn, MI

- Rosemary Orlando, St. Clair Shores Public Library, St. Clair Shores, MI

Health Reference Series *Update Policy*

The inaugural book in the *Health Reference Series* was the first edition of *Cancer Sourcebook* published in 1989. Since then, the *Series* has been enthusiastically received by librarians and in the medical community. In order to maintain the standard of providing high-quality health information for the layperson the editorial staff at Omnigraphics felt it was necessary to implement a policy of updating volumes when warranted.

Medical researchers have been making tremendous strides, and it is the purpose of the *Health Reference Series* to stay current with the most recent advances. Each decision to update a volume is made on an individual basis. Some of the considerations include how much new information is available and the feedback we receive from people who use the books. If there is a topic you would like to see added to the update list, or an area of medical concern you feel has not been adequately addressed, please write to:

Managing Editor
Health Reference Series
Omnigraphics
615 Griswold, Ste. 520
Detroit, MI 48226

Part One

What You Need to Know about Infectious Diseases

Chapter 1

Understanding Emerging Infectious Diseases

Infectious diseases emerging throughout history have included some of the most feared plagues of the past. New infections continue to emerge today, while many of the old plagues are with us still. These are global problems (William Foege, the former director at the Centers for Disease Control and Prevention (CDC) who is now at the Carter Center, terms them "global infectious disease threats"). As demonstrated by influenza epidemics, under suitable circumstances, a new infection first appearing anywhere in the world could traverse entire continents within days or weeks.

"Emerging infections" can be defined as those that have newly appeared in the population or those that have existed but are rapidly increasing in incidence or geographic range. Recent examples of emerging diseases in various parts of the world include human immunodeficiency virus (HIV)/acquired immunodeficiency syndrome (AIDS); classic cholera in South America and Africa; cholera due to *Vibrio cholerae* O139; Rift Valley fever; *Hantavirus* pulmonary syndrome (HPS); Lyme disease; and hemolytic uremic syndrome (HUS), a foodborne infection caused by certain strains of *Escherichia coli* (in the United States, serotype O157:H7).

This chapter includes text excerpted from "Factors in the Emergence of Infectious Diseases," Centers for Disease Control and Prevention (CDC), June 8, 2011. Reviewed May 2019.

Although these occurrences may appear inexplicable, emerging infections rarely appear without reason. Specific factors responsible for disease emergence can be identified in virtually all cases studied. It has been suggested that infectious disease emergence can be viewed operationally as a two-step process: 1. introduction of the agent into a new host population (whether the pathogen originated in the environment, possibly in another species, or as a variant of an existing human infection), followed by 2. establishment and further dissemination within the new host population. Whatever its origin, the infection emerges when it reaches a new population.

Factors that promote one or both of these steps will, therefore, tend to precipitate disease emergence. Most emerging infections, and even antibiotic-resistant strains of common bacterial pathogens, usually originate in one geographic location and then disseminate to new places.

Regarding the introduction step, the numerous examples of infections originating as zoonoses (infections transmitted to humans by animals) suggest that the zoonotic pool introductions of infections from other species is an important and potentially rich source of emerging diseases; periodic discoveries of new zoonoses suggest that the zoonotic pool appears by no means exhausted. Once introduced, an infection might then be disseminated through other factors, although rapid course and high mortality combined with low transmissibility are often limiting.

However, even if a zoonotic agent is not able to spread readily from person to person and establish itself, other factors (e.g., nosocomial infection) might transmit the infection. Additionally, if the reservoir host or vector becomes more widely disseminated, the microbe can appear in new places. Bubonic plague transmitted by rodent fleas and rat-borne *Hantavirus* infections are examples.

Most emerging infections appear to be caused by pathogens already present in the environment, brought out of obscurity or given a selective advantage by changing conditions and afforded an opportunity to infect new host populations (on rare occasions, a new variant may also evolve and cause a new disease). The process by which infectious agents may transfer from animals to humans or disseminate from isolated groups into new populations can be called "microbial traffic." A number of activities increase microbial traffic and, as a result, promote emergence and epidemics. In some cases, including many of the most novel infections, the agents are zoonotic, crossing from their natural hosts into the human population. In other cases, pathogens already present in geographically isolated populations are given an opportunity to disseminate further. Surprisingly often, disease emergence is caused by human actions, however inadvertently; natural causes, such as changes in climate, can also at times be responsible. Although this discussion is confined largely to human disease, similar considerations apply to emerging pathogens in other species.

Any categorization of the factors is, of course, somewhat arbitrary but should be representative of the underlying processes that cause emergence. According to the Institute of Medicine's (IOM) report on emerging infections and the CDC's emerging infections plan, responsible factors include ecological changes, such as those due to agricultural or economic development or to anomalies in climate; human demographic changes and behavior; travel and commerce; technology and industry; microbial adaptation and change; and breakdown of public health measures.

Ecological interactions can be complex, with several factors often working together or in sequence. For example, population movement from rural areas to cities can spread a once-localized infection. The strain on infrastructure in the overcrowded and rapidly growing cities may disrupt or slow public health measures, perhaps allowing establishment of the newly introduced infection. Finally, the city may also provide a gateway for further dissemination of the infection. Most successful emerging infections, including HIV, cholera, and dengue, have followed this route.

Consider HIV as an example. Although the precise ancestry of HIV-1 is still uncertain, it appears to have had a zoonotic origin. Ecological factors that would have allowed human exposure to a natural host carrying the virus that was the precursor to HIV-1 were, therefore, instrumental in the introduction of the virus into humans. This probably occurred in a rural area. A plausible scenario is suggested by the identification of an HIV-2-infected man in a rural area of Liberia whose virus strain resembled viruses isolated from the sooty mangabey monkey (an animal widely hunted for food in rural areas and the putative source of HIV-2) more closely than it did strains circulating in the city.

Such findings suggest that zoonotic introductions of this sort may occur on occasion in isolated populations but may go unnoticed so long as the recipients remain isolated. But with increasing movement from rural areas to cities, such isolation is increasingly rare. After its likely first move from a rural area into a city, HIV-1 spread regionally along highways, then by long-distance routes, including air travel, to more distant places. This last step was critical for HIV and facilitated today's global pandemic. Social changes that allowed the virus to reach a larger population and to be transmitted, despite its relatively low natural transmissibility, were instrumental in the success of the virus in its newfound human host. For HIV, the long duration of infectivity allowed this normally poorly transmissible virus many opportunities to be transmitted and to take advantage of such factors as human behavior (sexual transmission, intravenous drug use) and changing technology (early spread through blood transfusions and blood products).

Ecological Changes and Agricultural Development

Ecological changes, including those due to agricultural or economic development, are among the most frequently identified factors in emergence. They are especially frequent as factors in outbreaks of previously unrecognized diseases with high case-fatality rates, which often turn out to be zoonotic introductions. Ecological factors usually precipitate emergence by placing people in contact with a natural reservoir or host for an infection hitherto unfamiliar but usually already present (often a zoonotic or arthropod-borne infection), either by increasing proximity or, often, also by changing conditions so as to favor an increased population of the microbe or its natural host. The emergence of Lyme disease in the United States and Europe was probably due largely to reforestation, which increased the population of deer and the deer tick, the vector of Lyme disease. The movement of people into these areas placed a larger population in close proximity to the vector.

Agricultural development, one of the most common ways in which people alter and interpose themselves into the environment, is often a factor. Hantaan virus, the cause of Korean hemorrhagic fever, causes over 100,000 cases a year in China and has been known in Asia for centuries. The virus is a natural infection of the field mouse Apodemus agrarius. The rodent flourishes in rice fields; people usually contract the disease during the rice harvest from contact with infected rodents. Junin virus, the cause of Argentine hemorrhagic fever, is an unrelated virus with a history remarkably similar to that of Hantaan virus. Conversion of grassland to maize cultivation favored a rodent that was the natural host for this virus, and human cases increased in proportion with expansion of maize agriculture. Other examples, in addition to those already known, are likely to appear as new areas are placed under cultivation.

Perhaps most surprisingly, pandemic influenza appears to have an agricultural origin, integrated pig–duck farming in China. Strains causing the frequent annual or biennial epidemics generally result from mutation (antigenic drift), but pandemic influenza viruses do not generally arise by this process. Instead, gene segments from two influenza strains reassort to produce a new virus that can infect humans. Evidence amassed indicates that waterfowl, such as ducks, are major reservoirs of influenza and that pigs can serve as mixing vessels for new mammalian influenza strains. Pandemic influenza viruses have generally come from China. Scholtissek and Naylor suggested that integrated pig-duck agriculture, an extremely efficient food production system traditionally practiced in certain parts of China for several centuries, puts these two species in contact and provides a natural laboratory for making new influenza recombinants. Webster has suggested that, with high-intensity agriculture and movement of livestock across borders, suitable conditions may now also be found in Europe.

Water is also frequently associated with disease emergence. Infections transmitted by mosquitoes or other arthropods, which include some of the most serious and widespread diseases, are often stimulated by the expansion of standing water, simply because many of the mosquito vectors breed in water. There are many cases of diseases transmitted by water-breeding vectors, most involving dams, water for irrigation, or stored drinking water in cities. The incidence of Japanese encephalitis, another mosquito-borne disease that accounts for almost 30,000 human cases and approximately 7,000 deaths annually in Asia, is closely associated with flooding of fields for rice growing. Outbreaks of Rift Valley fever in some parts of Africa have been associated with dam building, as well as with periods of heavy rainfall. In the outbreaks of Rift Valley fever in Mauritania in 1987, the human cases occurred in villages near dams on the Senegal River. The same effect has been documented with other infections that have aquatic hosts, such as schistosomiasis.

Because humans are important agents of ecological and environmental change, many of these factors are anthropogenic. Of course, this is not always the case, and natural environmental changes, such as climate or weather anomalies, can have the same effect. The outbreak of *Hantavirus* pulmonary syndrome in the southwestern United States in 1993 is an example. It is likely that the virus has long been present in mouse populations, but an unusually mild and wet winter and spring in that area led to an increased rodent population in the spring and summer and, thus, to greater opportunities for people to come in contact with infected rodents (and, hence, with the virus); it has been suggested that the weather anomaly was due to large-scale climatic effects. The same causes may have been responsible for outbreaks of *Hantavirus* disease in Europe at approximately the same time. With cholera, it has been suggested that certain organisms in marine environments are natural reservoirs for cholera vibrios, and that large scale effects on ocean currents may cause local increases in the reservoir organism with consequent flare-ups of cholera.

Changes in Human Demographics and Behavior

Human population movements or upheavals, caused by migration or war, are often important factors in disease emergence. In many parts of the world, economic conditions are encouraging the mass movement of workers from rural areas to cities. The United Nations has estimated that, largely as a result of continuing migration, by the year 2025, 65 percent of the world population (also expected to be larger in absolute numbers), including 61 percent of the population in developing regions, will live in cities. As discussed above for HIV, rural urbanization allows infections arising in isolated rural areas, which may once have remained obscure and localized, to reach larger populations. Once in a city, the newly introduced infection would have the opportunity to spread locally among the population and could also spread further along highways and interurban transport routes and by airplane.

HIV has been, and in Asia is becoming, the best known beneficiary of this dynamic, but many other diseases, such as dengue, stand to benefit. The frequency of the most severe form, dengue hemorrhagic fever, which is thought to occur when a person is sequentially infected by 2 types of dengue virus, is increasing as different dengue viruses have extended their range and now overlap. Dengue hemorrhagic fever is now common in some cities in Asia, where the high prevalence of infection is attributed to the proliferation of open containers needed for water storage (which also provide breeding grounds for the mosquito vector) as the population size exceeds the infrastructure. In urban environments, rain-filled tires or plastic bottles are often breeding grounds of choice for mosquito vectors. The resulting mosquito population boom is complemented by the high human population density in such situations, increasing the chances of stable transmission cycles between infected and susceptible persons. Even in industrialized countries (e.g., the United States) infections, such as tuberculosis, can spread through high-population density settings (e.g., daycare centers or prisons).

Human behavior can have important effects on disease dissemination. The best known examples are sexually transmitted diseases (STDs), and the ways in which sex or intravenous drug use have contributed to the emergence of HIV are now well known. Other factors responsible for disease emergence are influenced by a variety of human actions, so human behavior in the broader sense is also very important. Motivating appropriate individual behavior and constructive action, both locally and in a larger scale, will be essential for controlling emerging infections. Ironically, as AIDS prevention efforts have demonstrated, human behavior remains one of the weakest links in our scientific knowledge.

International Travel and Commerce

The dissemination of HIV through travel has already been mentioned. In the past, an infection introduced to people in a geographically isolated area might, on occasion, be brought to a new place through travel, commerce, or war. Trade between Asia and Europe, perhaps beginning with the silk route and continuing with the Crusades, brought the rat and one of its infections, the bubonic plague, to Europe. Beginning in the 16th and 17th centuries, ships bringing slaves from West Africa to the New World also brought yellow fever and its mosquito vector, *Aedes aegypti*, to the new territories. Similarly, smallpox escaped its Old World origins to wreak havoc in the New World. In the 19th century, cholera had similar opportunities to spread from its probable origin in the Ganges plain to the Middle East and, from there, to Europe and much of the remaining world. Each of these infections had once been localized and took advantage of opportunities to be carried to previously unfamiliar parts of the world.

Similar histories are being repeated nowadays, but opportunities in recent years have become far richer and more numerous, reflecting the increasing volume, scope, and speed of traffic in an increasingly mobile world. Rats have carried *Hantaviruses* virtually worldwide. *Aedes albopictus* (the Asian tiger mosquito) was introduced into the United States, Brazil, and parts of Africa in shipments of used tires from Asia. Since its introduction in 1982, this mosquito has established itself in at least 18 U.S. states and has acquired local viruses including Eastern equine encephalomyelitis, a cause of serious disease. Another mosquito-borne disease, malaria, is one of the most frequently imported diseases in nonendemic-disease areas, and cases of airport malaria are occasionally identified.

A classic bacterial disease, cholera, recently entered both South America (for the first time this century) and Africa. Molecular typing shows the South American isolates to be of the current pandemic strain, supporting the suggestion that the organism was introduced in contaminated bilge water from an Asian freighter. Other evidence indicates that cholera was only one of many organisms to travel in ballast water; dozens, perhaps hundreds, of species have been exchanged between distant places through this means of transport alone. New bacterial strains, such as the recently identified *Vibrio cholerae* O139, or an epidemic strain of Neisseria meningitidis (also examples of microbial adaptation and change) have disseminated rapidly along routes of trade and travel, as have antibiotic-resistant bacteria.

Technology and Industry

High-volume rapid movement characterizes not only travel but other industries in modern society as well. In operations, including food production, that process or use products of biological origin, modern production methods yield increased efficiency and reduced costs but can increase the chances of accidental contamination and amplify the effects of such contamination. The problem is further compounded by globalization, allowing the opportunity to introduce agents from far away. A pathogen present in some of the raw material may find its way into a large batch of final product, as happened with the contamination of hamburger meat by *Escherichia coli* (*E. coli*) strains causing hemolytic uremic syndrome (HUS). In the United States, the implicated *E. coli* strains are serotype O157:H7; additional serotypes have been identified in other countries. Bovine spongiform encephalopathy (BSE), which emerged in Britain within the last few years, was likely an interspecies transfer of scrapie from sheep to cattle that occurred when changes in rendering processes led to incomplete inactivation of scrapie agent in sheep byproducts fed to cattle.

The concentrating effects that occur with blood and tissue products have inadvertently disseminated infections unrecognized at the time, such as HIV and hepatitis B and C. Medical settings are also at the front line of exposure to new diseases, and a number of infections, including many emerging infections, have spread nosocomially in healthcare settings. Among the numerous examples—in the outbreaks of Ebola fever in Africa, many of the secondary cases were hospital acquired—most transmitted to other patients through contaminated hypodermic apparatus and some to the healthcare staff by contact. Transmission of Lassa fever to healthcare workers has also been documented.

On the positive side, advances in diagnostic technology can also lead to new recognition of agents that are already widespread. When such agents are newly recognized, they may at first often be labeled, in some cases incorrectly, as emerging infections. Human herpesvirus 6 (HHV-6) was identified only a few years ago, but the virus appears to be extremely widespread and has recently been implicated as the cause of roseola (exanthem subitum), a very common childhood disease. Because roseola has been known since at least 1910, HHV-6 is likely to have been common for decades and probably much longer. Another recent example is the bacterium *Helicobacter pylori*, a probable cause of gastric ulcers and some cancers. We have lived with these diseases for a long time without knowing their cause. Recognition of the agent is often advantageous, offering new promise of controlling a previously intractable disease, such as treating gastric ulcers with specific anti-microbial therapy.

Microbial Adaptation and Change

Microbes, as with all other living things, are constantly evolving. The emergence of antibiotic-resistant bacteria as a result of the ubiquity of antimicrobials in the environment is an evolutionary lesson on microbial adaptation, as well as a demonstration of the power of natural selection. Selection for antibiotic-resistant bacteria and drug-resistant parasites has become frequent, driven by the wide and sometimes inappropriate use of antimicrobial drugs in a variety of applications. Pathogens can also acquire new antibiotic resistance genes from other, often nonpathogenic, species in the environment, selected or perhaps even driven by the selection pressure of antibiotics.

Many viruses show a high mutation rate and can rapidly evolve to yield new variants. A classic example is influenza. Regular annual epidemics are caused by antigenic drift in a previously circulating influenza strain. A change in an antigenic site of a surface protein, usually the hemagglutinin (H) protein, allows the new variant to reinfect previously infected persons because the altered antigen is not immediately recognized by the immune system.

On rare occasions, perhaps more often with nonviral pathogens than with viruses, the evolution of a new variant may result in a new expression of disease. The epidemic of Brazilian purpuric fever in 1990, associated with a newly emerged clonal variant of Haemophilus influenzae, biogroup aegyptius, may fall into this category. It is possible, but not yet clear, that some recently described manifestations of disease by group A Streptococcus, such as rapidly invasive infection or necrotizing fasciitis, may also fall into this category.

Breakdown of Public-Health Measures and Deficiencies in Public-Health Infrastructure

Classical public health and sanitation measures have long served to minimize dissemination and human exposure to many pathogens spread by traditional routes, such as water, or preventable by immunization or vector control. The pathogens themselves often still remain, albeit in reduced numbers, in reservoir hosts or in the environment, or in small pockets of infection; therefore, they are often able to take advantage of the opportunity to reemerge if there are breakdowns in preventive measures.

Reemerging diseases are those, such as cholera, that were once decreasing but are now rapidly increasing again. These are often conventionally understood and well-recognized public health threats for which (in most cases) previously active public health measures had been allowed to lapse, a situation that unfortunately now applies all too often in both developing countries and the inner cities of the industrialized world. The appearance of reemerging diseases may, therefore, often be a sign of the breakdown of public health measures and should be a warning against complacency in the war against infectious diseases.

Cholera, for example, has recently been raging in South America (for the first time in this century) and Africa. The rapid spread of cholera in South America may have been abetted by recent reductions in chlorine levels used to treat water supplies. The success of cholera and other enteric diseases is often due to the lack of a reliable water supply. These problems are more severe in developing countries but are not confined to these areas. The U.S. outbreak of waterborne *Cryptosporidium* infection in Milwaukee, Wisconsin, in the spring of 1993, with over 400,000 estimated cases, was in part due to a nonfunctioning water filtration plant; similar deficiencies in water purification have been found in other cities in the United States.

For Our Future

The history of infectious diseases has been a history of microbes on the march, often in our wake, and of microbes that have taken advantage of the rich opportunities offered them to thrive, prosper, and spread. And yet, the historical processes that have given rise to the emergence of new infections throughout history continue nowadays with unabated force; in fact, they are accelerating because the conditions of modern life ensure that the factors responsible for disease emergence are more prevalent than ever before. Speed of travel and global reach are further borne out by studies modeling the spread of influenza epidemics and HIV.

Humans are not powerless, however, against this relentless march of microbes. Knowledge of the factors underlying disease emergence can help focus resources on the key situations and areas worldwide and develop more effective prevention strategies. If we are to protect ourselves against emerging diseases, the essential first step is effective global disease surveillance to give early warning of emerging infections. This must be tied to incentives, such as national development, and eventually be backed by a system for an appropriate rapid response. World surveillance capabilities are critically deficient. Efforts—such as the CDC plan, now underway in the United States and internationally—to remedy this situation are the essential first steps and deserve strong support. Research, both basic and applied, will also be vital.

Chapter 2

The Immune System and Its Functions

Functions of Immune System

The overall function of the immune system is to prevent or limit infection. An example of this principle is found in immune-compromised people, including those with genetic immune disorders; immune-debilitating infections, such as human immunodeficiency virus (HIV); and even pregnant women, who are susceptible to a range of microbes that typically do not cause infection in healthy individuals.

The immune system can distinguish between normal, healthy cells and unhealthy cells by recognizing a variety of danger cues called "danger-associated molecular patterns" (DAMPs). Cells may be unhealthy because of infection or because of cellular damage caused by noninfectious agents, such as sunburn or cancer. Infectious microbes, such as viruses and bacteria, release another set of signals recognized by the immune system called "pathogen-associated molecular patterns" (PAMPs).

This chapter contains text excerpted from the following sources: Text beginning with the heading "Functions of Immune System" is excerpted from "Overview of the Immune System," National Institute of Allergy and Infectious Diseases (NIAID), December 30, 2013. Reviewed May 2019; Text under the heading "Features of an Immune Response" is excerpted from "Immune System Research," National Institute of Allergy and Infectious Diseases (NIAID), July 11, 2016.

When the immune system first recognizes these signals, it responds to address the problem. If an immune response cannot be activated when there is sufficient need, problems arise, such as infection. On the other hand, when an immune response is activated without a real threat or is not turned off once the danger passes, different problems arise, such as allergic reactions and autoimmune disease.

The immune system is complex and pervasive. There are numerous cell types that either circulate throughout the body or reside in a particular tissue. Each cell type plays a unique role, with different ways of recognizing problems, communicating with other cells, and performing their functions. By understanding all the details behind this network, researchers may optimize immune responses to confront specific issues, ranging from infections to cancer.

Location

All immune cells come from precursors in the bone marrow and develop into mature cells through a series of changes that can occur in different parts of the body.

Skin: The skin is usually the first line of defense against microbes. Skin cells produce and secrete important antimicrobial proteins, and immune cells can be found in specific layers of skin.

Bone marrow: The bone marrow contains stems cells that can develop into a variety of cell types. The common myeloid progenitor stem cell in the bone marrow is the precursor to innate immune cells— neutrophils, eosinophils, basophils, mast cells, monocytes, dendritic cells, and macrophages—that are important first-line responders to infection.

The common lymphoid progenitor stem cell leads to adaptive immune cells—B cells and T cells—that are responsible for mounting responses to specific microbes based on previous encounters (immunological memory). Natural killer (NK) cells also are derived from the common lymphoid progenitor and share features of both innate and adaptive immune cells, as they provide immediate defenses, similar to innate cells but also may be retained as memory cells, similar to adaptive cells. B, T, and NK cells also are called "lymphocytes."

Bloodstream: Immune cells constantly circulate throughout the bloodstream, patrolling for problems. When blood tests are used to monitor white blood cells, another term for immune cells, a snapshot

16

of the immune system is taken. If a cell type is either scarce or over-abundant in the bloodstream, this may reflect a problem.

Thymus: T cells mature in the thymus, a small organ located in the upper chest.

Lymphatic system: The lymphatic system is a network of vessels and tissues composed of lymph, an extracellular fluid, and lymphoid organs, such as lymph nodes. The lymphatic system is a conduit for travel and communication between tissues and the bloodstream. Immune cells are carried through the lymphatic system and converge in lymph nodes, which are found throughout the body.

Lymph nodes are a communication hub where immune cells sample information brought in from the body. For instance, if adaptive immune cells in the lymph node recognize pieces of a microbe brought in from a distant area, they will activate, replicate, and leave the lymph node to circulate and address the pathogen. Thus, doctors may check patients for swollen lymph nodes, which may indicate an active immune response.

Spleen: The spleen is an organ located behind the stomach. While it is not directly connected to the lymphatic system, it is important for processing information from the bloodstream. Immune cells are enriched in specific areas of the spleen, and upon recognizing bloodborne pathogens, they will activate and respond accordingly.

Mucosal tissue: Mucosal surfaces are prime entry points for pathogens, and specialized immune hubs are strategically located in mucosal tissues, such as the respiratory tract and gut. For instance, Peyer's patches are important areas in the small intestine where immune cells can access samples from the gastrointestinal tract.

Features of an Immune Response

An immune response is generally divided into innate and adaptive immunity. Innate immunity occurs immediately, when circulating innate cells recognize a problem. Adaptive immunity occurs later, as it relies on the coordination and expansion of specific adaptive immune cells. Immune memory follows the adaptive response, when mature adaptive cells, highly specific to the original pathogen, are retained for later use.

Innate Immunity

Innate immune cells express genetically encoded receptors, called "Toll-like receptors" (TLRs), which recognize general danger or pathogen-associated patterns. Collectively, these receptors can broadly recognize viruses, bacteria, fungi, and even noninfectious problems. However, they cannot distinguish between specific strains of bacteria or viruses.

There are numerous types of innate immune cells with specialized functions. They include neutrophils, eosinophils, basophils, mast cells, monocytes, dendritic cells, and macrophages. Their main feature is the ability to respond quickly and broadly when a problem arises, typically leading to inflammation. Innate immune cells also are important for activating adaptive immunity. Innate cells are critical for host defense, and disorders in innate cell function may cause chronic susceptibility to infection.

Adaptive Immunity

Adaptive immune cells are more specialized, with each adaptive B or T cell bearing unique receptors, B-cell receptors (BCRs) and T-cell receptors (TCRs), that recognize specific signals rather than general patterns. Each receptor recognizes an antigen, which is simply any molecule that may bind to a BCR or TCR. Antigens are derived from a variety of sources including pathogens, host cells, and allergens. Antigens are typically processed by innate immune cells and presented to adaptive cells in the lymph nodes.

The genes for BCRs and TCRs are randomly rearranged at specific cell maturation stages, resulting in unique receptors that may potentially recognize anything. Random generation of receptors allows the immune system to respond to new or unforeseen problems. This concept is especially important because environments may frequently change, for instance when seasons change or a person relocates, and pathogens are constantly evolving to survive. Because BCRs and TCRs are so specific, adaptive cells may only recognize one strain of a particular pathogen, unlike innate cells, which recognize broad classes of pathogens. In fact, a group of adaptive cells that recognize the same strain will likely recognize different areas of that pathogen.

If a B or T cell has a receptor that recognizes an antigen from a pathogen and also receives cues from innate cells that something is wrong, the B or T cell will activate, divide, and disperse to address the problem. B cells make antibodies, which neutralize pathogens, rendering them harmless. T cells carry out multiple functions, including killing infected cells and activating or recruiting other immune cells. The adaptive response has a system of checks and balances to prevent unnecessary activation that could cause damage to the host. If a B or T cell is autoreactive, meaning its receptor recognizes antigens from the body's own cells, the cell will be deleted. Also, if a B or T cell does not receive signals from innate cells, it will not be optimally activated.

Immune memory is a feature of the adaptive immune response. After B or T cells are activated, they expand rapidly. As the problem resolves, cells stop dividing and are retained in the body as memory cells. The next time this same pathogen enters the body, a memory cell is already poised to react and can clear away the pathogen before it establishes itself.

Vaccination

Vaccination, or immunization, is a way to train your immune system against a specific pathogen. Vaccination achieves immune memory without an actual infection, so the body is prepared when the virus or bacterium enters. Saving time is important to prevent a pathogen from establishing itself and infecting more cells in the body.

An effective vaccine will optimally activate both the innate and adaptive response. An immunogen is used to activate the adaptive immune response so that specific memory cells are generated. Because BCRs and TCRs are unique, some memory cells are simply better at eliminating the pathogen. The goal of vaccine design is to select immunogens that will generate the most effective and efficient memory response against a particular pathogen. Adjuvants, which are important for activating innate immunity, can be added to vaccines to optimize the immune response. Innate immunity recognizes broad patterns, and without innate responses, adaptive immunity cannot be optimally achieved.

Immune Cells

Granulocytes include basophils, eosinophils, and neutrophils. Basophils and eosinophils are important for host defense against parasites. They also are involved in allergic reactions. Neutrophils, the most numerous innate immune cell, patrol for problems by circulating in the bloodstream. They can phagocytose, or ingest, bacteria, degrading them inside special compartments called "vesicles."

Immune Tolerance

Tolerance is the prevention of an immune response against a particular antigen. For instance, the immune system is generally tolerant of self-antigens, so it does not usually attack the body's own cells, tissues, and organs. However, when tolerance is lost, disorders such as an autoimmune disease or a food allergy may occur.

Disorders of the Immune System

Complications arise when the immune system does not function properly. Some issues are less pervasive, such as pollen allergy, while others are extensive, such as genetic disorders that wipe out the presence or function of an entire set of immune cells.

Chapter 3

Immunodeficiency and Infectious Diseases

Primary immune deficiency diseases (PIDDs) are rare, genetic disorders that impair the immune system. Without a functional immune response, people with PIDDs may be subject to chronic, debilitating infections, such as Epstein-Barr virus (EBV), which can increase the risk of developing cancer. Some PIDDs can be fatal. PIDDs may be diagnosed in infancy, childhood, or adulthood, depending on disease severity.

There are more than 200 different forms of primary immune deficiency diseases affecting approximately 500,000 people in the United States. These rare genetic diseases may be chronic, debilitating, and costly.

Types of Primary Immune Deficiency Diseases

The National Institute of Allergy and Infectious Diseases (NIAID) conducts research across all PIDDs, as well as among the individual diseases that make up this broad category.

This chapter contains text excerpted from the following sources: Text in this chapter begins with excerpts from "Primary Immune Deficiency Diseases (PIDDs)," National Institute of Allergy and Infectious Diseases (NIAID), June 21, 2016; Text beginning with the heading "Why Are Immunization and Infectious Diseases Important?" is excerpted from "Immunization and Infectious Diseases," National Heart, Lung, and Blood Institute (NHLBI), March 15, 2010. Reviewed May 2019.

Autoimmune Lymphoproliferative Syndrome

Autoimmune lymphoproliferative syndrome (ALPS) is a rare immune disorder first described by scientists at the National Institutes of Health (NIH) in the mid-1990s that can cause numerous autoimmune problems, such as low levels of red blood cells, clot-forming platelets, and infection-fighting white blood cells. These problems can increase the risk of infection and hemorrhage.

Autoimmune Polyglandular Syndrome Type 1

Autoimmune polyglandular syndrome type 1 (APS-1), also called "autoimmune polyendocrinopathy-candidiasis-ectodermal dystrophy" (APECED), causes a diverse range of symptoms, including autoimmunity against different types of organs and increased susceptibility to candidiasis, a fungal infection caused by Candida yeast.

BENTA Disease

B cell expansion with NF-κB and T cell anergy (BENTA) disease is a rare genetic disorder of the immune system caused by mutations in the gene CARD11. The disease is characterized by high levels of certain immune cells starting in infancy; an enlarged spleen; enlarged lymph nodes; immunodeficiency; and an elevated risk of lymphoma, a type of cancer.

Caspase Eight Deficiency State

Caspase eight deficiency state, or CEDS, is a very rare genetic disorder of the immune system caused by mutations in the CASP8 gene. CEDS is characterized by an enlarged spleen and lymph nodes, recurrent sinus and lung infections, recurrent viral infections, and a low level of infection-fighting antibodies. The NIH researchers first described this condition in two siblings in 2002.

CARD9 Deficiency and Other Syndromes of Susceptibility to Candidiasis

The National Institute of Allergy and Infectious Diseases (NIAID) researchers are studying how CARD9 deficiency and other genetic disorders result in susceptibility to candidiasis. People with CARD9 deficiency are particularly susceptible to Candida infections of the central nervous system.

Chronic Granulomatous Disease

Chronic granulomatous disease (CGD) occurs when white blood cells called "phagocytes" are unable to kill certain bacteria and fungi, making people highly susceptible to some bacterial and fungal infections. Mutations in one of five different genes can cause this disease.

Common Variable Immunodeficiency

Common variable immunodeficiency (CVID) is caused by a variety of different genetic abnormalities that result in a defect in the capability of immune cells to produce normal amounts of protective antibodies. People with CVID experience frequent bacterial and viral infections of the upper airway, sinuses, and lungs.

Congenital Neutropenia Syndromes

Congenital neutropenia syndromes are a group of disorders present from birth that are characterized by low levels of neutrophils, a type of white blood cell necessary for fighting infections.

Cytotoxic T-Lymphocyte-Associated Protein 4 Deficiency

Cytotoxic T-lymphocyte-associated protein 4 (CTLA4) deficiency is a rare disorder that severely impairs the normal regulation of the immune system, resulting in conditions, such as intestinal disease, respiratory infections, autoimmune problems, and enlarged lymph nodes, liver, and spleen. NIAID scientists and their collaborators identified the disease in 2014.

DOCK8 Deficiency

DOCK8 immunodeficiency syndrome is a rare immune disorder named after the mutated gene responsible for the disease. The disorder causes decreased numbers of immune cells, as well as poor ability of immune cells to move across dense tissues, such as the skin. These abnormalities resulting from this disease lead to recurrent viral infections of the skin and respiratory system.

GATA2 Deficiency

GATA2 deficiency is a rare disorder of the immune system with wide-ranging effects. First identified in 2011, the disorder is characterized by immunodeficiency, lung disease, problems of the vascular and lymphatic systems, and myelodysplastic syndrome (a condition characterized by ineffective blood cell production).

Glycosylation Disorders with Immunodeficiency

Glycosylation refers to the attachment of sugars to proteins, a normal process required for the function of healthy cells. Defects in glycosylation can disrupt the immune system, resulting in immunodeficiency and potentially causing extensive and severe symptoms.

Hyperimmunoglobulin E Syndrome

People with autosomal dominant hyperimmunoglobulin E syndrome (HIES) have recurrent bacterial infections of the skin and lungs, and they typically also have eczema, distinct facial features, and a tendency to experience bone fractures. The disease has several other names, including "Job syndrome," "signal transducer and activator of transcription 3 (STAT3) deficiency," and "Buckley syndrome."

Hyper-Immunoglobulin M Syndromes

Hyper-immunoglobulin M (IgM) syndromes are rare, inherited conditions in which the immune system fails to produce normal levels of the antibodies IgA, IgG, and IgE but can produce normal or elevated levels of IgM. Various gene defects that impair communication between T cells and antibody-producing B cells can lead to hyper-IgM syndromes. Hyper-IgM syndromes can cause severe respiratory infections in infancy and a higher risk of rare infections throughout life. Treatment includes regular intravenous or subcutaneous antibody replacement therapy, anti-fungal prophylactics, and, in some cases, bone marrow transplant from a healthy donor.

Interferon Gamma, Interleukin 12, and Interleukin 23 Deficiencies

Interferon gamma, interleukin 12, and interleukin 23 deficiencies are rare, inherited immune disorders in which the body fails to produce one or more of these signaling molecules, which allow infection-fighting immune cells to communicate. Deficiencies in these molecules lead to increased susceptibility to bacterial and viral infections. Many people with these deficiencies develop granulomas, or inflammatory lesions that form in tissues and organs because of recurring infections. While many of these deficiencies begin to cause symptoms in infancy or childhood, some symptoms appear later in life. Treatment includes antibiotic therapy to prevent infections and, in some cases, bone marrow transplant from a healthy donor.

Leukocyte Adhesion Deficiency

Leukocyte adhesion deficiency (LAD) is a rare, inherited immune disorder in which immune cells called "phagocytes" are unable to move to the site of an infection to fight off invading pathogens. People with LAD experience recurrent, life-threatening infections and poor wound healing. LAD is caused by a mutation in the gene ITGB2, which provides instructions for the phagocyte surface molecule CD18. Treatments for LAD include antibiotics to prevent and treat infection and, in some cases, bone marrow transplants from a healthy donor.

Lipopolysaccharide-Responsive and Beige-Like Anchor Protein Deficiency

Lipopolysaccharide-responsive and beige-like anchor protein (LRBA) deficiency is a rare genetic disorder of the immune system caused by mutations in the LRBA gene. This disease impairs normal immune system function and results in autoimmunity; recurrent infections; and an increased risk of lymphoma, a type of cancer. People with LRBA deficiency have excessive numbers of immune cells called "lymphocytes," which sometimes enter and accumulate in organs where lymphocytes typically are not present in large numbers, such as the gut, lungs, and brain. This can cause a variety of symptoms.

PI3 Kinase Disease

PI3 Kinase disease is caused by genetic mutations that overactivate an important immune-system signaling pathway. This causes a chain reaction of problems, disrupting the normal development of infection-fighting B and T cells. People with the disease have a weakened immune system and experience frequent bacterial and viral infections.

PLCG2-Associated Antibody Deficiency and Immune Dysregulation

PLCG2-associated antibody deficiency and immune dysregulation (PLAID) and PLAID-like diseases are rare immune disorders with overlapping features, and an allergic response to cold, called "cold urticaria," is the most distinct symptom.

Severe Combined Immunodeficiency

Severe combined immunodeficiency (SCID) is a group of rare, life-threatening disorders caused by mutations in different genes involved in the development and function of infection-fighting T and B cells. Infants with SCID appear healthy at birth but are highly susceptible to severe infections.

Signal Transducer and Activator of Transcription 3 Gain-of-Function Disease

Signal transducer and activator of transcription 3 (STAT3) gain-of-function disease is a rare genetic disorder of the immune system caused by a malfunction in the STAT3 gene that leads to overactive STAT3 protein. Symptoms of this disease begin early in life and include swelling of the lymph nodes, low blood cell counts, and autoimmunity that can affect multiple organs and tissues. People with STAT3 gain-of-function disease may experience recurrent infections, eczema, and growth problems.

Warts, Hypogammaglobulinemia, Infections, and Myelokathexis Syndrome

People with warts, hypogammaglobulinemia, infections, and myelo-kathexis (WHIM) syndrome have low levels of infection-fighting white blood cells, especially neutrophils, predisposing them to frequent infections and persistent warts.

Wiskott-Aldrich Syndrome

Wiskott-Aldrich syndrome (WAS) is a rare genetic disorder of the immune system that primarily affects boys. WAS is an X-linked recessive disease caused by mutations in the WAS gene, which provides instructions for production of Wiskott-Aldrich syndrome protein. The disorder is characterized by abnormal immune function and a reduced ability to form blood clots. This can result in prolonged episodes of bleeding, recurrent bacterial and fungal infections, and increased risk of cancers and autoimmune diseases.

X-Linked Agammaglobulinemia

X-linked agammaglobulinemia (XLA) is caused by an inability to produce B cells or immunoglobulins (antibodies), which are made by B cells. People with XLA develop frequent infections of the ears, throat, lungs, and sinuses.

X-Linked Lymphoproliferative Disease

X-linked lymphoproliferative disease (XLP) primarily affects boys and is characterized by a life-long vulnerability to Epstein-Barr virus (EBV), a common type of herpesvirus. People with XLP are healthy until they are exposed to EBV. Then, they can become seriously ill and experience swollen lymph nodes; an enlarged liver and spleen; hepatitis and lymphoma, a type of cancer.

X-Linked Immunodeficiency Disease with Magnesium Defect, Epstein-Barr Virus Infection, and Neoplasia

X-linked immunodeficiency with magnesium defect, Epstein-Barr virus infection, and neoplasia (XMEN) disease is a rare genetic disorder of the immune system. It is characterized by low levels of infection-fighting CD4+ cells; chronic EBV infection; and EBV-related lymphoproliferative disease, in which excessive numbers of immune cells are produced. The NIH investigators first described XMEN disease in 2011.

How Is National Institute of Allergy and Infectious Diseases Addressing This Critical Topic?

Since the 1970s, NIAID-supported investigators have been examining the causes and complications of PIDDs to improve the lives of patients and families. NIAID aims to improve diagnosis, explore new treatments, and preventions for PIDDs, and facilitate genetic counseling. NIAID is home to the Primary Immune Deficiency Clinic, which provides diagnoses and disease management recommendations to patients and families whose lives are touched by PIDDs.

Why Are Immunization and Infectious Diseases Important?

People in the United States continue to get diseases that are vaccine preventable. Viral hepatitis, influenza, and tuberculosis (TB) remain among the leading causes of illness and death in the United States and account for substantial spending on the related consequences of infection.

The infectious disease public health infrastructure, which carries out disease surveillance at the federal, state, and local levels, is an essential tool in the fight against newly emerging and reemerging infectious diseases. Other important defenses against infectious diseases include:

- Proper use of vaccines

- Antibiotics

- Screening and testing guidelines

- Scientific improvements in the diagnosis of infectious disease-related health concerns

Respiratory Diseases

Acute respiratory infections, including pneumonia and influenza, are the eighth leading cause of death in the United States, accounting for 56,000 deaths annually. Pneumonia mortality in children fell by 97 percent in the last century, but respiratory infectious diseases continue to be leading causes of pediatric hospitalization and outpatient visits in the United States. On average, influenza leads to more than 200,000 hospitalizations and 36,000 deaths each year. The 2009 H1N1 influenza pandemic caused an estimated 270,000 hospitalizations and 12,270 deaths (1,270 of which were of people younger than the age of 18) between April 2009 and March 2010.

Hepatitis and Tuberculosis

Viral hepatitis and TB can be prevented, yet healthcare systems often do not make the best use of their available resources to support prevention efforts. Because the U.S. healthcare system focuses on the treatment of illnesses rather than health promotion, patients do not always receive information about prevention and healthy lifestyles. This includes advancing effective and evidence-based viral hepatitis and TB prevention priorities and interventions.

Emerging Issues in Immunization and Infectious Diseases

In the coming decade, the United States will continue to face new and emerging issues in the area of immunization and infectious diseases. The public-health infrastructure must be capable of responding to emerging threats. State-of-the-art technology and highly skilled professionals need to be in place to provide rapid response to the threat of epidemics. A coordinated strategy is necessary to understand, detect, control, and prevent infectious diseases.

The following are some specific emerging issues:

- Providing culturally appropriate preventive healthcare is an immediate responsibility that will grow over the decade. As the demographics of the population continue to shift, public health and healthcare systems will need to expand their capacity to protect the growing needs of a diverse and aging population.

- New infectious agents and diseases continue to be detected. Infectious diseases must be looked at in a global context due to increasing:

- International travel and trade

- Migration

- Importation of foods and agricultural practices

- Threats of bioterrorism

- Inappropriate use of antibiotics and environmental changes multiply the potential for worldwide epidemics of all types of infectious diseases.

Infectious diseases are a critical public health, humanitarian, and security concern; coordinated efforts will protect people across the nation and around the world.

Chapter 4

Common Variable Immune Deficiency

Common variable immunodeficiency (CVID) is a group of disorders characterized by low levels of a type of protein known as "immunoglobulins" (Ig). Because of low level of Ig, the immune system cannot make antibodies that fight bacteria, viruses, or other toxins in the body. This leads to frequent infections, particularly in the sinuses, lungs, and digestive tract.

Symptoms most commonly begin in early adulthood but can occur at any age. While in most cases the cause of CVID is unknown, a genetic change has been found in about one-third of cases. This condition is diagnosed based on the symptoms, specific laboratory testings, and exclusion of other disorders. Treatment for CVID includes Ig replacement therapy, which stops the cycle of recurrent infections. The long-term outlook for people with CVID varies depending on the severity of the symptoms and any underlying conditions.

Symptoms

The symptoms of common variable immunodeficiency may be different from person to person. Some people may be more severely affected

This chapter includes text excerpted from "Common Variable Immunodeficiency," Genetic and Rare Diseases Information Center (GARD), National Center for Advancing Translational Sciences (NCATS), April 19, 2019.

than others, even people who have the same form. Not everyone with common variable immunodeficiency will have the same symptoms.

The most common signs and symptoms of CVID include:

- Low levels of proteins that help the immune system work (immunoglobulins)

- Recurrent infections, especially of the lungs and digestive systems

- Autoimmunity (body attacks healthy organs and tissues)

- Liver involvement

- Increased risk for malignancy

About 20 to 30 percent of people with CVID will develop autoimmunity, and about 10 percent of people with CVID will have liver involvement.

Cause

Common variable immunodeficiency is thought to be the result of a combination of genetic and environmental factors. In most cases, the exact cause of CVID is unknown.

At least 20 different genes have been associated with CVID. Some families with this condition have a gene mutation that has not yet been found in any other family. Genes associated with CVID are generally involved in the development and function of immune system cells (B cells) which help protect against infection.

Inheritance

Most cases of common variable immunodeficiency are sporadic and occur in someone with no family history of the condition. Some cases of CVID are inherited in families, and the pattern varies depending on the specific gene change (mutation). Autosomal dominant, recessive, and X-linked inheritance have been reported.

Diagnosis

Common variable immunodeficiency is diagnosed based on symptoms (chronic, recurrent infections) and laboratory tests that look for decreased levels of specific immunoglobulins. Because there are many causes of immune deficiency, other conditions must be ruled out. Several groups have published criteria for diagnosing CVID and other immune deficiencies.

Treatment

The main treatment for common variable immunodeficiency is Ig replacement therapy, which stops the cycle of recurrent infections. Ig may be taken intravenously (through the vein) or subcutaneously (by injection). Adverse reactions to Ig must be monitored during therapy. In some people with CVID and severe autoimmune disease, steroids or other immunosuppressive drugs in addition to Ig therapy may be needed.

There are multiple forms of Ig replacement therapy available, and people with CVID should speak to their healthcare providers to determine which therapy may be best for their situation.

Prognosis

The long-term outlook (prognosis) and life expectancy for people with common variable immunodeficiency (CVID) varies. The prognosis largely depends on whether there is severe autoimmune disease, whether there are recurrent infections that cause structural lung damage, and the development of a malignancy (cancer). Other major factors that influence prognosis include the extent of end-organ damage and how successfully infections can be prevented.

Chapter 5

Transmission of Infectious Diseases

Germs are a part of everyday life and are found in our air, soil, water, and in and on our bodies. Some germs are helpful, others are harmful. Many germs live in and on our bodies without causing harm and some even help us to stay healthy. Only a small portion of germs are known to cause infection.

How Do Infections Occur?

An infection occurs when germs enter the body, increase in number, and cause a reaction of the body.

Three things are necessary for an infection to occur:

- **Source:** Places where infectious agents (germs) live (e.g., sinks, surfaces, human skin)

- **Susceptible person** with a way for germs to enter the body

- **Transmission:** A way germs are moved to the susceptible person

---

This chapter includes text excerpted from "How Infections Spread," Centers for Disease Control and Prevention (CDC), January 7, 2016

Source

A source is an infectious agent or germ and refers to a virus, bacteria, or other microbe.

In healthcare settings, germs are found in many places. People are one source of germs including:

- Patients

- Healthcare workers

- Visitors and household members

People can be sick with symptoms of an infection or colonized with germs (not have symptoms of an infection but able to pass the germs to others).

Germs are also found in the healthcare environment. Examples of environmental sources of germs include:

- Dry surfaces in patient care areas (e.g., bed rails, medical equipment, countertops, and tables)

- Wet surfaces, moist environments, and biofilms (e.g., cooling towers, faucets and sinks, and equipment such as ventilators)

- Indwelling medical devices (e.g., catheters and IV lines)

- Dust or decaying debris (e.g., construction dust or wet materials from water leaks)

Susceptible Person

A susceptible person is someone who is not vaccinated or otherwise immune, or a person with a weakened immune system who has a way for the germs to enter the body. For an infection to occur, germs must enter a susceptible person's body and invade tissues, multiply, and cause a reaction.

Devices like IV catheters and surgical incisions can provide an entryway, whereas a healthy immune system helps fight infection.

When patients are sick and receive medical treatment in healthcare facilities, the following factors can increase their susceptibility to infection.

- Patients in healthcare who have underlying medical conditions such as diabetes, cancer, and organ transplantation are at increased risk for infection because often these illnesses decrease the immune system's ability to fight infection.

- Certain medications used to treat medical conditions, such as antibiotics, steroids, and certain cancer-fighting medications increase the risk of some types of infections.

- Lifesaving medical treatments and procedures used in healthcare such as urinary catheters, tubes, and surgery increase the risk of infection by providing additional ways that germs can enter the body.

Recognizing the factors that increase patients' susceptibility to infection allows providers to recognize risks and perform basic infection prevention measures to prevent infection from occurring.

Transmission

Transmission refers to the way germs are moved to the susceptible person.

Germs do not move themselves. Germs depend on people, the environment, and/or medical equipment to move in healthcare settings.

There are a few general ways that germs travel in healthcare settings—through contact (i.e., touching), sprays and splashes, inhalation, and sharps injuries (i.e., when someone is accidentally stuck with a used needle or sharp instrument).

- Contact moves germs by touch (e.g., Methicillin-resistant *Staphylococcus aureus* (MRSA) or vancomycin-resistant enterococcus (VRE)). For example, healthcare provider hands become contaminated by touching germs present on medical equipment or high touch surfaces and then carry the germs on their hands and spread to a susceptible person when proper hand hygiene is not performed before touching the susceptible person.

- Sprays and splashes occur when an infected person coughs or sneezes, creating droplets which carry germs short distances (within approximately six feet). These germs can land on a susceptible person's eyes, nose, or mouth and can cause infection (example: pertussis or meningitis).

- Close range inhalation occurs when a droplet containing germs is small enough to breathe in but not durable over distance.

- Inhalation occurs when germs are aerosolized in tiny particles that survive on air currents over great distances and time and reach a susceptible person. Airborne transmission can occur when infected patients cough, talk, or sneeze germs into the air (e.g., Tuberculosis (TB) or measles), or when germs are aerosolized by medical equipment or by dust from a construction zone (e.g., Nontuberculous mycobacteria or aspergillus).

- Sharps injuries can lead to infections (e.g., human immunodeficiency virus (HIV), hepatitis B virus (HBV), and hepatitis C virus (HCV)) when bloodborne pathogens enter a person through a skin puncture by a used needle or sharp instrument.

Chapter 6

Biofilms: Microbial Life on Surfaces

For most of the history of microbiology, microorganisms have primarily been characterized as planktonic, freely suspended cells and described on the basis of their growth characteristics in nutritionally rich culture media. The rediscovery of a microbiologic phenomenon, first described by scientist Antonie van Leeuwenhoek, that microorganisms attach to and grow universally on exposed surfaces led to studies that revealed surface-associated microorganisms (biofilms) exhibited a distinct phenotype with respect to gene transcription and growth rate. These biofilm microorganisms have been shown to elicit specific mechanisms for initial attachment to a surface, development of a community structure and ecosystem, and detachment.

A Historical Basis

A biofilm is an assemblage of surface-associated microbial cells that is enclosed in an extracellular polymeric substance matrix. Van Leeuwenhoek, using his simple microscopes, first observed microorganisms on tooth surfaces and can be credited with the discovery of microbial biofilms. Researchers Hovhannes Heukelekian and Andrew A. Heller observed the "bottle effect" for marine microorganisms, i.e., bacterial

This chapter includes text excerpted from "Biofilms: Microbial Life on Surfaces," Centers for Disease Control and Prevention (CDC), June 26, 2012. Reviewed May 2019.

growth and activity were substantially enhanced by the incorporation of a surface to which these organisms could attach. Researcher Claude E. ZoBell observed that the number of bacteria on surfaces was dramatically higher than in the surrounding medium (in this case, seawater). However, a detailed examination of biofilms would await the electron microscope, which allowed high-resolution photomicroscopy at much higher magnifications than did the light microscope. Researchers Donald S. Dwyer, Katherine C. Gordon, and Brad Jones used scanning and transmission electron microscopy to examine biofilms on trickling filters in a wastewater treatment plant and showed them to be composed of a variety of organisms (based on cell morphology). By using a specific polysaccharide-stain called "Ruthenium red" and coupling this with osmium tetroxide fixative, these researchers were also able to show that the matrix material surrounding and enclosing cells in these biofilms was polysaccharide. As early as 1973, researcher Gregory W. Characklis studied microbial slimes in industrial water systems and showed that they were not only very tenacious but also highly resistant to disinfectants, such as chlorine. In 1978, based on observations of the dental plaque and sessile communities in mountain streams, researcher William Costerton et al. put forth a theory of biofilms that explained the mechanisms whereby microorganisms adhere to living and nonliving materials and the benefits accrued by this ecologic niche. Since that time, the studies of biofilms in industrial and ecologic settings and in environments more relevant for public health have basically paralleled each other. Much of the work in the last two decades has relied on tools, such as scanning electron microscopy (SEM) or standard microbiologic culture techniques, for biofilm characterization. Two major thrusts in the last decade have dramatically impacted our understanding of biofilms:

- The utilization of the confocal laser scanning microscope to characterize biofilm ultrastructure

- An investigation of the genes involved in cell adhesion and biofilm formation

Biofilm Defined

A biofilm is an assemblage of microbial cells that is irreversibly associated (not removed by gentle rinsing) with a surface and enclosed in a matrix of primarily polysaccharide material. Depending on the environment in which the biofilm has developed, noncellular materials, such as mineral crystals, corrosion particles, clay or silt particles, or blood components, may also be found in the biofilm matrix. Biofilm-associated organisms also differ from their planktonic (freely suspended) counterparts with respect to the genes that are transcribed. Biofilms may form on a wide variety of surfaces, including living tissues, indwelling medical devices, industrial or potable water system piping, or natural aquatic systems. The variable nature of biofilms can be illustrated from scanning electron micrographs of biofilms from an industrial water system and a medical device. The water system biofilm is highly complex, containing corrosion products, clay material, freshwater diatoms, and filamentous bacteria. The biofilm on the medical device, on the other hand, appears to be composed of a single, coccoid organism and the associated extracellular polymeric substance (EPS) matrix.

Attachment

The solid-liquid interface between a surface and an aqueous medium (e.g., water, blood) provides an ideal environment for the attachment and growth of microorganisms. A clear picture of attachment cannot be obtained without considering the effects of the substratum, conditioning films forming on the substratum, hydrodynamics of the aqueous medium, characteristics of the medium, and various properties of the cell surface. Each of these factors will be considered in detail.

Substratum Effects

The solid surface may have several characteristics that are important in the attachment process. Characklis et al. noted that the extent of microbial colonization appears to increase as the surface roughness increases. This is because shear forces are diminished, and surface area is higher on rougher surfaces. The physicochemical properties of the surface may also exert a strong influence on the rate and extent of attachment. Most investigators have found that microorganisms attach more rapidly to hydrophobic, nonpolar surfaces, such as Teflon and other plastics, than to hydrophilic materials, such as glass or metals. Even though results of these studies have, at times, been contradictory because no standardized methods exist for determining surface hydrophobicity, some kind of hydrophobic interaction apparently occurs between the cell surface and the substratum that would enable the cell to overcome the repulsive forces active within a certain distance from the substratum surface and irreversibly attach.

41

Conditioning Films

A material surface exposed in an aqueous medium will inevitably and almost immediately become conditioned or coated by polymers from that medium, and the resulting chemical modification will affect the rate and extent of microbial attachment. Researchers George I. Loeb and Rex. A. Neihof were the first to report the formation of these conditioning films on surfaces exposed in seawater. These researchers found that films were organic in nature, formed within minutes of exposure, and continued to grow for several hours. The nature of conditioning films may be quite different for surfaces exposed in the human host. A prime example may be the proteinaceous conditioning film called "acquired pellicle," which develops on tooth enamel surfaces in the oral cavity. Pellicle comprises albumin, lysozyme, glycoproteins, phosphoproteins, lipids, and gingival crevice fluid; bacteria from the oral cavity colonize pellicle-conditioned surfaces within hours of exposure to these surfaces. Researcher Marc W. Mittelman noted that a number of host-produced conditioning films, such as blood, tears, urine, saliva, intervascular fluid, and respiratory secretions, influence the attachment of bacteria to biomaterials. Researchers Itzhak Ofek and Ronald J. Doyle also noted that the surface energy of the suspending medium may affect hydrodynamic interactions of microbial cells with surfaces by altering the substratum characteristics.

Hydrodynamics

In theory, the flow velocity immediately adjacent to the substratum/liquid interface is negligible. This zone of negligible flow is termed the "hydrodynamic boundary layer." Its thickness is dependent on linear velocity; the higher the velocity, the thinner the boundary layer. The region outside the boundary layer is characterized by substantial mixing or turbulence. For flow regimes characterized as "laminar" or "minimally turbulent," the hydrodynamic boundary layer may substantially affect cell-substratum interactions. Cells behave as particles in a liquid, and the rate of settling and association with a submerged surface will depend largely on the velocity characteristics of the liquid. Under very low linear velocities, the cells must traverse the sizeable hydrodynamic boundary layer, and association with the surface will depend in large part on cell size and cell motility. As the velocity increases, the boundary layer decreases, and cells will be subjected to increasingly greater turbulence and mixing. Higher linear velocities would, therefore, be expected to equate to more rapid association with the surface, at least until velocities become high enough to exert substantial shear forces on the attaching cells, resulting in detachment of these cells This finding has been confirmed in studies by researchers H.H. Rijnaarts et al. and S. Zheng et al.

Characteristics of the Aqueous Medium

Other characteristics of the aqueous medium, such as pH, nutrient levels, ionic strength, and temperature, may play a role in the rate of microbial attachment to a substratum. Several studies have shown a seasonal effect on bacterial attachment and biofilm formation in different aqueous systems. This effect may be due to water temperature or to other unmeasured, seasonally affected parameters. Researcher M.P. Fletcher found that an increase in the concentration of several cations (sodium, calcium, lanthanum, ferric iron) affected the attachment of *Pseudomonas fluorescens* to glass surfaces, presumably by reducing the repulsive forces between the negatively charged bacterial cells and the glass surfaces. Researcher S.T. Cowan et al. showed in a laboratory study that an increase in nutrient concentration correlated with an increase in the number of attached bacterial cells.

Chapter 7

Bioterrorism: Weaponized Infectious Diseases

Chapter Contents

Section 7.1

Overview of Weaponized Infectious Diseases

This section includes text excerpted from "Bioterrorism," Ready, Department of Homeland Security (DHS), July 31, 2017.

Biological agents are organisms or toxins that can kill or incapacitate people, livestock, and crops. A biological attack is the deliberate release of germs or other biological substances that can make you sick.

There are three basic groups of biological agents that could likely be used as weapons: bacteria, viruses, and toxins. Biological agents can be dispersed by spraying them into the air, person-to-person contact, infecting animals that carry the disease to humans, and by contaminating food and water.

Before a Biological Threat

A biological attack may or may not be immediately obvious. In most cases, local healthcare workers will report a pattern of unusual illness or there will be a wave of sick people seeking emergency medical attention. The public would be alerted through an emergency radio or TV broadcast, or some other signal used in your community, such as a telephone call or a home visit from an emergency response worker.

The following are things you can do to protect yourself, your family and your property from the effects of a biological threat:

- Build an emergency supply kit

- Make a family emergency plan

- Check with your doctor to ensure all required or suggested immunizations are up to date for yourself, your children, and elderly family members

- Consider installing a high-efficiency particulate air (HEPA) filter in your furnace return duct, which will filter out most biological agents that may enter your house

During a Biological Threat

The first evidence of an attack may be when you notice symptoms of the disease caused by exposure to an agent. In the event of a biological attack, public health officials may not immediately be able to provide information on what you should do. It will take time to determine exactly what the illness is, how it should be treated, and who is in danger.

Follow these guidelines during a biological threat:

- Watch TV, listen to the radio, or check the Internet for official news and information including signs and symptoms of the disease, areas in danger, if medications or vaccinations are being distributed and where you should seek medical attention if you become ill.

- If you become aware of an unusual and suspicious substance, quickly get away.

- Cover your mouth and nose with layers of fabric that can filter the air but still allow breathing. Examples include two to three layers of cotton, such as a T-shirt, handkerchief, or towel.

- Depending on the situation, wear a face mask to reduce inhaling or spreading germs.

- If you have been exposed to a biological agent, remove and bag your clothes and personal items. Follow official instructions for disposal of contaminated items.

- Wash yourself with soap and water, and put on clean clothes.

- Contact authorities, and seek medical assistance. You may be advised to stay away from others or even quarantined.

- If your symptoms match those described and you are in the group considered at risk, immediately seek emergency medical attention.

- Follow instructions of doctors and other public health officials.

- If the disease is contagious, expect to receive medical evaluation and treatment.

- For noncontagious diseases, expect to receive medical evaluation and treatment.

- In a declared biological emergency or developing epidemic, avoid crowds.

- Wash your hands with soap and water frequently.

- Do not share food or utensils.

After a Biological Threat

Pay close attention to all official warnings and instructions on how to proceed. The delivery of medical services for a biological event may be handled differently to respond to increased demand.

The basic public health procedures and medical protocols for handling exposure to biological agents are the same as for any infectious disease. It is important for you to pay attention to official instructions via radio, television, and emergency alert systems.

Section 7.2

Questions and Answers about the Strategic Stockpiling of Medicines

This section includes text excerpted from "Strategic National Stockpile (SNS)," Chemical Hazards Emergency Medical Management (CHEMM), U.S. Department of Health and Human Services (HHS), January 23, 2019.

Who Authorized the Strategic National Stockpile Program

- In 1998, the Congress appropriated funds for the Centers for Disease Control and Prevention (CDC) to acquire a pharmaceutical and vaccine stockpile to counter potential biological and chemical threats and threats from widespread diseases that could affect large numbers of persons in the civilian population.

- The program was originally called the "National Pharmaceutical Stockpile (NPS) program," but it has since been extended to involve much more than just drugs.

- On March 1, 2003, the NPS became the Strategic National Stockpile (SNS) program managed jointly by the U.S. Department of Homeland Security (DHS) and the U.S. Department of Health and Human Services (HHS).

- With the signing of the BioShield legislation, the SNS program was returned to the HHS for oversight and guidance.

- Effective October 1, 2018, the SNS is managed by the Office of the Assistant Secretary for Preparedness and Response (ASPR) in the HHS.

- The Strategic National Stockpile is designed to supplement and resupply state and local public health agencies in the event of a national emergency anywhere and at any time within the United States or its territories.

What Is in the Strategic National Stockpile?

- The Strategic National Stockpile is a national repository of antibiotics, chemical antidotes, antitoxins, life-support medications, intravenous (IV) administration, airway maintenance supplies, and medical/surgical items.

Who Manages the Strategic National Stockpile Program

- The Office of the ASPR in the HHS

- Federal agencies, primarily ASPR, are responsible for maintenance and delivery of SNS assets, but state and local authorities must plan to receive, store, stage, distribute, and dispense the assets.

When Would the Stockpile Be Used?

- The plan is to deliver critical medical resources to the site of a national emergency when local public health resources would likely become or have already been overwhelmed by the magnitude of the medical emergency.

- Examples might be emergencies resulting from a major earthquake; pandemic flu; a smallpox event; and terrorist events of chemical, biological, radiological/nuclear, or explosive incidents.

- Pre-event requests for SNS resources might include:
  - Actionable intelligence indicating an impending chemical, biological, radiological/nuclear, or large explosive attack or overwhelming public health disaster

- Analysis of data derived from syndromic or epidemiologic surveillance

- A sentinel event, such as a single case of smallpox

Who Can Request Assets of the Strategic National Stockpile?

- State departments of health, usually in conjunction with the state governor

- National agencies, such as the Federal Emergency Management Agency (FEMA) or the Federal Bureau of Investigation (FBI) in certain circumstances

- To receive SNS assets, the affected state's governor's office would directly request the deployment of the SNS assets from the HHS

Whose Decision Is It to Release Assets from the Strategic National Stockpile?

- The HHS and other federal agencies will evaluate the request, the situation, and determine a prompt course of action, releasing those assets that are most appropriate.

What Kinds of Things Are in the Stockpile?

- 12-hour push packs (less than 5 percent of the SNS inventory):

  - Broad-spectrum oral and intravenous antibiotics

  - Other medicines for emergency conditions

  - IV fluids and fluid administration kits

  - Airway equipment, such as endotracheal (ET) tubes, stylettes, oropharyngeal airways, Ambu bags, and carbon dioxide (CO_2) detectors

  - Bandages

- Managed inventories maintained by specific vendors or manufacturers, or the SNS:

  - Vaccines

  - Antitoxins (e.g., Botulinum)

- Ventilators
- Additional quantities of 12-hour push pack items

Where Are the Strategic National Stockpile Assets Stored

- This is not public information.
- The SNS maintains ownership of the inventory and is responsible for storing, monitoring, and maintaining the inventory, which is located in secure, environmentally controlled areas throughout the United States.

How Fast Can the Strategic National Stockpile Assets Be Deployed?

- The SNS program is committed to having 12-hour push packs delivered anywhere in the United States or its territories within 12 hours of a federal decision to deploy.
- The 12-hour push packs have been configured to be immediately loaded onto either trucks or commercial cargo aircraft for the most rapid transportation.
- At the same time assets from the SNS are deployed, the SNS program will deploy its Technical Advisory Response Unit (TARU) to coordinate with state and local officials so the SNS assets can be efficiently received and distributed on arrival at the site.

Are There Specific Agents Available in the Strategic National Stockpile for Chemical Emergencies?

- Yes, the SNS is in the process of forward deploying "CHEMPACK" to the states. The CHEMPACK contain nerve agent antidotes that can be used in the event of a nerve agent attack that overwhelms locally available resources.
- The SNS also contains nerve agent antidotes at this time.

Chapter 8

The United States' Preparedness for Public-Health Emergencies

State and local health departments must stand ready to handle many different types of emergencies that threaten the health and safety of families, communities, and the nation.

Public health emergencies occur every day across the United States. Tornadoes, hurricanes, wildfires, floods, infectious disease outbreaks, terrorist attacks, and other emergencies have all occurred in the United States within the past few years and will happen again.

Communities must be ready in the event of a public health emergency—both those they expect and those that come without warning. The terrorist and anthrax attacks of 2001 clearly demonstrated that states need expertise and resources in place before disaster strikes. Since 9/11, the Centers for Disease Control and Prevention's (CDC) Public Health Emergency Preparedness (PHEP) program has worked with states, cities, and territories to prepare and plan for emergencies.

The PHEP program provides:

- **Guidance:** Annual evidence-based guidance to ensure state, local, tribal, and territorial jurisdictions have the most current information to better protect their communities

This chapter includes text excerpted from "Ready to Respond to Public Health Emergencies," Centers for Disease Control and Prevention (CDC), August 27, 2018.

- **Technical assistance:** Operational know-how to ensure health departments are ready to respond

- **Evaluation:** Measurement and evaluation of state and local capabilities to prepare for any public health emergency

Why Preparedness Matters

Emergency preparedness is critical for the safety of people, communities, and the nation. Planning and exercising plans helps ensure that health departments are ready to respond and save lives when emergencies occur.

Preparedness in Action

Since 2002, the PHEP program has provided support to 50 states, 4 cities, and 8 territorial health departments across the nation to protect communities and save lives.

While we all hope that emergencies never occur, they are inevitable and the true test of any preparedness system. For example, in late 2016 and early 2017, Washington experienced an outbreak of mumps that affected more than 800 people of all ages. During this outbreak, the state and local health departments in Washington investigated new cases, advised local school districts on prevention measures, and developed culturally appropriate risk communication materials. Due to a robust preparedness system and the efforts of the health department staff and partners, approximately 5,000 more people were vaccinated for measles, mumps, and rubella than in previous years to prevent further spread of disease.

Part Two

Types of Emerging and Reemerging Infectious Diseases

Chapter 9

Viral Infectious Diseases

Chapter Contents

Section 9.1

Avian Influenza

This section includes text excerpted from "Bird Flu Basics," Centers for Disease Control and Prevention (CDC), April 10, 2017.

Avian influenza (AI) refers to the disease caused by infection with avian (bird) influenza (flu) type A viruses. These viruses occur naturally among wild aquatic birds worldwide and can infect domestic poultry and other bird and animal species. Avian flu viruses do not normally infect humans. However, sporadic human infections with avian flu viruses have occurred.

Influenza Type A Viruses

There are four types of influenza viruses: A, B, C, and D. Wild aquatic birds—particularly certain wild ducks, geese, swans, gulls, shorebirds, and terns—are the natural hosts for most influenza type A viruses.

Subtypes of Influenza A Viruses

Influenza A viruses are divided into subtypes on the basis of 2 proteins on the surface of the virus: hemagglutinin (HA) and neuraminidase (NA). There are 18 known HA subtypes and 11 known NA subtypes. Many different combinations of HA and NA proteins are possible. For example, an "H7N2 virus" designates an influenza A virus subtype that has an HA 7 protein and an NA 2 protein. Similarly, an "H5N1" virus has an HA 5 protein and an NA 1 protein.

All known subtypes of influenza A viruses can infect birds, except subtypes H17N10 and H18N11, which have only been found in bats. Only two influenza A virus subtypes (i.e., H1N1, and H3N2) are currently in general circulation among people. Some subtypes are found in other infected animal species. For example, H7N7 and H3N8 viral infections can cause illness in horses, and H3N8 virus infection cause illness in horses and dogs.

Lineages of Influenza A Viruses

Avian influenza viruses have evolved into distinct genetic lineages in different geographic locations. These different lineages can be distinguished by studying the genetic makeup of these viruses. For example, AI viruses circulating in birds in Asia, called "Asian lineage AI viruses," can be recognized as genetically different from AI viruses that circulate among birds in North America (called "North American lineage AI viruses"). These broad lineage classifications can be further narrowed by genetic comparisons that allow researchers to group the most closely related viruses together. Thus, the North American lineage of H7N9 viruses could be further broken down into the North American wild bird lineage versus the North American poultry lineage. The host, time period, and geographical location are often used in the lineage name to help further delineate one lineage from another.

Highly Pathogenic and Low Pathogenic Avian Influenza A Viruses

Avian influenza A viruses are designated as highly pathogenic avian influenza (HPAI) or low pathogenicity avian influenza (LPAI), based on molecular characteristics of the virus and the ability of the virus to cause disease and mortality in chickens in a laboratory setting. HPAI and LPAI designations do not refer to the severity of illness in cases of human infection with these viruses; both LPAI and HPAI viruses have caused severe illness in humans.

Poultry infected with LPAI viruses may show no signs of disease or only exhibit mild illness (such as ruffled feathers and a drop in egg production) which may not be detected. Infection of poultry with HPAI viruses can cause severe disease with high mortality. Both HPAI and LPAI viruses can spread rapidly through poultry flocks. HPAI virus infection can cause disease that affects multiple internal organs with mortality up to 90 to 100 percent in chickens, often within 48 hours. However, ducks can be infected without any signs of illness. There are genetic and antigenic differences between the influenza A virus subtypes that typically infect only birds and those that can infect birds and people.

Avian influenza viruses rarely infect people. The most frequently identified subtypes of avian influenza that have caused human infections are H5, H7, and H9 viruses. Other viruses, such as H10N8, H10N7, and H6N8, have been detected in people also, but to a lesser extent.

Influenza A H5

There are 9 known subtypes of H5 viruses (H5N1, H5N2, H5N3, H5N4, H5N5, H5N6, H5N7, H5N8, and H5N9). Most H5 viruses identified worldwide in wild birds and poultry are LPAI, but HPAI viruses have occasionally been detected. Sporadic H5 virus infection of humans has occurred, such as with Asian lineage HPAI H5N1 viruses circulating among poultry in Asia and the Middle East. Human infection of H5N1 viral infections have been reported in 16 countries, often resulting in severe pneumonia and greater than 50 percent mortality.

Influenza A H7

There are nine known subtypes of H7 viruses (H7N1, H7N2, H7N3, H7N4, H7N5, H7N6, H7N7, and H7N9). Most H7 viruses identified worldwide in wild birds and poultry are LPAI viruses. H7 virus infection in humans is uncommon. The most frequently identified H7 viruses associated with human infection are Asian lineage avian influenza A(H7N9) viruses, which were first detected in China in 2013. While human infections are rare, these have commonly resulted in severe respiratory illness and death. In addition to Asian lineage H7N9 viruses, H7N2, H7N3, H7N7 viral infections have been reported. These viruses have primarily caused mild to moderate illness in people, with symptoms that include conjunctivitis and/or upper respiratory tract symptoms.

Influenza A H9

There are nine known subtypes of H9 viruses (H9N1, H9N2, H9N3, H9N4, H9N5, H9N6, H9N7, H9N8, and H9N9); all H9 viruses identified worldwide in wild birds and poultry are LPAI viruses. H9N2 virus has been detected in bird populations in Asia, Europe, the Middle East, and Africa. Rare, sporadic H9N2 viral infections in people have been reported to generally cause mild upper respiratory tract illness; one infection has resulted in death.

Avian Influenza A Viral Infections in Humans

Although avian influenza A viruses usually do not infect people, rare cases of human infection with these viruses have been reported. Infected birds shed avian influenza virus in their saliva, mucus, and feces. Human infections with bird flu viruses can happen when enough of the virus gets into a person's eyes, nose or mouth, or is inhaled. This can happen when the virus is in the air (in droplets or possibly dust) and a person breathes it in, or when a person touches something that has the virus on it then touches their mouth, eyes, or nose. Rare human infections with some avian viruses have occurred most often after unprotected contact with infected birds or surfaces contaminated with avian influenza viruses. However, some infections have been identified where direct contact was not known to have occurred. Illness in people has ranged from mild to severe.

The spread of avian influenza A viruses from one ill person to another has been reported very rarely; when it has been reported, it has been limited, inefficient, and not sustained. However, because of the possibility that avian influenza A viruses could change and gain the ability to spread easily between people, monitoring for human infection and person-to-person spread is extremely important for public health.

Signs and Symptoms of Avian Influenza A Viral Infections in Humans

The reported signs and symptoms of avian influenza A viral infections in humans have ranged from mild to severe and included conjunctivitis; influenza-like illness (e.g., fever, cough, sore throat, muscle aches), sometimes accompanied by nausea, abdominal pain, diarrhea, and vomiting; severe respiratory illness (e.g., shortness of breath, difficulty breathing, pneumonia, acute respiratory distress, viral pneumonia, respiratory failure); neurologic changes (altered mental status, seizures); and the involvement of other organ systems. Asian lineage H7N9 and HPAI Asian lineage H5N1 viruses have been responsible for most human illness worldwide to date, including most serious illnesses and highest mortality.

Detecting Avian Influenza A Virus Infection in Humans

Avian influenza A virus infection in people cannot be diagnosed by clinical signs and symptoms alone—laboratory testing is needed. Avian influenza A virus infection is usually diagnosed by collecting a swab from the upper respiratory tract (nose or throat) of the sick person. (Testing is more accurate when the swab is collected during the first few days of illness.) This specimen is sent to a laboratory; the laboratory looks for avian influenza A virus either by using a molecular test, by trying to grow the virus, or both. (Growing avian influenza A viruses should only be done in laboratories with high levels of biosafety.)

For critically ill patients, collection and testing of lower respiratory tract specimens also may lead to the diagnosis of avian influenza viral infection. However, for some patients who are no longer very sick or who have fully recovered, it may be difficult to detect the avian influenza A virus in the specimen. Sometimes, it may still be possible to diagnose avian influenza A virus infection by looking for evidence of antibodies the body has produced in response to the virus. This is not always an option because it requires two blood specimens (one taken during the first week of illness and another taken three to four weeks later). Also, it can take several weeks to verify the results, and testing must be performed in a special laboratory, such as at the Centers for Disease Control and Prevention (CDC).

The CDC has posted guidance for clinicians and public-health professionals in the United States on appropriate testing, specimen collection, and processing of samples from patients who may be infected with avian influenza A viruses.

Treating Avian Influenza A Viral Infections in Humans

The CDC recommends a neuraminidase inhibitor for treatment of human infection with avian influenza A viruses. Analyses of available avian influenza viruses circulating worldwide suggest that most viruses are susceptible to oseltamivir, peramivir, and zanamivir. However, some evidence of antiviral resistance has been reported in Asian H5N1 and Asian H7N9 viruses isolated from some human cases. Monitoring for antiviral resistance among avian influenza A viruses is crucial and ongoing.

Preventing Human Infection with Avian Influenza A Viruses

The best way to prevent infection with avian influenza A viruses is to avoid sources of exposure. Most human infections with avian influenza A viruses have occurred following direct or close contact with infected poultry.

People who have had contact with infected birds may be given influenza antiviral drugs preventatively. While antiviral drugs are most often used to treat influenza, they also can be used to prevent infection in someone who has been exposed to influenza viruses. When used to prevent seasonal influenza, antiviral drugs are 70 to 90 percent effective. Seasonal influenza vaccination will not prevent infection with avian influenza A viruses, but it can reduce the risk of coinfection with human and avian influenza A viruses. It is also possible to make a vaccine that can protect people against avian influenza viruses. For example, the United States government maintains a stockpile of vaccines to protect against some Asian avian influenza A H5N1 viruses.

The stockpiled vaccine could be used if similar H5N1 viruses were to begin transmitting easily from person to person. Since influenza viruses change, the CDC continues to make new candidate vaccine viruses as needed. Creating a candidate vaccine virus is the first step in producing a vaccine.

Transmission of Avian Influenza A Viruses Between Animals and People

Influenza A viruses have infected many different animals, including ducks, chickens, pigs, whales, horses, and seals. However, certain subtypes of influenza A virus are specific to certain species, except for birds, which are hosts to all known subtypes of influenza A viruses. Currently circulating Influenza A subtypes in humans are the H3N2 and H1N1 viruses. Examples of different influenza A virus subtypes that have infected animals to cause outbreaks include the H1N1 and H3N2 viral infections of pigs, and H7N7 and H3N8 viral infections of horses.

Influenza A viruses that typically infect and transmit among one animal species sometimes can cross over and cause illness in another species. For example, until 1998, only H1N1 viruses circulated widely in the United States pig population. However, in 1998, H3N2 viruses from humans were introduced into the pig population and caused widespread disease among pigs. More recently, H3N8 viruses from horses have crossed over and caused outbreaks in dogs.

Avian influenza A viruses may be transmitted from animals to humans in two main ways:

- Directly from birds or from avian influenza A virus-contaminated environments to people

- Through an intermediate host, such as a pig

Influenza A viruses have eight separate gene segments. The segmented genome allows influenza A viruses from different species to mix and create a new virus if influenza A viruses from two different species infect the same person or animal. For example, if a pig were infected with a human influenza A virus and an avian influenza A virus at the same time, the new replicating viruses could mix existing genetic information (reassortment) and produce a new influenza A virus that had most of the genes from the human virus, but a hemagglutinin gene and/or neuraminidase gene and other genes from the avian virus. The resulting new virus might then be able to infect humans and spread easily from person to person, but it would have surface proteins (hemagglutinin and/or neuraminidase) different than those currently found in influenza viruses that infect humans.

This type of major change in the influenza A viruses is known as "antigenic shift." Antigenic shift results when a new influenza A virus subtype to which most people have little or no immune protection infects humans. If this new influenza A virus causes illness in people and is transmitted easily from person to person in a sustained manner, an influenza pandemic can occur.

It is possible that the process of genetic reassortment could occur in a person who is coinfected with an avian influenza A virus and a human influenza A virus. The genetic information in these viruses could reassort to create a new influenza A virus with a hemagglutinin gene from the avian virus and other genes from the human virus. Influenza A viruses with a hemagglutinin against which humans have little or no immunity that have reassorted with a human influenza virus are more likely to result in sustained human-to-human transmission and pose a major public health threat of pandemic influenza. Therefore, careful evaluation of influenza A viruses recovered from humans who are infected with avian influenza A viruses is very important to identify reassortment if it occurs.

Although it is unusual for people to get influenza viral infections directly from animals, sporadic human infections and outbreaks caused by certain avian influenza A viruses and swine influenza A viruses have been reported.

Examples of Human Infections with Avian Influenza A Viruses with Possible Limited, Nonsustained Human-to-Human Transmission

Human infections with avian influenza A viruses are rare and have most often occurred after people had exposure to infected poultry (e.g., direct contact with chickens, or visiting a live poultry market). However, some clusters in which limited, nonsustained person-to-person spread of avian influenza A viruses was suspected or is believed to have occurred have been reported in several countries. There is no test to confirm human-to-human spread of avian influenza A viruses. Rather, a determination that human-to-human transmission likely occurred is based upon the findings of detailed epidemiologic and laboratory investigations.

For example:

- In 1997, when the first human cases of Asian H5N1 virus infection were identified in Hong Kong, there was serologic evidence of limited, nonsustained transmission of Asian H5N1 virus to a very small number of healthcare workers and household contacts, but the virus did not spread further.

- In 2003, in the Netherlands, there was evidence of possible transmission of H7N7 virus from two poultry workers to three family members. All three family members had conjunctivitis, and one also had an influenza-like illness.

- In 2004, in Thailand, there was evidence of probable human-to-human spread of Asian H5N1 virus in a family cluster. Transmission was associated with prolonged very close unprotected contact between an ill child with H5N1 virus infection and her mother and her aunt. Further transmission did not occur.

- In 2005, in Indonesia, limited, nonsustained person-to-person transmission of Asian H5N1 virus could not be excluded among two clusters of patients who had no known contact with poultry or other animals.

- In 2006, in Indonesia, limited, nonsustained person-to-person transmission of Asian H5N1 virus may have occurred among a family cluster of 8 probable or confirmed Asian H5N1 cases.

- In December 2007, in China, limited, nonsustained Asian H5N1 virus transmission is thought to have occurred between a sick son and his father through prolonged very close unprotected exposure while the son was in the hospital.

- Also in 2007, in Pakistan, limited, nonsustained human-to-human H5N1 virus transmission is thought to have occurred among brothers.

- In 2013, human infections with an Asian lineage avian influenza A(H7N9) virus were first reported in China. Annual epidemics of human infections with Asian H7N9 viruses in China driven mostly by exposure to infected poultry at live poultry markets have been reported since 2013. A small percentage of reported cases have been associated with possible limited, nonsustained human-to-human transmission, mostly occurring between family members. However, limited, nonsustained transmission of Asian H7N9 has been reported in a few cases in hospitals.

It is possible for human-to-human transmission of other nonhuman (animal-origin) influenza A viruses to range along a continuum: from occasional, limited, nonsustained human-to-human transmission of one or more generations without further spread ("dead-end transmission"), to efficient and sustained human-to-human transmission. Efficient and sustained (ongoing) transmission of nonhuman influenza A viruses (including avian influenza A viruses) among people in the community is needed for an influenza pandemic to begin.

Prevention and Treatment of Avian Influenza A Viruses in People
The Best Prevention Is to Avoid Sources of Exposure

The best way to prevent infection with avian influenza A viruses is to avoid sources of exposure whenever possible. Infected birds shed avian influenza virus in their saliva, mucus, and feces. Human infections with bird flu viruses can happen when enough of the virus gets into a person's eyes, nose or mouth, or is inhaled. This can happen when the virus is in the air (in droplets or possibly dust) and a person breathes it in, or when a person touches something that has the virus on it then touches their mouth, eyes, or nose. Rare human infections with some avian viruses have occurred most often after unprotected contact with infected birds or surfaces contaminated with avian influenza viruses. However, some infections have been identified where direct contact was not known to have occurred.

People who work with poultry or who respond to avian influenza outbreaks are advised to follow recommended biosecurity and infection control practices; these include use of appropriate personal protective equipment and careful attention to hand hygiene. Additionally, the CDC recommends that people responding to poultry outbreaks should get a seasonal influenza vaccination every year, preferably at least two weeks before engaging in an outbreak response. Seasonal influenza vaccination will not prevent infection with avian influenza A viruses, but can reduce the risk of coinfection with human and avian influenza A viruses. These people should also be monitored for illness during and after responding to avian influenza outbreaks among poultry.

What to Do If You Find a Dead Bird

State and local agencies have different policies for collecting and testing birds, so check with your state health department, state veterinary diagnostic laboratory, or state wildlife agency for information about reporting dead birds in your area. Wildlife agencies routinely investigate sick or dead bird events if large numbers are impacted.

This type of reporting could help with the early detection of illnesses like West Nile virus or avian influenza. If local authorities tell you to simply dispose of the bird's carcass (body), do not handle it with your bare hands. Use gloves or an inverted plastic bag to place the carcass in a garbage bag, which can then be disposed of in your regular trash.

To report unusual signs in birds you have seen in the wild, call 866-4USDA-WS (866-487-3297).

Preparing Food

- The United States poultry industry maintains rigorous health and safety standards, including routine monitoring for avian influenza.

- It is safe to eat properly handled and cooked poultry in the United States.

- However, consumers are reminded to handle raw poultry hygienically and cook all poultry and poultry products (including eggs) thoroughly before eating.

- Raw poultry can be associated with many infections, including salmonella.

- While there is no evidence that any human cases of avian influenza have ever been acquired by eating properly cooked poultry products, uncooked poultry and poultry products (such as blood) have been linked to human infections with organisms other than influenza. Proper cooking kills influenza viruses.

Traveling to Other Countries

- The CDC does not recommend any travel restrictions to any of the countries affected by avian influenza viruses in poultry or people.

- The CDC does recommend that travelers to countries with avian influenza A outbreaks in poultry or people observe the following:

  - Avoid visiting poultry farms, bird markets, and other places where live poultry are raised, kept, or sold.

  - Avoid preparing or eating raw or undercooked poultry products.

  - Practice hygiene and cleanliness.

  - Visit a doctor if you become sick during or after travel.

If You Have Had Direct Contact with Infected Birds

- People who have had direct contact with infected bird(s) should be watched to see if they become ill. They may be given influenza antiviral drugs to prevent illness.

- While antiviral drugs are most often used to treat flu, they also can be used to prevent infection in someone who has been exposed to influenza viruses. When used to prevent seasonal influenza, antiviral drugs are 70 to 90 percent effective.

- Close contacts (family members, etc.) of people who have been exposed to avian influenza viruses are being asked to monitor their health and report any flu-like symptoms.

Section 9.2

B-Virus Infection

This section includes text excerpted from "B Virus," Centers for Disease Control and Prevention (CDC), January 31, 2019.

B virus infection is extremely rare, but it can lead to severe brain damage or death if you do not get treatment immediately. People typically get infected with B virus if they are bitten or scratched by an infected macaque monkey, or have contact with the monkey's eyes, nose, or mouth. Only one case has been documented of an infected person spreading B virus to another person.

Cause and Frequency

B virus infections in people are usually caused by macaque monkeys. These kinds of monkeys are commonly infected with B virus, but they usually do not have symptoms or just have mild disease. Other primates, such as chimpanzees and capuchin monkeys, can become infected with B virus and will frequently die from these infections. There have not been documented cases of such primates spreading B virus except to macaques.

B virus infections in people are rare. Since B virus was identified in 1932, only 50 people have been documented to have infections; 21 of them died. Most of these people got infected after they were bitten or scratched by a monkey, or when tissue or fluids from a monkey got on their broken skin, such as by needle stick or cut. In 1997, a researcher died from B virus infection after bodily fluid from an infected monkey splashed into her eye.

Hundreds of bites and scratches occur every year in monkey facilities in the United States, but people rarely get infected with B virus. A study of more than 300 animal-care workers showed that none had B virus infection, including the 166 workers who had possible exposures to monkeys.

Signs and Symptoms

Symptoms typically start within one month of being exposed to B virus but could appear in as little as three to seven days.

The first indications of B virus infection are typically flu-like symptoms:

- Fever and chills
- Muscle ache
- Fatigue
- Headache

Then, you may develop small blisters in the wound or area on your body that had contact with the monkey.

Other symptoms may include:

- Shortness of breath
- Nausea and vomiting
- Abdominal pain
- Hiccups

As the disease progresses, the virus spreads to and causes inflammation (swelling) of the brain and spinal cord. This can lead to:

- Neurologic and inflammatory symptoms (pain, numbness, itching) near the wound site
- Problems with muscle coordination

- Brain damage and severe damage to the nervous system

- Death

Problems with breathing and death can occur one day to three weeks after symptoms appear. It may be possible for people to have mild B virus infection or no symptoms. However, there are no studies or evidence of this.

Transmission

B virus can spread from infected macaque monkeys to people. Macaque monkeys commonly have this virus, and it can be found in their saliva, feces, urine, or brain or spinal cord tissue. The virus may also be found in cells coming from an infected monkey in a lab. B virus can survive for hours on surfaces, particularly when moist.

Most people will not come in contact with monkeys, so their risk of getting infected with B virus is very low. However, laboratory workers, veterinarians, and others who may be exposed to monkeys or their specimens have a higher risk of getting B virus infection. In recent years, many macaque attacks have been reported by people visiting temple parks in some countries in Asia, where macaques commonly roam freely. About 70 to 80 percent of these macaques have been found to be B virus positive, but there have not been any documented cases of B virus spreading to humans.

You can get infected with B virus if you:

- Are bitten or scratched by an infected monkey

- Get an infected monkey's tissue or fluid on your broken skin or in your eyes, nose, or mouth

- Have a needle stick by a contaminated syringe

- Scratch or cut yourself on a contaminated cage or other sharp-edged surface

- Are exposed to the brain (especially), spinal cord, or skull of an infected monkey

- Only one case has been documented of an infected person spreading B virus to another person

Prevention

There are no vaccines that can protect you against B virus infection.

If you are in a place where there are macaque monkeys, you should stay away from them so that you do not get bitten or scratched. You should not touch or feed monkeys.

Section 9.3

Chikungunya Virus

This section includes text excerpted from
"Chikungunya Virus," Centers for Disease Control
and Prevention (CDC), December 17, 2018.

Chikungunya virus is spread to people by the bite of an infected mosquito. The most common symptoms of infection are fever and joint pain. Other symptoms may include headache, muscle pain, joint swelling, or rash. Outbreaks have occurred in countries in Africa, Asia, and Europe, and in the Indian and Pacific Oceans. In late 2013, chikungunya virus was found for the first time in the Americas on islands in the Caribbean. There is a risk that the virus will be imported to new areas by infected travelers. There is no vaccine to prevent or medicine to treat chikungunya virus infection. Travelers can protect themselves by preventing mosquito bites. When traveling to countries with chikungunya virus, use insect repellent, wear long sleeves and pants, and stay in places with air conditioning or that use window and door screens.

Symptoms

- Most people infected with chikungunya virus will develop some symptoms.

- Symptoms usually begin three to seven days after being bitten by an infected mosquito.

- The most common symptoms are fever and joint pain.

- Other symptoms may include headache, muscle pain, joint swelling, or rash.

- Chikungunya disease does not often result in death, but the symptoms can be severe and disabling.

71

- Most patients feel better within a week. In some people, the joint pain may persist for months.

- People at risk for more severe disease include newborns infected around the time of birth; older adults (older than 65 years of age); and people with medical conditions, such as high blood pressure, diabetes, or heart disease.

- Once a person has been infected, she or he is likely to be protected from future infections.

Diagnosis

- The symptoms of chikungunya are similar to those of dengue and Zika, diseases spread by the same mosquitoes that transmit chikungunya.

- See your healthcare provider if you develop the symptoms described above and have visited an area where chikungunya is found.

- If you have recently traveled, tell your healthcare provider when and where you traveled.

- Your healthcare provider may order blood tests to look for chikungunya or other similar viruses, such as dengue and Zika.

Treatment

- There is no vaccine to prevent or medicine to treat chikungunya virus.

- Treat the symptoms:
  - Get plenty of rest.
  - Drink fluids to prevent dehydration.
  - Take medicine, such as acetaminophen (Tylenol®) or paracetamol, to reduce fever and pain.
  - Do not take aspirin and other nonsteroidal anti-inflammatory drugs (NSAIDs) until dengue can be ruled out to reduce the risk of bleeding.

- If you are taking medicine for another medical condition, talk to your healthcare provider before taking additional medication.

- If you have chikungunya, prevent mosquito bites for the first week of your illness.

  - During the first week of infection, chikungunya virus can be found in the blood and passed from an infected person to a mosquito through mosquito bites.

  - An infected mosquito can then spread the virus to other people.

Transmission
Through Mosquito Bites

- Chikungunya virus is transmitted to people through mosquito bites. Mosquitoes become infected when they feed on a person already infected with the virus. Infected mosquitoes can then spread the virus to other people through bites.

- Chikungunya virus is most often spread to people by *Aedes aegypti* and *Aedes albopictus* mosquitoes. These are the same mosquitoes that transmit dengue virus. They bite during the day and at night.

Rarely, from Mother to Child

- Chikungunya virus is transmitted rarely from mother to newborn around the time of birth.

- To date, no infants have been found to be infected with chikungunya virus through breastfeeding. Because of the benefits of breastfeeding, mothers are encouraged to breastfeed even in areas where chikungunya virus is circulating.

Rarely, through Infected Blood

- In theory, the virus could be spread through a blood transfusion. To date, there are no known reports of this happening.

Prevention

The most effective way to prevent infection from chikungunya virus is to prevent mosquito bites. Mosquitoes bite during the day and night. Use insect repellent, wear long-sleeved shirts and pants, treat clothing and gear, and take steps to control mosquitoes indoors and outdoors.

Use Insect Repellent

Use U.S. Environmental Protection Agency (EPA)-registered insect repellents with one of the active ingredients below. When used as directed, EPA-registered insect repellents are proven safe and effective, even for pregnant and breastfeeding women.

- N,N-diethyl-meta-toluamide (DEET)
- Picaridin (known as "KBR 3023" and "icaridin" outside the United States)
- IR3535
- Oil of lemon eucalyptus (OLE)
- Para-menthane-diol (PMD)
- 2-undecanone

Find the right insect repellent for you by using the EPA's online search tool offered by the EPA.

Tips for Babies and Children

- Always follow instructions when applying insect repellent to children.
- Do not use insect repellent on babies younger than two months of age.
- Instead, dress your child in clothing that covers their arms and legs.
- Cover strollers and baby carriers with mosquito netting.
- Do not use products containing OLE or PMD on children under three years of age.
- Do not apply insect repellent to a child's hands, eyes, mouth, cuts, or irritated skin.
- Adults: Spray insect repellent onto your hands and then apply to a child's face.

Tips for Everyone

- Always follow the product label instructions.
- Reapply insect repellent as directed.

- Do not spray repellent on the skin under clothing.
- If you are also using sunscreen, apply sunscreen first and insect repellent second.

Natural Insect Repellents (Repellents Not Registered with U.S. Environmental Protection Agency)

- We do not know the effectiveness of non-EPA registered insect repellents, including some natural repellents.
- To protect yourself against diseases spread by mosquitoes, the Centers for Disease Control and Prevention (CDC) and EPA recommend using an EPA-registered insect repellent.
- Choosing an EPA-registered repellent ensures the EPA has evaluated the product for effectiveness.

Wear Long-Sleeved Shirts and Long Pants
Treat Clothing and Gear

- Use permethrin to treat clothing and gear (such as boots, pants, socks, and tents), or buy permethrin-treated clothing and gear.
  - Permethrin is an insecticide that kills or repels mosquitoes.
  - Permethrin-treated clothing provides protection after multiple washings.
  - Read product information to find out how long the protection will last.

If treating items yourself, follow the product instructions.

- Do not use permethrin products directly on skin.

Take Steps to Control Mosquitoes Indoors and Outdoors

- Use screens on windows and doors. Repair holes in screens to keep mosquitoes outdoors.
- Use air conditioning, if available.
- Stop mosquitoes from laying eggs in or near water.
- Once a week, empty and scrub, turn over, cover, or throw out items that hold water, such as tires, buckets, planters, toys, pools, birdbaths, flowerpots, or trash containers.
- Check indoors and outdoors.

Prevent Mosquito Bites When Traveling Overseas

- Choose a hotel or lodging with air conditioning or screens on windows and doors.

- Sleep under a mosquito bed net if you are outside or in a room that does not have screens.

  - Buy a bed net at your local outdoor store or online before traveling overseas.

  - Choose a World Health Organization Pesticide Evaluation Scheme (WHOPES)-approved bed net: compact, white, rectangular, with 156 holes per square inch, and long enough to tuck under the mattress.

  - Permethrin-treated bed nets provide more protection than untreated nets.

    - Do not wash bed nets or expose them to sunlight. This will break down the insecticide more quickly.

Section 9.4

Coronaviruses

This section includes text excerpted from *"Coronavirus,"* Centers for Disease Control and Prevention (CDC), November 9, 2017.

Human Coronavirus *Types*

Coronaviruses are named for the crown-like spikes on their surface. There are four main subgroupings of *coronaviruses*, known as "alpha," "beta," "gamma," and "delta."

Human *coronaviruses* were first identified in the mid-1960s. The six *coronaviruses* that can infect people are:

Common Human Coronaviruses

- 229E (alpha *coronavirus*)

- NL63 (alpha *coronavirus*)

- OC43 (beta *coronavirus*)

- HKU1 (beta *coronavirus*)

Other Human Coronaviruses

- MERS-CoV (the beta *coronavirus* that causes Middle East respiratory syndrome, or MERS)

- SARS-CoV (the beta *coronavirus* that causes severe acute respiratory syndrome, or SARS)

People around the world commonly get infected with human *coronaviruses* 229E, NL63, OC43, and HKU1.

Sometimes, new *coronaviruses* can emerge and make people sick. Two examples of this are MERS-CoV and SARS-CoV, which are known to frequently cause severe illness.

Severe Acute Respiratory Syndrome Coronavirus

Severe acute respiratory syndrome *coronavirus* (SARS-CoV) was first recognized in China in November 2002. It caused a worldwide outbreak in 2003 with 8,098 probable cases, including 774 deaths from 2002 to 2003. Since 2004, there have not been any known cases of SARS-CoV infection reported anywhere in the world.

Middle East Respiratory Syndrome Coronavirus

Middle East respiratory syndrome *coronavirus* (MERS-CoV) was first reported in Saudi Arabia in 2012. It has since caused illness in people from dozens of other countries. All cases to date have been linked to countries in and near the Arabian Peninsula. The Centers for Disease Control and Prevention (CDC) continues to closely monitor the Middle East respiratory syndrome (MERS) situation globally and work with partners to better understand the risks of this virus, including the source, how it spreads, and how infections might be prevented.

Symptoms
Common Human Coronaviruses

Common human *coronaviruses*, including types 229E, NL63, OC43, and HKU1, usually cause mild to moderate upper respiratory tract illnesses, such as the common cold. Most people get infected with these viruses at some point in their lives. These illnesses usually only last for a short amount of time. Symptoms may include:

- Runny nose
- Headache
- Cough
- Sore throat
- Fever
- A general feeling of being unwell

Coronaviruses can sometimes cause lower respiratory tract illnesses, such as pneumonia or bronchitis. This is more common in people with cardiopulmonary disease, people with weakened immune systems, infants, and older adults.

Other Human Coronaviruses

Two other *coronaviruses*, MERS-CoV and SARS-CoV have been known to frequently cause severe symptoms. MERS symptoms usually include fever, cough, and shortness of breath, which often progress to pneumonia or kidney failure; many people with MERS have died. SARS symptoms often included fever, chills, and body aches, which usually progressed to pneumonia. No human cases of SARS have been reported anywhere in the world since 2004. Sporadic MERS cases continue to occur, primarily in the Arabian Peninsula.

Diagnosis

Your healthcare provider may order laboratory tests on respiratory specimens and serum (part of your blood) to detect human *coronavirus*. This is especially likely if you have severe disease or are suspected of having MERS.

You should always tell your healthcare provider if you have recently traveled or had contact with animals. Most MERS-CoV infections have been reported from countries in the Arabian Peninsula. Therefore, reporting a travel history or contact with camels is very important when trying to diagnose MERS.

Transmission

The ways that common human *coronaviruses* spread have not been studied very much. However, human *coronaviruses* likely spread from an infected person to others through:

- The air by coughing and sneezing
- Close personal contact, such as touching or shaking hands
- Touching an object or surface with germs on it, then touching your mouth, nose, or eyes before washing your hands
- Rarely, fecal contamination

In the United States, people usually get infected with common human *coronaviruses* in the fall and winter. However, you can get infected at any time of the year. Most people will get infected with one or more of the common human *coronaviruses* in their lifetime. Young children are most likely to get infected. However, people can have multiple infections in their lifetime.

Prevention
How to Protect Yourself

There are currently no vaccines available to protect you against human *coronavirus* infection. You may be able to reduce your risk of infection by doing the following:

- Wash your hands often with soap and water.
- Avoid touching your eyes, nose, or mouth with unwashed hands.
- Avoid close contact with people who are sick.

How to Protect Others

If you have cold-like symptoms, you can help protect others by doing the following:

- Stay home while you are sick.
- Avoid close contact with others.
- Cover your mouth and nose with a tissue when you cough or sneeze, then throw the tissue in the trash and wash your hands.
- Clean and disinfect objects and surfaces.

Treatment

There are no specific treatments for illnesses caused by human *coronaviruses*. Most people with common human *coronavirus* illness will recover on their own. However, you can do some things to relieve your symptoms:

- Take pain and fever medications (caution: do not give aspirin to children).

- Use a room humidifier or take a hot shower to help ease a sore throat and cough.

If you are mildly sick, you should:

- Drink plenty of liquids.

- Stay home and rest.

If you are concerned about your symptoms, you should see your healthcare provider.

Section 9.5

Dengue

This section includes text excerpted from "Dengue,"
Centers for Disease Control and Prevention (CDC), May 3, 2019.

Dengue viruses are spread to people through the bite of an infected *Aedes* species (*Ae. aegypti* or *Ae. albopictus*) mosquito. Dengue is common in more than 100 countries around the world. Forty percent of the world's population, about 3 billion people, live in areas with a risk of dengue. Dengue is often a leading cause of illness in areas with risk.

- Dengue viruses are spread to people through the bite of an infected Aedes species (*Ae. aegypti* or *Ae. albopictus*) mosquito. These mosquitoes also spread Zika, chikungunya, and other viruses.

- Dengue is common in more than 100 countries around the world.

- Forty percent of the world's population, about 3 billion people, live in areas with a risk of dengue. Dengue is often a leading cause of illness in areas with risk.

- Each year, up to 400 million people get infected with dengue. Approximately 100 million people get sick from infection, and 22,000 die from severe dengue.

- Dengue is caused by one of any of four related viruses: Dengue virus 1, 2, 3, and 4. For this reason, a person can be infected with a dengue virus as many as four times in his or her lifetime.

Symptoms and Treatment
Symptoms of Mild Symptoms

Mild symptoms of dengue can be confused with other illnesses that cause fever, aches and pains, or a rash.

The most common symptom of dengue is fever with any of the following:

- Nausea, vomiting

- Rash

- Aches and pains (eye pain, typically behind the eyes; muscle, joint, or bone pain)

- Any warning sign

Symptoms of dengue typically last two to seven days. Most people will recover after about a week.

Treatment of Mild Dengue

- There is no specific medication to treat dengue.

- Treat the symptoms of dengue and see your healthcare provider.

If You Think You Have Dengue

- See a healthcare provider if you develop a fever or have symptoms of dengue. Inform your provider about your travel.

- Rest as much as possible.

- Take acetaminophen (also known as "paracetamol" outside of the United States) to control fever and relieve pain.

- Do not take aspirin or ibuprofen!

- Drink plenty of fluids such as water or drinks with added electrolytes to stay hydrated.

Symptoms of dengue can become severe within a few hours. Severe dengue is a medical emergency.

Severe Dengue

- About 1 in 20 people who get sick with dengue will develop severe dengue.
- Severe dengue is a more serious form of disease that can result in shock, internal bleeding, and even death.
- You are more likely to develop severe dengue if you have had a dengue infection before.
- Infants and pregnant women are at increased risk for developing severe dengue.

Symptoms of Severe Dengue
Warning Signs of Severe Dengue

Watch for signs and symptoms of severe dengue. Warning signs generally begin in the 24 to 48 hours after your fever has gone away.

If you or a family member develops any of the following symptoms, immediately go to a local clinic or emergency room:

- Stomach or belly pain, tenderness
- Vomiting (at least 3 times in 24 hours)
- Bleeding from the nose or gums
- Vomiting blood, or blood in the stool
- Feeling tired, restless, or irritable

Treatment of Severe Dengue

- If you develop any warning signs, see a healthcare provider or go to the emergency room immediately.
- Severe dengue is a medical emergency and requires immediate medical attention or hospitalization.
- If you are traveling, find healthcare abroad.

Testing

- See your healthcare provider if you have symptoms of dengue and live in or have recently traveled to an area with risk of dengue.

- If you have recently traveled to an area with risk of dengue, tell your healthcare provider.

- A blood test is the only way to confirm the diagnosis.

- Your healthcare provider may order blood tests to look for dengue or other similar viruses such as Zika or chikungunya.

Transmission
Through Mosquito Bites

Dengue viruses are spread to people through the bites of infected Aedes species mosquitoes (*Ae. aegypti* or *Ae. albopictus*). These are the same types of mosquitoes that spread Zika and chikungunya viruses.

- These mosquitoes typically lay eggs near standing water in containers that hold water, such as buckets, bowls, animal dishes, flower pots, and vases.

- These mosquitoes prefer to bite people, and live both indoors and outdoors near people.

- Mosquitoes that spread dengue, chikungunya, and Zika bite during the day and night.

- Mosquitoes become infected when they bite a person infected with the virus. Infected mosquitoes can then spread the virus to other people through bites.

From Mother to Child

- A pregnant woman already infected with dengue can pass the virus to her fetus during pregnancy or around the time of birth.

- To date, there has been one documented report of dengue spread through breast milk. Because of the benefits of breastfeeding, mothers are encouraged to breastfeed even in areas with risk of dengue.

Through Infected Blood, Laboratory, or Healthcare Setting Exposures

Rarely, dengue can be spread through blood transfusion, organ transplant, or through a needle-stick injury.

Section 9.6

Ebola Virus Disease

This section includes text excerpted from "Ebola,"
Centers for Disease Control and Prevention (CDC),
September 18, 2018.

What Is Ebola Virus Disease?

Ebola virus disease (EVD) is a rare and deadly disease most commonly affecting people and nonhuman primates (monkeys, gorillas, and chimpanzees). It is caused by an infection with a group of viruses within the genus Ebolavirus:

- Ebola virus (species Zaire ebolavirus)

- Sudan virus (species Sudan ebolavirus)

- Taï Forest virus (species Taï Forest ebolavirus, formerly Côte d'Ivoire ebolavirus)

- Bundibugyo virus (species Bundibugyo ebolavirus)

- Reston virus (RESTV) (species Reston ebolavirus)

- Bombali virus (species Bombali ebolavirus)

Of these, only four (Ebola, Sudan, Taï Forest, and Bundibugyo viruses) are known to cause disease in people. Reston virus is known to cause disease in nonhuman primates and pigs, but not in people. It is unknown if the Bombali virus, which was recently identified in bats, causes disease in either animals or people.

Ebola virus was first discovered in 1976 near the Ebola river in what is now the Democratic Republic of Congo. Since then, the virus has been infecting people from time to time, leading to outbreaks in several African countries. Scientists do not know where the Ebola virus comes from. However, based on the nature of similar viruses, they believe the virus is animal-borne, with bats being the most likely source. The bats carrying the virus can transmit it to other animals, such as apes, monkeys, duikers, and humans.

Ebola virus spreads to people through direct contact with bodily fluids of a person who is sick with or has died from EVD. This can occur when a person touches the infected body fluids (or objects that are contaminated with them), and the virus gets in through broken skin or mucous membranes in the eyes, nose, or mouth. The virus can also spread to people through direct contact with the blood, body fluids, and tissues of infected fruit bats or primates. People can get the virus through sexual contact as well.

Ebola survivors may experience difficult side effects after their recovery, such as tiredness, muscle aches, eye and vision problems, and stomach pain. Survivors may also experience stigma as they re-enter their communities.

History of Ebola Virus Disease
Emergence of Ebola in Humans

Ebola virus disease, one of the deadliest viral diseases, was discovered in 1976 when two consecutive outbreaks of fatal hemorrhagic fever occurred in different parts of Central Africa. The first outbreak occurred in the Democratic Republic of Congo (formerly Zaire) in a village near the Ebola river, which gave the virus its name. The second outbreak occurred in what is now South Sudan, approximately 500 miles (850 km) away.

Initially, public health officials assumed these outbreaks were a single event associated with an infected person who traveled between the two locations. However, scientists later discovered that the two outbreaks were caused by two genetically distinct viruses: Zaire ebolavirus and Sudan ebolavirus. After this discovery, scientists concluded that the virus came from two different sources and spread independently to people in each of the affected areas.

Viral and epidemiologic data suggest that Ebola virus existed long before these recorded outbreaks occurred. Factors such as population growth, encroachment into forested areas, and direct interaction with wildlife (such as bushmeat consumption) may have contributed to the spread of the Ebola virus.

Identifying a Host

Following the discovery of the virus, scientists (called "reservoir among virologists," people who study viruses) studied thousands of animals, insects, and plants in search of its source. Gorillas, chimpanzees, and other mammals may be implicated when the first cases of an EVD outbreak in people occur. However, they—like people—are "dead-end" hosts, meaning the organism dies following the infection and does not survive and spread the virus to other animals. As with other viruses of its kind, it is possible that the reservoir host animal of Ebola virus does not experience acute illness despite the virus being present in its organs, tissues, and blood. Thus, the virus is likely maintained in the environment by spreading from host to host or through intermediate hosts or vectors.

African fruit bats are likely involved in the spread of the Ebola virus and may even be the source animal (reservoir host). Scientists continue to search for conclusive evidence of the bat's role in the transmission of Ebola. The most recent Ebola virus to be detected, Bombali virus, was identified in samples from bats collected in Sierra Leone.

History of Ebola Outbreaks

Since its discovery in 1976, the majority of cases and outbreaks of Ebola virus disease have occurred in Africa. The 2014 to 2016 Ebola outbreak in West Africa began in a rural setting of southeastern Guinea, spread to urban areas and across borders within weeks, and became a global epidemic within months.

Understanding Pathways of Transmission

The use of contaminated needles and syringes during the earliest outbreaks enabled transmission and amplification of Ebola virus. During the first outbreak in Zaire (now Democratic Republic of Congo— DRC), nurses in the Yambuku mission hospital reportedly used 5 syringes for 300 to 600 patients a day. Close contact with infected blood, reuse of contaminated needles, and improper nursing techniques were the source for much of the human-to-human transmission during early Ebola outbreaks.

In 1989, Reston ebolavirus was discovered in research monkeys imported from the Philippines into the United States. Later, scientists confirmed that the virus spread throughout the monkey population through droplets in the air (aerosolized transmission) in the facility. However, such airborne transmission is not proven to be a significant factor in human outbreaks of Ebola. The discovery of the Reston virus in these monkeys from the Philippines revealed that Ebola was no longer confined to African settings, but was present in Asia as well.

By the 1994 Cote d'Ivoire outbreak, scientists and public health officials had a better understanding of how Ebola virus spreads and progress was made to reduce transmission through the use of face masks, gloves, and gowns for healthcare personnel. In addition, the use of disposable equipment, such as needles, was introduced.

During the 1995 Kikwit, Zaire (now DRC) outbreak, the international public health community played a strong role, as it was now widely agreed that containment and control of Ebola virus were paramount in ending outbreaks. The local community was educated on how the disease spreads; the hospital was properly staffed and stocked with necessary equipment; and healthcare personnel was trained on disease reporting, patient case identification, and methods for reducing transmission in the healthcare setting.

In the 2014 to 2015 Ebola outbreak in West Africa, healthcare workers represented only 3.9 percent of all confirmed and probable cases of EVD in Sierra Leone, Liberia, and Guinea combined. In comparison, healthcare workers accounted for 25 percent of all infections during the 1995 outbreak in Kikwit. During the 2014 to 2015 West Africa outbreak, the majority of transmission events were between family members (74%). Direct contact with the bodies of those who died from EVD proved to be one of the most dangerous—and effective—methods of transmission. Changes in behaviors related to mourning and burial, along with the adoption of safe burial practices, were critical in controlling that epidemic.

Signs and Symptoms

Symptoms of Ebola virus disease include:

- Fever

- Severe headache

- Muscle pain

- Weakness

- Fatigue

- Diarrhea

- Vomiting

- Abdominal (stomach) pain

- Unexplained hemorrhage (bleeding or bruising)

Symptoms may appear anywhere from 2 to 21 days after contact with the virus, with an average of 8 to 10 days. Many common illnesses can have these same symptoms, including influenza (flu) or malaria.

Ebola virus disease is a rare but severe and often deadly disease. Recovery from EVD depends on good supportive clinical care and the patient's immune response. Studies show that survivors of Ebola virus infection have antibodies (molecules that are made by the immune system to label invading pathogens for destruction) that can be detected in the blood up to 10 years after recovery.

Diagnosis

Diagnosing Ebola virus disease shortly after infection can be difficult. Early symptoms of EVD, such as fever, headache, and weakness, are not specific to Ebola virus infection and often are seen in patients with other more common diseases, like malaria and typhoid fever.

To determine whether Ebola virus infection is a possible diagnosis, there must be a combination of symptoms suggestive of EVD and possible exposure to EVD within 21 days before the onset of symptoms. An exposure may include contact with:

- Blood or body fluids from a person sick with or who died from EVD
- Objects contaminated with blood or body fluids of a person sick with or who died from EVD
- Infected fruit bats and primates (apes or monkeys)
- Semen from a man who has recovered from EVD

If a person shows early signs of EVD and has had a possible exposure, she or he should be isolated (separated from other people) and public health authorities notified. Blood samples from the patient should be collected and tested to confirm infection. Ebola virus can be detected in blood after onset of symptoms, most notably fever. It may take up to three days after symptoms start for the virus to reach detectable levels. A positive laboratory test means that Ebola infection is confirmed. Public health authorities will conduct a public health investigation, including tracing of all possibly exposed contacts.

Treatment

Symptoms of Ebola virus disease are treated as they appear. When used early, basic interventions can significantly improve the chances of survival. These include:

- Providing fluids and electrolytes (body salts) through infusion into the vein (intravenously)
- Offering oxygen therapy to maintain oxygen status
- Using medication to support blood pressure, reduce vomiting and diarrhea and to manage fever and pain

- Treating other infections, if they occur

Recovery from EVD depends on good supportive care and the patient's immune response. Those who do recover develop antibodies that can last 10 years, possibly longer. It is not known if people who recover are immune for life or if they can later become infected with a different species of Ebola virus. Some survivors may have long-term complications, such as joint and vision problems.

Antiviral Drugs

There is currently no antiviral drug licensed by the FDA to treat EVD in people. Drugs that are being developed to treat EVD work by stopping the virus from making copies of itself.

Blood transfusions from survivors and mechanical filtering of blood from patients are also being explored as possible treatments for EVD.

Survivors

In the wake of the 2014 West African outbreak, the largest outbreak of Ebola virus disease to date, there are now more EVD survivors than ever before. This large number of survivors provides a chance to better understand how Ebola virus affects people who have recovered, and to advise survivors on how to take care of themselves and their communities.

Recovery from Ebola

Recovery from EVD depends on good supportive care and the patient's immune response. Antibodies to the virus have been detected in some survivors up to 10 years after recovery. Scientists do not know if people who recover from EVD are immune for life or if they may be susceptible to infection from a different species of Ebola virus.

Health Concerns for Survivors of Ebola

In most cases, people who have completely recovered from EVD do not go through a comeback of the illness. However, many survivors suffer from health issues after recovery from Ebola.

The most commonly reported complications are:

- Tiredness
- Headaches

- Muscle and joint pain
- Eye and vision problems (blurry vision, pain, redness, and light sensitivity)
- Weight gain
- Stomach pain or loss of appetite

Other health problems can include memory loss, neck swelling, dry mouth, tightness of the chest, hair loss, hearing problems (ringing in the ears and hearing loss), pain or tingling in the hands and feet, inflammation of the pericardium (tissue around the heart), inflammation of one or both testicles, changes in menstruation, impotence, decreased or lost interest in sex, difficulty falling or remaining asleep, depression, anxiety, and posttraumatic stress disorder (PTSD).

The timing of onset, severity, and duration of complications among EVD survivors are variable.

Persistence of Ebola Virus

There is no known risk of getting EVD through casual contact with an Ebola survivor. However, the virus can remain in areas of the body that are immunologically privileged sites for several months after acute infection. These are sites where viruses and pathogens, such as the Ebola virus, are shielded from the survivor's immune system, even after being cleared elsewhere in the body. These areas include the testes, interior of the eyes, and central nervous system (CNS), particularly the cerebrospinal fluid (CSF). Whether the virus is present in these body parts and for how long varies by survivor.

Scientists continue to study the long-term effects of Ebola virus infection, including viral persistence, to better understand how to provide treatment and care to EVD survivors.

Transmission

Scientists think people are initially infected with Ebola virus through contact with an infected animal, such as a fruit bat or non-human primate. This is called a "spillover event." After that, the virus spreads from person to person, potentially affecting a large number of people.

The virus spreads through direct contact (such as through broken skin or mucous membranes in the eyes, nose, or mouth) with:

- Blood or body fluids (urine, saliva, sweat, feces, vomit, breast milk, and semen) of a person who is sick with or has died from Ebola virus disease

- Objects (such as needles and syringes) contaminated with body fluids from a person sick with EVD or the body of a person who died from EVD

- Infected fruit bats or nonhuman primates (such as apes and monkeys)

- Semen from a man who recovered from EVD (through oral, vaginal, or anal sex). The virus can remain in certain bodily fluids (including semen) of a patient who has recovered from EVD, even if they no longer have symptoms of severe illness.

When someone gets infected with Ebola, they will not show signs or symptoms of illness right away. The Ebola virus cannot spread to others until a person develops signs or symptoms of EVD. After a person infected with Ebola develops symptoms of illness, they can spread Ebola to others.

Additionally, the Ebola virus usually is not transmitted by food. However, in certain parts of the world, Ebola virus may spread through the handling and consumption of bushmeat (wild animals hunted for food). There is also no evidence that mosquitoes or other insects can transmit Ebola virus.

Persistence of the Virus

There is no known risk of becoming infected with Ebola virus through casual contact with a survivor. However, the virus can remain in certain bodily fluids and continue to spread to others after a person has recovered from the infection. The virus can persist in semen, breast milk, ocular (eye) fluid, and spinal column fluid. Areas of the body that contain these fluids are known as "immunologically privileged sites." These are sites of the body where viruses and pathogens, such as Ebola virus, can remain undetected even after the immune system has cleared the virus from other sites of the body. Scientists are now studying how long the virus stays in these body fluids among Ebola survivors.

During an Ebola outbreak, the virus can spread quickly within healthcare settings (such as clinics or hospitals). Clinicians and other healthcare personnel providing care should use dedicated medical equipment, preferably disposable. Proper cleaning and disposal of instruments, such as needles and syringes, are important. If instruments are not disposable, they must be sterilized before additional use.

Ebola virus is killed using a U.S. Environmental Protection Agency (EPA)-registered hospital disinfectant with a label claim for a nonenveloped virus. On dry surfaces, such as doorknobs and countertops, the virus can survive for several hours. However, in body fluids, such as blood, the virus can survive up to several days at room temperature.

Pets and Livestock

Serologic studies show that Ebola virus has been detected in dogs and cats living in areas affected by an Ebola outbreak, but there are no reports of dogs or cats becoming sick with EVD, or spreading the Ebola virus to people or other animals. However, certain exotic or unusual pets (monkeys, apes, or pigs) have a higher risk of being infected with the virus and spreading it, if they are exposed to it.

Pigs are the only species of livestock known to be at risk of infection by an Ebola virus. In the Philippines and China, pigs are naturally infected with Ebola Reston virus, which does not cause illness in people. While pigs have developed illness when infected with an extremely high dose of Ebola virus (Zaire ebolavirus) in a laboratory setting, they are not known to become naturally infected with this virus strain, and there is no indication they are involved in the spread of this virus.

Prevention

In the United States, Ebola virus disease is a very rare disease that has only occurred because of cases that were acquired in other countries, eventually followed by the human-to-human transmission. The reservoir of the virus does not exist in the United States. EVD is more common in some parts of sub-Saharan Africa, with occasional outbreaks occurring in people. In these areas, the Ebola virus is believed to circulate at low rates in certain animal populations (enzootic). Occasionally, people become sick with Ebola after coming into contact with these infected animals, which can then lead to Ebola outbreaks where the virus spreads between people.

When living in or traveling to a region where Ebola virus is present, there are a number of ways to protect yourself and prevent the spread of EVD.

While in an area affected by Ebola, it is important to avoid the following:

- Contact with blood and body fluids (such as urine, feces, saliva, sweat, vomit, breast milk, semen, and vaginal fluids)
- Items that may have come in contact with an infected person's blood or body fluids (such as clothes, bedding, needles, and medical equipment)
- Funeral or burial rituals that require handling the body of someone who died from EVD
- Contact with bats and nonhuman primates or blood, fluids and raw meat prepared from these animals (bushmeat), or meat from an unknown source
- Contact with semen from a man who had EVD until you know the virus is gone from the semen

These same prevention methods apply when living in or traveling to an area affected by an Ebola outbreak. After returning from an area affected by Ebola, monitor your health for 21 days and seek medical care immediately if you develop symptoms of EVD.

Ebola Vaccine

There is currently no vaccine licensed by the U.S. Food and Drug Administration (FDA) to protect people from the Ebola virus.

An experimental vaccine called "rVSV-ZEBOV was found to be highly protective against the virus in a trial conducted by the World Health Organization (WHO) and other international partners in Guinea in 2015. FDA licensure for the vaccine is expected in 2019. In the meantime, 300,000 doses have been committed for an emergency use stockpile under the appropriate regulatory mechanism (investigational new drug application (IND) or Emergency Use Authorization (EUA)) in the event an outbreak occurs before FDA approval is received. Scientists continue to study the safety of this vaccine in populations such as children and people with HIV.

Another Ebola vaccine candidate, the recombinant adenovirus type-5 Ebola vaccine, was evaluated in a phase 2 trial in Sierra Leone in 2015. An immune response was stimulated by this vaccine within 28 days of vaccination, the response decreased over six months after injection. Research on this vaccine is ongoing.

Handwashing

Ebola virus spreads through direct contact with the blood or body fluids of an infected person. The virus from blood and body fluids can enter the body through broken skin or mucous membranes in the eyes, nose, or mouth. In most cases, this happens by touching the face with contaminated hands.

Hand hygiene is the most effective way to prevent the spread of dangerous germs, such as Ebola virus. Correct hand hygiene lowers the number of germs on the hands and limits the opportunity for spread.

Proper hand hygiene methods are described below:

- Use alcohol-based hand sanitizer when hands are not visibly dirty. These products usually contain 60 to 95 percent ethanol or isopropanol. Alcohol-based hand sanitizer should not be used when hands are visibly soiled with dirt, blood, or other body fluids.

- Use soap and water when hands are visibly soiled with dirt, blood, or other body fluids and as an alternative to alcohol-based hand sanitizer. Antimicrobial soaps are not proven to offer benefits over washing hands with plain soap (not containing antimicrobial compounds) and water.

- Use mild (0.05%) chlorine solution in settings where hand sanitizer and soap are not available. Repeated use of 0.05 percent chlorine solution may cause skin irritation.

Section 9.7

Foot and Mouth Disease

This section includes text excerpted from "Hand, Foot, and Mouth Disease (HFMD)," Centers for Disease Control and Prevention (CDC), February 22, 2019.

Hand, foot, and mouth disease is caused by viruses that belong to the Enterovirus genus (group), which includes polioviruses, coxsackieviruses, echoviruses, and other enteroviruses.

- Coxsackievirus A16 is typically the most common cause of hand, foot, and mouth disease in the United States, but other coxsackieviruses can also cause the illness.

- Enterovirus 71 (EV71) has also been associated with cases and outbreaks of hand, foot, and mouth disease, mostly in children in East and Southeast Asia. Less often, enterovirus 71 has been associated with severe disease, such as encephalitis.

- Several types of enteroviruses may be identified in outbreaks of hand, foot, and mouth disease, but most of the time, only one or two enteroviruses are identified.

Signs and Symptoms

Hand, foot, and mouth disease is a common viral illness that usually affects infants and children younger than five years of age. However, it can sometimes occur in older children and adults. It usually starts with a fever, reduced appetite, sore throat, and a general feeling of being unwell (malaise).

One or two days after the fever starts, painful sores can develop in the mouth (herpangina). They usually begin as small red spots, often in the back of the mouth, that blister and can become painful.

A skin rash on the palms of the hands and soles of the feet may also develop over one or two days as flat, red spots, sometimes with blisters. It may also appear on the knees, elbows, buttocks, or genital area.

Some people, especially young children, may get dehydrated if they are not able to swallow enough liquids because of painful mouth sores. You should seek medical care in these cases.

Not everyone will get all of these symptoms. Some people, especially adults, may become infected and show no symptoms at all, but they can still pass the virus to others.

Most people who get hand, foot, and mouth disease will have mild illness or no symptoms at all. But, a small proportion of cases can be more severe.

Complications

Health complications from hand, foot, and mouth disease are not common:

- Viral or "aseptic" meningitis can occur with hand, foot, and mouth disease, but it is rare. It causes fever, headache, stiff neck, or back pain and may require the infected person to be hospitalized for a few days.

- Encephalitis (inflammation of the brain) or polio-like paralysis can occur, but this is even rarer.

- Fingernail and toenail loss have been reported, occurring mostly in children within a few weeks after having a hand, foot, and mouth disease. At this time, we do not know whether the nail loss was a result of the disease in reported cases. However, in the reports reviewed, the nail loss was temporary, and the nail grew back without medical treatment.

Transmission

The viruses that cause hand, foot, and mouth disease can be found in an infected person's:

- Nose and throat secretions (such as saliva, sputum, or nasal mucus)
- Blister fluid
- Feces

You can be exposed to the viruses that cause hand, foot, and mouth disease through:

- Close personal contact, such as hugging an infected person
- The air when an infected person coughs or sneezes
- Contact with feces, such as changing diapers of an infected person, then touching your eyes, nose, or mouth before washing your hands
- Contact with contaminated objects and surfaces, such as touching a doorknob that has viruses on it, then touching your eyes, mouth, or nose before washing your hands

It is also possible to become infected with the viruses that cause hand, foot, and mouth disease if you swallow recreational water, such as water in swimming pools. However, this is not very common. This can happen if the water is not properly treated with chlorine and becomes contaminated with feces from a person who has a hand, foot, and mouth disease.

Generally, a person with hand, foot, and mouth disease is most contagious during the first week of illness. People can sometimes be contagious for days or weeks after symptoms go away. Some people, especially adults, may become infected and not develop any symptoms, but they can still spread the virus to others. This is why people should always try to maintain good hygiene, such as frequent hand-washing, so they can minimize their chance of spreading or getting infections.

You should stay home while you are sick with hand, foot, and mouth disease. Talk with your healthcare provider if you are not sure when you should return to work or school. The same applies to children returning to daycare.

Hand, foot, and mouth disease is not transmitted to or from pets or other animals.

Diagnosis

Hand, foot, and mouth disease is one of the many infections that causes mouth sores. Healthcare providers can usually identify mouth sores caused by hand, foot, and mouth disease by considering:

- How old the patient is

- What symptoms the patient has

- How the rash and mouth sores look

A healthcare professional may sometimes collect samples from the patient's throat or feces then send them to a laboratory to test for the virus.

Prevention and Treatment
Prevention

There is currently no vaccine in the United States to protect against the viruses that cause hand, foot, and mouth disease. But, researchers are working to develop vaccines to help prevent hand, foot, and mouth disease in the future.

You can lower your risk of being infected by doing the following

- Wash your hands often with soap and water for at least 20 seconds, especially after changing diapers and using the toilet.

- Clean and disinfect frequently touched surfaces and soiled items, including toys.

- Avoid close contact, such as kissing, hugging, or sharing eating utensils or cups, with people with hand, foot, and mouth disease.

Treatment

There is no specific treatment for hand, foot, and mouth disease. However, you can do some things to relieve symptoms:

- Take over-the-counter (OTC) medications to relieve pain and fever. (Caution: Aspirin should not be given to children.)

- Use mouthwashes or sprays that numb mouth pain.

If a person has mouth sores, it might be painful for them to swallow. However, it is important for people with hand, foot, and mouth disease to drink enough liquids to prevent dehydration (loss of body fluids). If a person cannot swallow enough liquids to avoid dehydration, they may need to receive them through an IV in their vein.

Section 9.8

Hantavirus *Infection*

This section includes text excerpted from
"Hantavirus," Centers for Disease Control and
Prevention (CDC), January 31, 2019.

Hantaviruses are a family of viruses spread mainly by rodents and can cause varied disease syndromes in people worldwide. Infection with any *Hantavirus* can produce *Hantavirus* disease in people. *Hantaviruses* in the Americas are known as "New World" *Hantaviruses* and may cause *Hantavirus* pulmonary syndrome (HPS). Other *Hantaviruses*, known as "Old World" *Hantaviruses*, are found mostly in Europe and Asia and may cause hemorrhagic fever with renal syndrome (HFRS).

Each *Hantavirus* serotype has a specific rodent host species and is spread to people via aerosolized virus that is shed in urine; feces; and saliva; and, less frequently, by a bite from an infected host. The most important *Hantavirus* in the United States that can cause HPS is the Sin Nombre virus, spread by the deer mouse.

Rodents in the United States That Carry Hantavirus
Cotton Rat (Sigmodon Hispidus)

The cotton rat (Sigmodon hispidus), found in the southeastern United States and down into Central and South America, has a bigger body than the deer mouse. The head and body measure approximately 5 to 7 inches (12.5 cm to 18 cm), with another 3 to 4 inches (7.5 cm to 10 cm) for the tail. The fur is longer and coarser, grayish-brown, even grayish-black, in color. The *Hantavirus* strain present in the cotton rat is Black Creek Canal virus (BCCV). The cotton rat inhabits overgrown areas with shrubs and tall grasses.

Deer Mouse (Peromyscus Maniculatus)

The deer mouse (Peromyscus maniculatus) is a deceptively cute animal, with big eyes and ears. Its head and body measure approximately 2 to 3 inches (5 cm to 7.5 cm) in length, and the tail adds another 2 to 3 inches. In color, the deer mouse ranges from grey to reddish brown, depending on age. The underbelly is always white, and the tail has clearly defined white sides. The *Hantavirus* strain present in deer mice is Sin Nombre (SNV). The deer mouse is found throughout North America, preferring woodlands, but also appearing in desert areas.

Rice Rat (Oryzomys Palustris)

The rice rat (Oryzomys palustris) is slightly smaller than the cotton rat, with a 5 to 6 inch (7.5 cm to 15 cm) head and a very long 4 to 7 inch (10 cm to 18 cm) tail. It has short, soft, grayish-brown fur on top, and gray or tawny underbellies. Their feet are whitish. The rice rat prefers marshy areas and is semi-aquatic. The *Hantavirus* strain present in the rice rat is Bayou virus (BAYV). It is found in the southeastern United States and Central America.

White-Footed Mouse (Peromyscus Leucopus)

The white-footed mouse (Peromyscus leucopus) closely resembles the deer mouse. The head and body together measure approximately four inches (10 cm). The tail is normally shorter than the body, typically 2 to 4 inches (5 cm to 10 cm). Its top fur ranges from pale to reddish brown, while its underside and feet are white. The virus strain present in the mouse is New York virus (NYV). The white-footed mouse is found throughout southern New England and the Mid-Atlantic and southern states, the midwestern and western states, and Mexico. It prefers wooded and brushy areas; although, it will sometimes inhabit more open ground.

Hantavirus *Pulmonary Syndrome*

Hantavirus pulmonary syndrome (HPS) is a severe, sometimes fatal, respiratory disease in humans caused by infection with *Hantaviruses*.

Anyone who comes into contact with rodents that carry *Hantaviruses* is at risk of HPS. Rodent infestation in and around the home remains the primary risk for *Hantavirus* exposure. Even healthy individuals are at risk for HPS infection if exposed to the virus.

To date, no cases of HPS have been reported in the United States in which the virus was transmitted from one person to another. In fact, in a study of healthcare workers who were exposed to either patients or specimens infected with related types of *Hantaviruses* (which cause a different disease in humans), none of the workers showed evidence of infection or illness.

In Chile and Argentina, rare cases of person-to-person transmission have occurred among close contacts of a person who was ill with a type of *Hantavirus* called "Andes virus."

Transmission
How People Get Hantavirus *Infection*
Where *Hantavirus* Is Found

Cases of human *Hantavirus* infection occur sporadically, usually in rural areas where forests, fields, and farms offer suitable habitat for the virus's rodent hosts. Areas around the home or work where rodents may live (for example, houses, barns, outbuildings, and sheds) are potential sites where people may be exposed to the virus. In the United States and Canada, the Sin Nombre *Hantavirus* is responsible for the majority of cases of *Hantavirus* infection. The host of the Sin Nombre virus is the deer mouse (Peromyscus maniculatus), which is present throughout the western and central United States and Canada.

Several other *Hantaviruses* are capable of causing *Hantavirus* infection in the United States. The New York *Hantavirus*, carried by the white-footed mouse, is associated with HPS cases in the northeastern United States. The Black Creek *Hantavirus*, carried by the cotton rat, is found in the southeastern United States Cases of HPS have been confirmed elsewhere in the Americas, including Canada, Argentina, Bolivia, Brazil, Chile, Panama, Paraguay, and Uruguay.

How People Become Infected with *Hantaviruses*

In the United States, deer mice (along with cotton rats, rice rats, and the white-footed mouse) are reservoirs of the *Hantaviruses*. The rodents shed the virus in their urine, droppings, and saliva. The virus is mainly transmitted to people when they breathe in air contaminated with the virus.

When fresh rodent urine, droppings, or nesting materials are stirred up, tiny droplets containing the virus get into the air. This process is known as "airborne transmission."

There are several other ways rodents may spread *Hantavirus* to people:

- If a rodent with the virus bites someone, the virus may be spread to that person, but this type of transmission is rare.

- Scientists believe that people may be able to get the virus if they touch something that has been contaminated with rodent urine, droppings, or saliva, and then touch their nose or mouth.

- Scientists also suspect people can become sick if they eat food contaminated by urine, droppings, or saliva from an infected rodent.

The *Hantaviruses* that cause human illness in the United States cannot be transmitted from one person to another. For example, you cannot get these viruses from touching or kissing a person who has HPS or from a healthcare worker who has treated someone with the disease.

People at Risk for *Hantavirus* Infection

Anyone who comes into contact with rodents that carry *Hantavirus* is at risk of HPS. Rodent infestation in and around the home remains the primary risk for *Hantavirus* exposure. Even healthy individuals are at risk for HPS infection if exposed to the virus.

Any activity that puts you in contact with rodent droppings, urine, saliva, or nesting materials can place you at risk for infection. *Hantavirus* is spread when virus-containing particles from rodent urine, droppings, or saliva are stirred into the air. It is important to avoid actions that raise dust, such as sweeping or vacuuming. Infection occurs when you breathe in virus particles.

Potential Risk Activities for Hantavirus *Infection*
Opening and Cleaning Previously Unused Buildings

Opening or cleaning cabins; sheds; and outbuildings, including barns, garages and storage facilities that have been closed during the winter is a potential risk for *Hantavirus* infections, especially in rural settings.

Housecleaning Activities

Cleaning in and around your own home can put you at risk if rodents have made it their home too. Many homes can expect to shelter rodents, especially as the weather turns cold.

Work-Related Exposure

Construction, utility, and pest control workers can be exposed when they work in crawl spaces, under houses, or in vacant buildings that may have a rodent population.

Campers and Hikers

Campers and hikers can also be exposed when they use infested trail shelters or camp in other rodent habitats.

The chance of being exposed to *Hantavirus* is greatest when people work, play, or live in closed spaces where rodents are actively living. However, recent research results show that many people who have become ill with HPS were infected with the disease after continued contact with rodents and/or their droppings. In addition, many people who have contracted HPS reported that they had not seen rodents or their droppings before becoming ill. Therefore, if you live in an area where the carrier rodents, such as the deer mouse, are known to live, take sensible precautions even if you do not see rodents or their droppings.

Signs and Symptoms

Due to the small number of HPS cases, the "incubation time" is not positively known. However, on the basis of limited information, it appears that symptoms may develop between one and eight weeks after exposure to fresh urine, droppings, or saliva of infected rodents.

Early Symptoms

Early symptoms include fatigue, fever and muscle aches, especially in the large muscle groups—thighs, hips, back, and sometimes shoulders. These symptoms are universal.

There may also be headaches; dizziness; chills; and abdominal problems, such as nausea, vomiting, diarrhea, and abdominal pain. About half of all HPS patients experience these symptoms.

Late Symptoms

4 to 10 days after the initial phase of illness, the late symptoms of HPS appear. These include coughing and shortness of breath, with the sensation of, as one survivor put it, a "…tight band around my chest and a pillow over my face" as the lungs fill with fluid.

Diagnosis and Treatment
Diagnosing Hantavirus Pulmonary Syndrome

Diagnosing HPS in an individual who has only been infected for a few days is difficult because early symptoms, such as fever, muscle aches, and fatigue, are easily confused with influenza. However, if the individual is experiencing fever and fatigue and has a history of potential rural rodent exposure, along with shortness of breath, it would be strongly suggestive of HPS. If the individual is experiencing these symptoms, they should see their physician immediately and mention their potential rodent exposure.

Treating Hantavirus Pulmonary Syndrome

There is no specific treatment, cure, or vaccine for *Hantavirus* infection. However, we do know that if infected individuals are recognized early and receive medical care in an intensive care unit, they may do better. In intensive care, patients are intubated and given oxygen therapy to help them through the period of severe respiratory distress.

The earlier the patient is brought in to intensive care, the better. If a patient is experiencing full distress, it is less likely the treatment will be effective.

Therefore, if you have been around rodents and have symptoms of fever, deep muscle aches, and severe shortness of breath, see your doctor immediately. Be sure to tell your doctor that you have been around rodents—this will alert your physician to look closely for any rodent-carried disease, such as HPS.

Prevention

Eliminate or minimize contact with rodents in your home, workplace, or campsite. If rodents do not find that where you are is a good place for them to be, then you are less likely to come into contact with them. Seal up holes and gaps in your home or garage. Place traps in and around your home to decrease rodent infestation. Clean up any easy to get food.

Research results show that many people who became ill with HPS developed the disease after having been in frequent contact with rodents and/or their droppings around a home or a workplace. On the other hand, many people who became ill reported that they had not seen rodents or rodent droppings at all. Therefore, if you live in an area where the carrier rodents are known to live, try to keep your home, vacation place, workplace, or campsite clean.

Reported Cases of Hantavirus *Disease*
Hantavirus *Infection in the United States*

Hantavirus disease surveillance in the United States began in 1993 during an outbreak of severe respiratory illness in the Four Corners region. *Hantavirus* pulmonary syndrome became a nationally notifiable disease in 1995 and is now reported through the Nationally Notifiable Disease Surveillance System (NNDSS) when fever is present in a patient with laboratory-confirmed evidence of *Hantavirus* infection.

In 2014, the Council of State and Territorial Epidemiologists (CSTE) expanded the national reporting of laboratory-confirmed *Hantavirus* infections to include HPS and nonpulmonary *Hantavirus* infection. Reporting of nonpulmonary *Hantavirus* cases began in 2015.

Hemorrhagic Fever with Renal Syndrome
What Is Hemorrhagic Fever with Renal Syndrome?

Hemorrhagic fever with renal syndrome (HFRS) is a group of clinically similar illnesses caused by *Hantaviruses* from the family Bunyaviridae. HFRS includes diseases such as Korean hemorrhagic fever, epidemic hemorrhagic fever, and nephropathia epidemica. The viruses that cause HFRS include Hantaan, Dobrava, Saaremaa, Seoul, and Puumala.

Where Is Hemorrhagic Fever with Renal Syndrome Found?

Hemorrhagic fever with renal syndrome is found throughout the world. Haantan virus is widely distributed in eastern Asia, particularly in China, Russia, and Korea. Puumala virus is found in Scandinavia, western Europe, and western Russia. Dobrava virus is found primarily in the Balkans, and Seoul virus is found worldwide. Saaremaa is found in central Europe and Scandinavia. In the Americas, *Hantaviruses* cause a different disease known as "*hantavirus* pulmonary syndrome."

How Do Humans Get Hemorrhagic Fever with Renal Syndrome?

Hantaviruses are carried and transmitted by rodents. People can become infected with these viruses and develop HFRS after exposure to aerosolized urine, droppings, or saliva of infected rodents or after exposure to dust from their nests. Transmission may also occur when infected urine or these other materials are directly introduced into broken skin or onto the mucous membranes of the eyes, nose, or mouth. In addition, individuals who work with live rodents can be exposed to *Hantaviruses* through rodent bites from infected animals. Transmission from one human to another may occur, but is extremely rare.

Which Rodents Carry the Hantaviruses That Cause Hemorrhagic Fever with Renal Syndrome in Humans?

Rodents are the natural reservoir for *Hantaviruses*. Known carriers include the striped field mouse (Apodemus agrarius), the reservoir for both the Saaremaa and Hantaan virus; the brown or Norway rat (Rattus norvegicus), the reservoir for Seoul virus; the bank vole (Clethrionomys glareolus), the reservoir for Puumala virus; and the yellow-necked field mouse (Apodemus flavicollis), which carries Dobrava virus.

What Are the Symptoms of Hemorrhagic Fever with Renal Syndrome?

Symptoms of HFRS usually develop within one to two weeks after exposure to infectious material, but in rare cases, they may take up to eight weeks to develop. Initial symptoms begin suddenly and include intense headaches, back and abdominal pain, fever, chills, nausea, and blurred vision. Individuals may have flushing of the face, inflammation or redness of the eyes, or a rash. Later symptoms can include low blood pressure, acute shock, vascular leakage, and acute kidney failure, which can cause severe fluid overload. The severity of the disease varies depending upon the virus causing the infection. Hantaan and Dobrava virus infections usually cause severe symptoms, while Seoul,

Saaremaa, and Puumala virus infections are usually more moderate. Complete recovery can take weeks or months.

How Is Hemorrhagic Fever with Renal Syndrome Diagnosed?

Several laboratory tests are used to confirm a diagnosis of HFRS in patients with a clinical history compatible with the disease. Such patients are determined to have HFRS if they have serologic test results positive for *Hantavirus* infection, evidence of *Hantavirus* antigen in tissue by immunohistochemical staining and microscope examination, or evidence of *Hantavirus* RNA sequences in blood or tissue.

How Is Hemorrhagic Fever with Renal Syndrome Treated?

Supportive therapy is the mainstay of care for patients with *Hantavirus* infections. Care includes careful management of the patient's fluid (hydration) and electrolyte (e.g., sodium, potassium, chloride) levels, maintenance of correct oxygen and blood pressure levels, and appropriate treatment of any secondary infections. Dialysis may be required to correct severe fluid overload. Intravenous ribavirin, an antiviral drug, has been shown to decrease illness and death associated with HFRS if used very early in the disease.

Is Hemorrhagic Fever with Renal Syndrome Ever Fatal?

Depending upon which virus is causing the HFRS, death occurs in less than 1 percent to as many as 15 percent of patients. Fatality ranges from 5 to 15 percent for HFRS caused by Hantaan virus, and it is less than 1 percent for disease caused by Puumala virus.

How Is Hemorrhagic Fever with Renal Syndrome Prevented?

Rodent control is the primary strategy for preventing *Hantavirus* infections. Rodent populations near human communities should be controlled, and rodents should be excluded from homes. Individuals should avoid contact with rodent urine, droppings, saliva, and nesting materials.

Section 9.9

Kyasanur Forest Disease Virus

This section includes text excerpted from "Kyasanur Forest Disease (KFD)," Centers for Disease Control and Prevention (CDC), December 23, 2013. Reviewed May 2019.

Kyasanur Forest disease (KFD) is caused by Kyasanur Forest disease virus (KFDV), a member of the virus family Flaviviridae. KFDV was identified in 1957 when it was isolated from a sick monkey from the Kyasanur Forest in Karnataka (formerly Mysore) state, India. Since then, between 400 to 500 humans cases per year have been reported.

Hard ticks (Hemaphysalis spinigera) are the reservoir of KFD virus and once infected, remain so for life. Rodents, shrews, and monkeys are common hosts for KFDV after being bitten by an infected tick. KFDV can cause epizootics with high fatality in primates.

Signs and Symptoms

After an incubation period of three to eight days, the symptoms of KFD begin suddenly with chills, fever, and headache. Severe muscle pain with vomiting, gastrointestinal symptoms, and bleeding problems may occur three to four days after initial symptom onset. Patients may experience abnormally low blood pressure and low platelet, red blood cell, and white blood cell counts.

After one to two weeks of symptoms, some patients recover without complication. However, the illness is biphasic for a subset of patients (10 to 20%) who experience a second wave of symptoms at the beginning of the third week. These symptoms include fever and signs of neurological manifestations, such as severe headache, mental disturbances, tremors, and vision deficits.

The estimated case fatality rate (CFR) is from three to five percent for KFD.

Risk of Exposure

Kyasanur Forest disease has historically been limited to the western and central districts of Karnataka state, India. However, in November 2012, samples from humans and monkeys tested positive for KFDV in the southernmost district of the state that neighbors Tamil Nadu state and Kerala state, indicating the possibility of wider distribution of KFDV. Additionally, a virus very similar to KFD virus (Alkhurma hemorrhagic fever virus) has been described in Saudi Arabia.

People with recreational or occupational exposure to rural or outdoor settings (e.g., hunters, herders, forest workers, farmers) within Karnataka state are potentially at risk for infection by contact with infected ticks. Seasonality is another important risk factor as more cases are reported during the dry season, from November through June.

Diagnosis

Diagnosis can be made in the early stage of illness by molecular detection by polymerase chain reaction (PCR) or virus isolation from blood. Later, serologic testing using enzyme-linked immunosorbent serologic assay (ELISA) can be performed.

Transmission

Transmission to humans may occur after a tick bite or contact with an infected animal, most significantly a sick or recently dead monkey. No person-to-person transmission has been described.

Large animals, such as goats, cows, and sheep, may become infected with KFD but play a limited role in the transmission of the disease. These animals provide the blood meals for ticks and it is possible for infected animals with viremia to infect other ticks, but transmission of KFDV to humans from these larger animals is extremely rare. Furthermore, there is no evidence of disease transmission via the unpasteurized milk of any of these animals.

Treatment

There is no specific treatment for KFD, but early hospitalization and supportive therapy is important. Supportive therapy includes the maintenance of hydration and the usual precautions for patients with bleeding disorders.

Prevention

A vaccine does exist for KFD and is used in endemic areas of India. Additional preventative measures include insect repellents and wearing protective clothing in areas where ticks are endemic.

Section 9.10

Lassa Fever

This section includes text excerpted from "Lassa Fever,"
Centers for Disease Control and Prevention (CDC), January 31, 2019.

Lassa fever is an animal-borne, or zoonotic, acute viral illness. It is endemic in parts of West Africa, including Sierra Leone, Liberia, Guinea, and Nigeria. Neighboring countries are also at risk, as the animal vector for Lassa virus, the multimammate rat (Mastomys natalensis) is distributed throughout the region.

The illness was discovered in 1969 and is named after the town in Nigeria where the first cases occurred.

An estimated 100,000 to 300,000 infections of Lassa fever occur annually, with approximately 5,000 deaths. Surveillance for Lassa fever is not standardized; therefore, these estimates are crude. In some areas of Sierra Leone and Liberia, it is known that 10 to 16 percent of people admitted to hospitals annually have Lassa fever, demonstrating the serious impact the disease has on the region.

Signs and Symptoms

Signs and symptoms of Lassa fever typically occur 1 to 3 weeks after the patient comes into contact with the virus. For the majority of Lassa fever virus infections (approximately 80%), symptoms are mild and undiagnosed. Mild symptoms include a slight fever, general malaise and weakness, and headache. In 20 percent of infected individuals, however, disease may progress to more serious symptoms, including hemorrhaging (in the gums, eyes, or nose, as examples); respiratory distress; repeated vomiting; facial swelling; pain in the chest, back, and abdomen; and shock. Neurological problems have also been described, including hearing loss, tremors, and encephalitis. Death may occur within 2 weeks after symptom onset due to multi-organ failure.

The most common complication of Lassa fever is deafness. Various degrees of deafness occur in approximately one-third of infections, and in many cases hearing loss is permanent. Severity of the disease does not affect this complication; deafness may develop in mild cases, as well as in severe cases.

Approximately 15 to 20 percent of patients hospitalized for Lassa fever die from the illness. However, only 1 percent of all Lassa virus infections result in death. The death rates for women in the third trimester of pregnancy are particularly high. Spontaneous abortion is a serious complication of infection, with an estimated 95 percent mortality in fetuses of infected pregnant mothers.

Because the symptoms of Lassa fever are so varied and nonspecific, clinical diagnosis is often difficult. Lassa fever is also associated with occasional epidemics, in which case fatality rate can reach 50 percent in hospitalized patients.

Risk of Exposure

Individuals at greatest risk of Lassa virus infection are those who live in or visit endemic regions, including Sierra Leone, Liberia, Guinea, and Nigeria and have exposure to the multimammate rat. Risk of exposure may also exist in other West African countries where Mastomys rodents exist. Hospital staff are not at great risk for infection as long as protective measures and proper sterilization methods are used.

Diagnosis

Lassa fever is most often diagnosed by using enzyme-linked immunosorbent serologic assays (ELISA), which detect Immunoglobulin M (IgM) and Immunoglobulin G (IgG) antibodies, as well as Lassa antigen. Reverse transcription-polymerase chain reaction (RT-PCR) can be used in the early stage of disease. The virus itself may be cultured in 7 to 10 days, but this procedure should only be done in a high containment laboratory with good laboratory practices. Immunohistochemistry, performed on formalin-fixed tissue specimens, can be used to make a postmortem diagnosis.

Treatment

Ribavirin, an antiviral drug, has been used with success in Lassa fever patients. It has been shown to be most effective when given early in the course of the illness. Patients should also receive supportive care consisting of maintenance of appropriate fluid and electrolyte balance, oxygenation and blood pressure, as well as treatment of any other complicating infections.

Transmission

The reservoir, or host, of Lassa virus is a rodent known as the "multimammate rat" (Mastomys natalensis). Once infected, this rodent is able to excrete the virus in urine for an extended time period, maybe for the rest of its life. Mastomys rodents breed frequently, produce large numbers of offspring, and are numerous in the savannas and forests of west, central, and east Africa. In addition, Mastomys readily colonize human homes and areas where food is stored. All of these factors contribute to the relatively efficient spread of Lassa virus from infected rodents to humans.

Transmission of Lassa virus to humans occurs most commonly through ingestion or inhalation. Mastomys rodents shed the virus in urine and droppings and direct contact with these materials, through touching soiled objects, eating contaminated food, or exposure to open cuts or sores, can lead to infection.

Because Mastomys rodents often live in and around homes and scavenge on leftover human food items or poorly stored food, direct contact transmission is common. Mastomys rodents are sometimes consumed as a food source, and infection may occur when rodents are caught and prepared. Contact with the virus may also occur when a person inhales tiny particles in the air contaminated with infected rodent excretions. This aerosol or airborne transmission may occur during cleaning activities, such as sweeping.

Direct contact with infected rodents is not the only way in which people are infected; person-to-person transmission may occur after exposure to virus in the blood, tissue, secretions, or excretions of a Lassa virus-infected individual. Casual contact (including skin-to-skin contact without exchange of body fluids) does not spread Lassa virus. Person-to-person transmission is common in healthcare settings (called "nosocomial transmission") where proper personal protective equipment (PPE) is not available or not used. Lassa virus may be spread in contaminated medical equipment, such as reused needles.

Prevention

Primary transmission of the Lassa virus from its host to humans can be prevented by avoiding contact with Mastomys rodents, especially in the geographic regions where outbreaks occur. Putting food away in rodent-proof containers and keeping the home clean help to discourage rodents from entering homes. Using these rodents as a food source is not recommended. Trapping in and around homes can help reduce rodent populations; however, the wide distribution of Mastomys in Africa makes complete control of this rodent reservoir impractical.

When caring for patients with Lassa fever, further transmission of the disease through person-to-person contact or nosocomial routes can be avoided by taking preventive precautions against contact with patient secretions (called "viral hemorrhagic fever (VHF) isolation precautions" or "barrier nursing methods"). Such precautions include wearing protective clothing, such as masks, gloves, gowns, and goggles; using infection control measures, such as complete equipment sterilization; and isolating infected patients from contact with unprotected persons until the disease has run its course.

Further, educating people in high-risk areas about ways to decrease rodent populations in their homes will aid in the control and prevention of Lassa fever. Other challenges include developing more rapid diagnostic tests and increasing the availability of the only known drug treatment, ribavirin. Research is presently underway to develop a vaccine for Lassa fever.

Section 9.11

Measles

This section includes text excerpted from
"Measles (Rubeola)," Centers for Disease Control and
Prevention (CDC), February 5, 2018.

Measles starts with fever, runny nose, cough, red eyes, and sore throat. It's followed by a rash that spreads over the body. Measles is highly contagious and spreads through coughing and sneezing. Make sure you and your child are protected with the measles, mumps, and rubella (MMR) vaccine.

Signs and Symptoms

The symptoms of measles generally appear about 7 to 14 days after a person is infected.

Measles typically begins with:

- High fever

- Cough

- Runny nose (coryza)
- Red, watery eyes (conjunctivitis)

Two or three days after symptoms begin, tiny white spots (Koplik spots) may appear inside the mouth.

Complications of Measles
Complications

Measles can be a serious in all age groups. However, children younger than 5 years of age and adults older than 20 years of age are more likely to suffer from measles complications.

Common Complications

Common measles complications include ear infections and diarrhea.

- Ear infections occur in about 1 out of every 10 children with measles and can result in permanent hearing loss.
- Diarrhea is reported in less than 1 out of 10 people with measles.

Severe Complications

Some people may suffer from severe complications, such as pneumonia (infection of the lungs) and encephalitis (swelling of the brain). They may need to be hospitalized and could die.

- As many as 1 out of every 20 children with measles gets pneumonia, the most common cause of death from measles in young children.
- About 1 child out of every 1,000 who get measles will develop encephalitis (swelling of the brain) that can lead to convulsions and can leave the child deaf or with intellectual disability.
- For every 1,000 children who get measles, 1 or 2 will die from it.

Measles may cause pregnant woman to give birth prematurely or have a low-birth-weight baby.

The Measles chapter of the Epidemiology and Prevention of Vaccine Preventable Diseases (the "pink book") describes measles complications in more depth.

Long-term Complications

Subacute sclerosing panencephalitis (SSPE) is a very rare, but fatal disease of the central nervous system that results from a measles virus infection acquired earlier in life. SSPE generally develops 7 to 10 years after a person has measles, even though the person seems to have fully recovered from the illness. Since measles was eliminated in 2000, SSPE is rarely reported in the United States.

Among people who contracted measles during the resurgence in the United States in 1989 to 1991, 4 to 11 out of every 100,000 were estimated to be at risk for developing SSPE. The risk of developing SSPE may be higher for a person who gets measles before they are 2 years of age.

Transmission of Measles

Measles is a highly contagious virus that lives in the nose and throat mucus of an infected person. It can spread to others through coughing and sneezing. Also, measles virus can live for up to 2 hours in an airspace where the infected person coughed or sneezed. If other people breathe the contaminated air or touch the infected surface, then touch their eyes, noses, or mouths, they can become infected. Measles is so contagious that if one person has it, up to 90 percent of the people close to that person who are not immune will also become infected.

Infected people can spread measles to others from four days before through four days after the rash appears.

Measles is a disease of humans; measles virus is not spread by any other animal species.

Prevaccine Era

In the 9th century, a Persian doctor published one of the first written accounts of measles disease.

Francis Home, a Scottish physician, demonstrated in 1757 that measles is caused by an infectious agent in the blood of patients.

In 1912, measles became a nationally notifiable disease in the United States, requiring U.S. healthcare providers and laboratories to report all diagnosed cases. In the first decade of reporting, an average of 6,000 measles-related deaths were reported each year.

In the decade before 1963 when a vaccine became available, nearly all children got measles by the time they were 15 years of age. It is estimated that 3 to 4 million people in the United States were infected each year. Also each year, among reported cases, an estimated 400 to 500 people died, 48,000 were hospitalized, and 1,000 suffered encephalitis (swelling of the brain) from measles.

Vaccine Development

In 1954, John F. Enders and Dr. Thomas C. Peebles collected blood samples from several ill students during a measles outbreak in Boston, Massachusetts. They wanted to isolate the measles virus in the student's blood and create a measles vaccine. They succeeded in isolating measles in 13-year-old David Edmonston's blood.

In 1963, John Enders and colleagues transformed their Edmonston-B strain of measles virus into a vaccine and licensed it in the United States. In 1968, an improved and even weaker measles vaccine, developed by Maurice Hilleman and colleagues, began to be distributed. This vaccine, called the Edmonston-Enders (formerly "Moraten") strain has been the only measles vaccine used in the United States since 1968. Measles vaccine is usually combined with mumps and rubella (MMR), or combined with mumps, rubella and varicella (MMRV).

Measles Elimination

In 1978, CDC set a goal to eliminate measles from the United States by 1982. Although this goal was not met, widespread use of measles vaccine drastically reduced the disease rates. By 1981, the number of reported measles cases was 80 percent less compared with the previous year. However, a 1989 measles outbreaks among vaccinated school-aged children prompted the Advisory Committee on Immunization Practices (ACIP), the American Academy of Pediatrics (AAP), and the American Academy of Family Physicians (AAFP) to recommend a second dose of MMR vaccine for all children. Following widespread implementation of this recommendation and improvements in first-dose MMR vaccine coverage, reported measles cases declined even more.

Measles was declared eliminated (absence of continuous disease transmission for greater than 12 months) from the United States in 2000. This was thanks to a highly effective vaccination program in the United States, as well as better measles control in the Americas region.

Measles Vaccination

Measles is a very contagious disease caused by a virus. It spreads through the air when an infected person coughs or sneezes. Measles starts with fever. Soon after, it causes a cough, runny nose, and red eyes. Then a rash of tiny, red spots breaks out. It starts at the head and spreads to the rest of the body.

Measles can be prevented with MMR vaccine. The vaccine protects against three diseases: measles, mumps, and rubella. CDC recommends children get two doses of MMR vaccine, starting with the first dose at 12 through 15 months of age, and the second dose at 4 through 6 years of age. Teens and adults should also be up to date on their MMR vaccination.

The MMR vaccine is very safe and effective. Two doses of MMR vaccine are about 97 percent effective at preventing measles; one dose is about 93 percent effective.

Children may also get MMRV vaccine, which protects against measles, mumps, rubella, and varicella (chickenpox). This vaccine is only licensed for use in children who are 12 months through 12 years of age.

Before the measles vaccination program started in 1963, an estimated 3 to 4 million people got measles each year in the United States. Of these, approximately 500,000 cases were reported each year to CDC; of these, 400 to 500 died, 48,000 were hospitalized, and 1,000 developed encephalitis (brain swelling) from measles. Since then, widespread use of measles vaccine has led to a greater than 99 percent reduction in measles cases compared with the prevaccine era. However, measles is still common in other countries. Unvaccinated people continue to get measles while abroad and bring the disease into the United States and spread it to others.

Section 9.12

Middle East Respiratory Syndrome

This section includes text excerpted from "Middle East Respiratory Syndrome (MERS)," Centers for Disease Control and Prevention (CDC), May 29, 2018.

There have been no Middle East respiratory syndrome (MERS) cases in the United States since May 2014. The risk of MERS to the general public in this country remains very low. The Centers for

Disease Control and Prevention (CDC) and other public health partners continue to closely monitor the MERS situation.

Since MERS first emerged in the Arabian Peninsula in 2012, the
CDC has been working with global partners to better understand
the nature of the virus, including how it affects people, and how it
spreads. The CDC recognizes the potential for Middle East respiratory syndrome *coronavirus* (MERS-CoV) to spread further and cause
more cases in the United States and globally, and are taking actions
in preparation.

Middle East Respiratory Syndrome in the United States

Only two patients in the United States have ever tested positive for
MERS-CoV infection—both in May 2014—while more than 900 people
have tested negative. In May 2014, the CDC confirmed two cases of
MERS in the United States—one in Indiana, the other in Florida. Both
cases were among healthcare providers who lived and worked in Saudi
Arabia. Both traveled to the United States from Saudi Arabia, where
they are believed to have been infected. Both were hospitalized in the
United States and later discharged after fully recovering.

Understanding the Virus

The Middle East respiratory syndrome (MERS) is a viral respiratory illness that is new to humans. It was first reported in Saudi
Arabia in 2012. The virus that causes MERS is called "Middle East
respiratory syndrome *coronavirus*" (MERS-CoV). *Coronaviruses* are
common viruses that most people get some time in their life. Human
coronaviruses usually cause mild to moderate cold-like illnesses. However, MERS-CoV is different from any other *coronavirus* previously
found in people.

Middle East respiratory syndrome *coronavirus* likely came from
an animal source in the Arabian Peninsula. Researchers have found
MERS-CoV in camels from several countries. However, it is not known
whether camels are the source of the virus. Studies continue to provide
evidence that camel infections may play a role in human infection with
MERS-CoV, but more information is needed.

Middle East Respiratory Syndrome Symptoms

Some infected people had mild symptoms or no symptoms at all, but
most people infected with MERS-CoV developed a severe respiratory

illness. They had fever, cough, and shortness of breath. Others reported having gastrointestinal symptoms, such as diarrhea and nausea/vomiting, and kidney failure. MERS can even be deadly. Many people have died.

How Middle East Respiratory Syndrome Spreads

Middle East respiratory syndrome *coronavirus* is thought to spread from an infected person to others through respiratory secretions, such as coughing. However, the precise ways the virus spreads are not currently well understood.

Protect Yourself from Respiratory Illnesses

There is currently no vaccine to prevent MERS-CoV infection. The CDC routinely advises Americans to help protect themselves from respiratory illnesses by:

- Washing their hands often

- Avoiding close contact with people who are sick

- Avoiding touching their eyes, nose, and mouth with unwashed hands

- Disinfecting frequently touched surfaces

Middle East Respiratory Syndrome and Travel

The CDC does not recommend that anyone change their travel plans because of MERS. The CDC travel notice to countries in or near the Arabian Peninsula is an alert (level 2), which provides special precautions for travelers. Because the spread of MERS has occurred in healthcare settings, the alert advises travelers going to countries in or near the Arabian Peninsula to provide healthcare services to practice the CDC's recommendations for infection control of confirmed or suspected cases and to monitor their health closely. Travelers who are going to the area for other reasons are advised to follow standard precautions, such as hand washing and avoiding contact with people who are ill.

Section 9.13

Monkeypox

This section includes text excerpted from "Monkeypox," Centers for Disease Control and Prevention (CDC), January 28, 2019.

Monkeypox was first discovered in 1958 when two outbreaks of a pox-like disease occurred in colonies of monkeys kept for research, hence the name "monkeypox." The first human case of monkeypox was recorded in 1970 in the Democratic Republic of Congo during a period of intensified effort to eliminate smallpox. Since then, monkeypox has been reported in humans in other central and western African countries.

About Monkeypox

Monkeypox is a rare disease that is caused by infection with monkeypox virus. Monkeypox virus belongs to the Orthopoxvirus genus in the family Poxviridae. The Orthopoxvirus genus also includes variola virus (the cause of smallpox), vaccinia virus (used in the smallpox vaccine), and cowpox virus.

Human monkeypox infections have only been documented 3 times outside of Africa; in the United States in 2003 (47 cases), and in both the United Kingdom (3 cases) and Israel (1 case) in 2018.

The natural reservoir of monkeypox remains unknown. However, African rodent species are suspected to play a role in transmission.

There are two distinct genetic groups (clades) of monkeypox virus— Central African and West African. Human infections with the Central African monkeypox virus clade are typically more severe compared to those with the West African virus clade and have higher mortality. Person-to-person spread is well-documented for Central African monkeypox virus and limited with West African monkeypox.

Signs and Symptoms

In humans, the symptoms of monkeypox are similar to but milder than the symptoms of smallpox. Monkeypox begins with fever, headache, muscle aches, and exhaustion. The main difference between symptoms of smallpox and monkeypox is that monkeypox causes the lymph nodes to swell (lymphadenopathy), while smallpox does not. The incubation period (time from infection to symptoms) for monkeypox is usually 7 to 14 days but can range from 5 to 21 days.

The illness begins with:

- Fever

- Headache

- Muscle aches

- Backache

- Swollen lymph nodes

- Chills

- Exhaustion

Within one to three days (sometimes longer) after the appearance of fever, the patient develops a rash, often beginning on the face then spreading to other parts of the body.

Lesions progress through the following stages before falling off:

- Macules

- Papules

- Vesicles

- Pustules

- Scabs

The illness typically lasts for 2 to 4 weeks. In Africa, monkeypox has been shown to cause death in as many as 1 in 10 persons who contract the disease.

Treatment

Currently, there is no proven, safe treatment for monkeypox virus infection. For purposes of controlling a monkeypox outbreak in the United States, smallpox vaccine, antivirals, and vaccinia immune globulin (VIG) can be used.

Transmission

Transmission of monkeypox virus occurs when a person comes into contact with the virus from an animal, human, or materials contaminated with the virus. The virus enters the body through broken skin (even if not visible), respiratory tract, or the mucous membranes (eyes, nose, or mouth). Animal-to-human transmission may occur by bite or scratch; bushmeat preparation; direct contact with body fluids or lesion material; or indirect contact with lesion material, such as through contaminated bedding. Human-to-human transmission is thought to occur primarily through large respiratory droplets. Respiratory droplets generally cannot travel more than a few feet, so prolonged face-to-face contact is required. Other human-to-human methods of transmission include direct contact with body fluids or lesion material, and indirect contact with lesion material, such as through contaminated clothing or linens.

The reservoir host (main disease carrier) of monkeypox is still unknown although African rodents are suspected to play a part in transmission. The virus that causes monkeypox has only been recovered (isolated) twice from an animal in nature. In the first instance (1985), the virus was recovered from an apparently ill African rodent (rope squirrel) in the Equateur Region of the Democratic Republic of Congo. In the second (2012), the virus was recovered from a dead infant mangabey found in the Tai National Park, Cote d'Ivoire.

Prevention

There are number of measures that can be taken to prevent infection with monkeypox virus:

- Avoid contact with animals that could harbor the virus (including animals that are sick or that have been found dead in areas where monkeypox occurs).

- Avoid contact with any materials, such as bedding, that has been in contact with a sick animal.

- Isolate infected patients from others who could be at risk for infection.

- Practice good hand hygiene after contact with infected animals or humans. For example, washing your hands with soap and water or using an alcohol-based hand sanitizer.

- Use personal protective equipment (PPE) when caring for patients.

Section 9.14

Nipah Virus Infection

This section includes text excerpted from "Frequently Asked Questions: Nipah Virus," Centers for Disease Control and Prevention (CDC), May 30, 2018.

What Is Nipah Virus?

Nipah virus is a type of virus that can infect people and cause severe illness.

Where Is Nipah Virus Found?

Nipah virus was first discovered in 1999 following a large outbreak in Malaysia and Singapore. Sizeable outbreaks also occurred in West Bengal, India in 2001 and in Bangladesh in 2004. In 2018, an outbreak was reported in the Kerala state of India. Other countries thought to be at risk for Nipah virus include Australia, Cambodia, China, Indonesia, Madagascar, Taiwan, Thailand, Bhutan, Brunei, Laos, Madagascar, Myanmar, Nepal, Philippines, Papua New Guinea, and Vietnam.

How Do People Get Nipah Virus?

People can get Nipah virus from contact with the excrement or droppings of infected fruit bats, pigs, or from other people infected with Nipah virus. People can also get infected with Nipah virus when they consume raw date palm sap (a drink found in parts of Asia) that is contaminated with bat droppings.

Do Animals Get Sick from Nipah Virus?

The main reservoir or carrier animal of Nipah virus is a species of fruit bat found in Southeast Asia. Fruit bats do not get sick from the Nipah virus. However, they can pass the virus to other animals, such as pigs, which can get sick. These animals can then pass the virus along to people.

How Can People Spread Nipah Virus to Each Other?

Nipah virus is spread from person to person through contact with infectious body fluids from another person, such as nasal or respiratory droplets, urine, or blood.

How Can People Protect Themselves from Getting Nipah Virus?

People can protect themselves from getting Nipah virus by limiting their contact with fruit bats and sick pigs in affected areas of Southeast Asia, and by not drinking raw date palm sap. People should also avoid direct contact with body fluids from infected patients by wearing appropriate personal protective equipment (PPE), such as gloves, gowns, and facemasks, and practicing good hand hygiene.

What Are the Symptoms of Nipah Virus?

Typically, people become ill between 5 to 14 days after they are infected. Initial symptoms can include fever, headache, nausea and vomiting, shortness of breath, and may worsen to include drowsiness, confusion, and coma. Death can occur in as many as 80 percent of cases.

What Is the Treatment for Nipah Virus?

At this time, the only treatment for Nipah virus is supportive care. There are no antivirals or other medicines that have been found to conclusively treat Nipah virus infection in people.

Is There a Vaccine for Nipah Virus?

There is currently no vaccine available for Nipah virus.

Section 9.15

Severe Acute Respiratory Syndrome

This section includes text excerpted from "About Severe Acute Respiratory Syndrome (SARS)," Centers for Disease Control and Prevention (CDC), February 20, 2013. Reviewed May 2019.

Severe acute respiratory syndrome (SARS) is a viral respiratory illness caused by a *coronavirus* called "SARS-associated *coronavirus*"

(SARS-CoV). SARS was first reported in Asia in February 2003. The illness spread to more than two dozen countries in North America, South America, Europe, and Asia before the SARS global outbreak of 2003 was contained.

Currently, there is no known SARS transmission anywhere in the world. The most recent human cases of SARS-CoV infection were reported in China in April 2004 in an outbreak resulting from laboratory-acquired infections. The Centers for Disease Control and Prevention (CDC) and its partners, including the World Health Organization, continue to monitor the SARS situation globally. Any new updates on disease transmission and SARS preparedness activities will be posted on the CDC's website.

What Are the Symptoms and Signs of Severe Acute Respiratory Syndrome?

The illness usually begins with a high fever (a measured temperature greater than 100.4°F [greater than 38.0°C]). The fever is sometimes associated with chills or other symptoms, including headache, general feeling of discomfort, and body aches. Some people also experience mild respiratory symptoms at the outset. Diarrhea is seen in approximately 10 to 20 percent of patients. After 2 to 7 days, SARS patients may develop a dry, nonproductive cough that might be accompanied by or progress to a condition in which the oxygen levels in the blood are low (hypoxia). In 10 to 20 percent of cases, patients require mechanical ventilation. Most patients develop pneumonia.

What Is the Cause of Severe Acute Respiratory Syndrome?

Severe acute respiratory syndrome is caused by the previously unrecognized *coronavirus* SARS-CoV. It is possible that other infectious agents might have a role in some cases of SARS.

How Is Severe Acute Respiratory Syndrome Spread?

The primary way that SARS appears to spread is by close person-to-person contact. SARS-CoV is thought to be transmitted most readily by respiratory droplets (droplet spread) produced when an infected person coughs or sneezes. Droplet spread can happen when droplets from the cough or sneeze of an infected person have propelled a short distance (generally up to 3 feet) through the air and deposited on the mucous membranes of the mouth, nose, or eyes of persons who are nearby. The virus also can spread when a person touches a surface or object contaminated with infectious droplets and then touches her or his mouth, nose, or eye(s). In addition, it is possible that SARS-CoV might be spread more broadly through the air (airborne spread) or by other ways that are not now known.

What Does Close Contact Mean?

Close contact is defined as having cared for or lived with a person known to have SARS or having a high likelihood of direct contact with respiratory secretions and/or body fluids of a patient known to have SARS. Examples include kissing or embracing, sharing eating or drinking utensils, close conversation (within 3 feet), physical examination, and any other direct physical contact between people. Close contact does not include activities such as walking by a person or briefly sitting across a waiting room or office.

If I Were Exposed to Severe Acute Respiratory Syndrome-Related Coronavirus, How Long Would It Take for Me to Become Sick?

The time between exposure to SARS-CoV and the onset of symptoms is called the "incubation period." The incubation period for SARS is typically 2 to 7 days, although in some cases it may be as long as 10 days. In a very small proportion of cases, incubation periods of up to 14 days have been reported.

How Long Is a Person with Severe Acute Respiratory Syndrome Infectious to Others?

Available information suggests that persons with SARS are most likely to be contagious only when they have symptoms, such as fever or cough. Patients are most contagious during the second week of illness. However, as a precaution against spreading the disease, the CDC recommends that persons with SARS limit their interactions outside the home (for example, by not going to work or to school) until 10 days after their fever has gone away and their respiratory (breathing) symptoms have gotten better.

Is a Person with Severe Acute Respiratory Syndrome Contagious before Symptoms Appear?

To date, no cases of SARS have been reported among persons who were exposed to a SARS patient before the onset of the patient's symptoms.

What Medical Treatment Is Recommended for Patients with Severe Acute Respiratory Syndrome?

The Centers for Disease Control and Prevention recommends that patients with SARS receive the same treatment that would be used for a patient with any serious community-acquired atypical pneumonia. SARS-CoV is being tested against various antiviral drugs to see if effective treatment can be found.

If There Is Another Outbreak of Severe Acute Respiratory Syndrome, How Can I Protect Myself?

If transmission of SARS-CoV recurs, there are some common-sense precautions that you can take that apply to many infectious diseases. The most important is frequent hand washing with soap and water or use of an alcohol-based hand rub. You should also avoid touching your eyes, nose, and mouth with unclean hands and encourage people around you to cover their nose and mouth with a tissue when coughing or sneezing.

Laboratory Testing
Is There a Laboratory Test for Severe Acute Respiratory Syndrome?

Yes, several laboratory tests can be used to detect SARS-associated *coronavirus*. A reverse transcription polymerase chain reaction (RT-PCR) test can detect SARS-CoV in clinical specimens such as blood, stool, and nasal secretions. Serologic testing also can be performed to detect SARS-CoV antibodies produced after infection. Finally, viral culture has been used to detect SARS-CoV.

What Is a Polymerase Chain Reaction Test?

Polymerase chain reaction (PCR) is a laboratory method for detecting the genetic material of an infectious disease agent in specimens from patients. This type of testing has become an essential tool for detecting infectious disease agents.

What Does Serologic Testing Involve?

A serologic test is a laboratory method for detecting the presence and/or level of antibodies to an infectious agent in serum from a person. Antibodies are substances made by the body's immune system to fight a specific infection.

What Does Viral Culture and Isolation Involve?

For a viral culture, a small sample of tissue or fluid that may be infected is placed in a container along with cells in which the virus can grow. If the virus grows in the culture, it will cause changes in the cells that can be seen under a microscope.

Section 9.16

West Nile Virus

This section includes text excerpted from "West Nile Virus," Centers for Disease Control and Prevention (CDC), December 10, 2018.

West Nile virus (WNV) is the leading cause of mosquito-borne disease in the continental United States. It is most commonly spread to people by the bite of an infected mosquito. Cases of WNV occur during mosquito season, which starts in the summer and continues through fall. There are no vaccines to prevent or medications to treat WNV. Fortunately, most people infected with WNV do not feel sick. About 1 in 5 people who are infected develop a fever and other symptoms. About 1 out of 150 infected people develop a serious, sometimes fatal, illness. You can reduce your risk of WNV by using insect repellent and wearing long-sleeved shirts and long pants to prevent mosquito bites.

Symptoms

No symptoms in most people. Most people (8 out of 10) infected with West Nile virus do not develop any symptoms.

Febrile illness (fever) in some people. About 1 in 5 people who are infected develop a fever with other symptoms such as headache, body aches, joint pains, vomiting, diarrhea, or rash. Most people with this type of West Nile virus disease recover completely, but fatigue and weakness can last for weeks or months.

Serious symptoms in a few people. About 1 in 150 people who are infected develop a severe illness affecting the central nervous system, such as encephalitis (inflammation of the brain) or meningitis (inflammation of the membranes that surround the brain and spinal cord).

- Symptoms of severe illness include high fever, headache, neck stiffness, stupor, disorientation, coma, tremors, convulsions, muscle weakness, vision loss, numbness, and paralysis.

- Severe illness can occur in people of any age; however, people over 60 years of age are at greater risk. People with certain medical conditions, such as cancer, diabetes, hypertension, kidney disease, and people who have received organ transplants, are also at greater risk.

- Recovery from severe illness might take several weeks or months. Some effects on the central nervous system might be permanent.

- About 1 out of 10 people who develop severe illness affecting the central nervous system die.

Diagnosis

- See your healthcare provider if you develop the symptoms described above.

- Your healthcare provider can order tests to look for West Nile virus infection.

Treatment

- No vaccine or specific antiviral treatments for West Nile virus infection are available.

- Over-the-counter (OTC) pain relievers can be used to reduce fever and relieve some symptoms.

- In severe cases, patients often need to be hospitalized to receive supportive treatment, such as intravenous fluids, pain medication, and nursing care.

- If you think you or a family member might have West Nile virus disease, talk with your healthcare provider.

Transmission

West Nile virus is most commonly spread to people by the bite of an infected mosquito.

Mosquitoes become infected when they feed on infected birds. Infected mosquitoes then spread West Nile virus to people and other animals by biting them.

In a very small number of cases, West Nile virus has been spread through:

- Exposure in a laboratory setting

- Blood transfusion and organ donation

- Mother to baby, during pregnancy, delivery, or breastfeeding

West Nile virus is not spread:

- Through coughing, sneezing, or touching

- By touching live animals

- From handling live or dead infected birds. Avoid bare-handed contact when handling any dead animal. If you are disposing of a dead bird, use gloves or double plastic bags to place the carcass in a garbage can.

- Through eating infected birds or animals. Always follow instructions for fully cooking meat from either birds or mammals.

Prevention

The most effective way to prevent infection from West Nile virus is to prevent mosquito bites. Mosquitoes bite during the day and night. Use insect repellent, wear long-sleeved shirts and pants, treat clothing and gear, and take steps to control mosquitoes indoors and outdoors.

Protect Yourself and Your Family from Mosquito Bites
Use Insect Repellent

Use Environmental Protection Agency (EPA)-registered insect repellents with one of the active ingredients below. When used as directed, EPA-registered insect repellents are proven safe and effective, even for pregnant and breastfeeding women.

- (N,N-Diethyl-meta-toluamide) DEET
- Picaridin (known as "KBR 3023" and "icaridin" outside the United States)
- IR3535
- Oil of lemon eucalyptus (OLE)
- Para-menthane-diol (PMD)
- 2-undecanone

Tips for Babies and Children

- Always follow instructions when applying insect repellent to children.
- Do not use insect repellent on babies younger than two months of age.
- Instead, dress your child in clothing that covers arms and legs.
- Cover strollers and baby carriers with mosquito netting.
- Do not use products containing oil of lemon eucalyptus (OLE) or para-menthane-diol (PMD) on children under three years of age.
- Do not apply insect repellent to a child's hands, eyes, mouth, cuts, or irritated skin.
- Adults: Spray insect repellent onto your hands and then apply to a child's face.

Tips for Everyone

- Always follow the product label instructions.
- Reapply insect repellent as directed.
- Do not spray repellent on the skin under clothing.
- If you are also using sunscreen, apply sunscreen first and insect repellent second.

Natural Insect Repellents

- We do not know the effectiveness of non-EPA registered insect repellents, including some natural repellents.

- To protect yourself against diseases spread by mosquitoes, the CDC and EPA recommend using an EPA-registered insect repellent.

- Choosing an EPA-registered repellent ensures the EPA has evaluated the product for effectiveness.

Wear Long-Sleeved Shirts and Long Pants
Treat Clothing and Gear

- Use permethrin to treat clothing and gear (such as boots, pants, socks, and tents) or buy permethrin-treated clothing and gear.

- Permethrin is an insecticide that kills or repels mosquitoes.

- Permethrin-treated clothing provides protection after multiple washings.

- Read product information to find out how long the protection will last.

- If treating items yourself, follow the product instructions.

- Do not use permethrin products directly on skin.

Take Steps to Control Mosquitoes Indoors and Outdoors

- Use screens on windows and doors. Repair holes in screens to keep mosquitoes outdoors.

- Use air conditioning, if available.

- Stop mosquitoes from laying eggs in or near water.

- Once a week, empty and scrub, turn over, cover, or throw out items that hold water, such as tires, buckets, planters, toys, pools, birdbaths, flowerpots, or trash containers.

- Check indoors and outdoors.

Prevent Mosquito Bites When Traveling Overseas

- Choose a hotel or lodging with air conditioning or screens on windows and doors.

- Sleep under a mosquito bed net if you are outside or in a room that does not have screens.

- Buy a bed net at your local outdoor store or online before traveling overseas.

- Choose a World Health Organization Pesticide Evaluation Scheme (WHOPES)-approved bed net: compact, white, rectangular, with 156 holes per square inch, and long enough to tuck under the mattress.

- Permethrin-treated bed nets provide more protection than untreated nets.

- Do not wash bed nets or expose them to sunlight. This will break down the insecticide more quickly.

Section 9.17

Yellow Fever

This section includes text excerpted from "Yellow Fever,"
Centers for Disease Control and Prevention (CDC), January 15, 2019.

The yellow fever virus is found in tropical and subtropical areas of Africa and South America. The virus is spread to people by the bite of an infected mosquito. Yellow fever is a very rare cause of illness in U.S. travelers. Illness ranges from a fever with aches and pains to severe liver disease with bleeding and yellowing skin (jaundice). A yellow fever infection is diagnosed based on laboratory testing, and a person's symptoms and travel history. There is no medicine to treat or cure this infection. To prevent getting sick from yellow fever, use insect repellent, wear long-sleeved shirts and long pants, and get vaccinated.

Symptoms

The majority of people infected with yellow fever virus will either not have symptoms or have mild symptoms and completely recover.

For people who develop symptoms, the time from infection until illness is typically three to six days.

Because there is a risk of severe disease, all people who develop symptoms of yellow fever after traveling to or living in an area at risk for the virus should see their healthcare provider. Once you have been infected, you are likely to be protected from future infections.

- Most people will not have symptoms.

- Some people will develop yellow fever illness with initial symptoms including:

  - Sudden onset of fever

  - Chills

  - Severe headache

  - Back pain

  - General body aches

  - Nausea

  - Vomiting

  - Fatigue (feeling tired)

  - Weakness

- Most people with the initial symptoms improve within one week.

- For some people who recover, weakness and fatigue (feeling tired) might last several months.

- A few people will develop a more severe form of the disease.

  - For one out of seven people who have the initial symptoms, there will be a brief remission (a time during which you feel better) that may last only a few hours or for a day, followed by a more severe form of the disease.

- Severe symptoms include:

  - High fever

  - Yellow skin (jaundice)

  - Bleeding

  - Shock

  - Organ failure

- Severe yellow fever disease can be deadly. If you develop any of these symptoms, see a healthcare provider immediately.

- Among those who develop severe disease, 30 to 60 percent die.

Diagnosis

Yellow fever infection is diagnosed based on laboratory testing, and a person's symptoms and travel history.

Treatment

- There is no medicine to treat or cure infection from yellow fever.

- Rest, drink fluids, and use pain relievers and medication to reduce fever and relieve aching.

- Avoid certain medications, such as aspirin or other nonsteroidal anti-inflammatory drugs, for example ibuprofen (Advil, Motrin), or naproxen (Aleve), which may increase the risk of bleeding.

- People with severe symptoms of yellow fever infection should be hospitalized for close observation and supportive care.

- If after returning from travel you have symptoms of yellow fever (usually about a week after being bitten by an infected mosquito), protect yourself from mosquito bites for up to five days after symptoms begin. This will help prevent spreading yellow fever to uninfected mosquitoes that can spread the virus to other people.

Transmission

The yellow fever virus is a ribonucleic acid (RNA) virus that belongs to the genus Flavivirus. It is related to West Nile, St. Louis encephalitis, and Japanese encephalitis viruses. Yellow fever virus is transmitted to people primarily through the bite of infected Aedes or Haemagogus species mosquitoes. Mosquitoes acquire the virus by feeding on infected primates (human or nonhuman) and then can transmit the virus to other primates (human or nonhuman). People infected with yellow fever virus are infectious to mosquitoes (referred to as being "viremic") shortly before the onset of fever and up to five days after onset.

Yellow fever virus has three transmission cycles: jungle (sylvatic), intermediate (savannah), and urban.

- The jungle (sylvatic) cycle involves transmission of the virus between nonhuman primates (e.g., monkeys) and mosquito species found in the forest canopy. The virus is transmitted by mosquitoes from monkeys to humans when humans are visiting or working in the jungle.

- In Africa, an intermediate (savannah) cycle exists that involves transmission of virus from mosquitoes to humans living or working in jungle border areas. In this cycle, the virus can be transmitted from monkey to human or from human to human via mosquitoes.

- The urban cycle involves transmission of the virus between humans and urban mosquitoes, primarily *Aedes aegypti*. The virus is usually brought to the urban setting by a viremic human who was infected in the jungle or savannah.

Prevention

The most effective way to prevent infection from Yellow Fever virus is to prevent mosquito bites. Mosquitoes bite during the day and night. Use insect repellent, wear long-sleeved shirts and pants, treat clothing and gear, and get vaccinated before traveling, if vaccination is recommended for you.

Prevent Mosquito Bites
Use Insect Repellent

Use U.S. Environmental Protection Agency (EPA)-registered insect repellents with one of the active ingredients below. When used as directed, EPA-registered insect repellents are proven safe and effective, even for pregnant and breastfeeding women.

- DEET (N,N-diethyl-meta-toluamide)

- Picaridin (known as "KBR 3023" and "icaridin" outside the United States)

- IR3535

- Oil of lemon eucalyptus (OLE)

- Para-menthane-diol (PMD)

- 2-undecanone

Tips for Babies and Children

- Always follow instructions when applying insect repellent to children.

- Do not use insect repellent on babies younger than two months old.

  - Instead, dress your child in clothing that covers arms and legs.

  - Cover strollers and baby carriers with mosquito netting.

- Do not use products containing oil of lemon eucalyptus (OLE) or para-menthane-diol (PMD) on children under three years old.

- Do not apply insect repellent to a child's hands, eyes, mouth, cuts, or irritated skin.

  - Adults: Spray insect repellent onto your hands and then apply to a child's face.

Tips for Everyone

- Always follow the product label instructions.

- Reapply insect repellent as directed.

  - Do not spray repellent on the skin under clothing.

  - If you are also using sunscreen, apply sunscreen first and insect repellent second.

Natural Insect Repellents

- We do not know the effectiveness of non-EPA registered insect repellents, including some natural repellents.

- To protect yourself against diseases spread by mosquitoes, the CDC and EPA recommend using an EPA-registered insect repellent.

- Choosing an EPA-registered repellent ensures the EPA has evaluated the product for effectiveness.

Wear Long-Sleeved Shirts and Long Pants
Treat Clothing and Gear

- Use permethrin to treat clothing and gear (such as boots, pants, socks, and tents) or buy permethrin-treated clothing and gear.

- Permethrin is an insecticide that kills or repels mosquitoes.
- Permethrin-treated clothing provides protection after multiple washings.
- Read product information to find out how long the protection will last.
- If treating items yourself, follow the product instructions.
- Do not use permethrin products directly on skin.

Take Steps to Control Mosquitoes Indoors and Outdoors

- Use screens on windows and doors. Repair holes in screens to keep mosquitoes outdoors.
- Use air conditioning, if available.
- Stop mosquitoes from laying eggs in or near water.
- Once a week, empty and scrub, turn over, cover, or throw out items that hold water, such as tires, buckets, planters, toys, pools, birdbaths, flowerpots, or trash containers.

Prevent Mosquito Bites When Traveling Overseas

- Choose a hotel or lodging with air conditioning or screens on windows and doors.
- Sleep under a mosquito bed net if you are outside or in a room that does not have screens.
  - Buy a bed net at your local outdoor store or online before traveling overseas.
  - Choose a World Health Organization Pesticide Evaluation Scheme (WHOPES)-approved bed net: compact, white, rectangular, with 156 holes per square inch, and long enough to tuck under the mattress.
  - Permethrin-treated bed nets provide more protection than untreated nets.
    - Do not wash bed nets or expose them to sunlight. This will break down the insecticide more quickly.

Section 9.18

Zika Fever

This section contains text excerpted from the following
sources: Text in this section begins with excerpts from "Zika,"
Centers for Disease Control and Prevention (CDC), December 11,
2018; Text under the heading "Transmission Methods" is excerpted
from "Zika Virus," Centers for Disease Control and
Prevention (CDC), January 9, 2019.

Mosquitoes can spread many diseases, including Zika. Although most people with Zika do not have symptoms, infection during pregnancy can cause serious birth defects.

Zika virus spreads primarily through the bite of an infected Aedes mosquito (*Aedes aegypti* or *Ae. albopictus*). Zika can also be transmitted through sex with a Zika-infected partner.

The mosquitoes that carry Zika can be found in many countries, and outbreaks of Zika are still occurring in parts of the world. Everyone can take steps to protect themselves and pregnant women in the United States.

Signs and Symptoms of Zika

Many people infected with Zika virus will not know they have it because they do not have symptoms. Symptoms are usually mild and can last for several days to a week. People usually do not get sick enough to go to the hospital, and they very rarely die of Zika. The most common symptoms of Zika include:

- Fever

- Rash

- Headache

- Joint pain

- Conjunctivitis (red eyes)

- Muscle pain

See your doctor or other healthcare provider if you have the symptoms described above and have visited an area with risk of Zika. This is especially important if you are pregnant. Be sure to tell your doctor or other healthcare provider where you traveled. Even if you do not feel sick, you should take steps to prevent mosquito bites for three weeks after travel so you do not spread Zika to uninfected mosquitoes.

Zika Can Cause Birth Defects

Zika infection during pregnancy is a cause of microcephaly (a condition in which a baby's head is smaller than expected when compared to babies of the same sex and age) and other birth defects. Because of the risk for birth defects, pregnant women should not travel to areas with risk of Zika. Pregnant women who travel to or live in areas with risk of Zika should take steps to prevent mosquito bites and use condoms or not have sex during their pregnancy to avoid getting Zika from their partner.

Women and their partners thinking about pregnancy should talk to a healthcare provider before traveling to areas with risk of Zika. If a couple decides to travel to an area with risk of Zika, they should consider waiting to get pregnant. If the couple travels together or only the male partner travels, they should consider using condoms or not having sex for at least three months after travel. If only the female partner travels, the couple should consider waiting at least two months after travel.

Protect Yourself, Your Family, and Your Community from Zika

There is no vaccine to protect against Zika. If you are traveling to an area with risk of Zika, the best way to prevent Zika is to take steps to prevent mosquito bites and sexual transmission of Zika during and after travel.

Take these steps to prevent mosquito bites:

- Wear long-sleeved shirts and long pants.

- Stay in places with air conditioning or window and door screens to keep mosquitoes outside. Make sure to check for and fix any holes in screens.

- Sleep under a mosquito bed net if air-conditioned or screened rooms are not available or if sleeping outdoors.

- Use U.S. Environmental Protection Agency (EPA)-registered insect repellents with one of the following active ingredients: (N,N-diethyl-meta-toluamide) DEET, picaridin, IR3535, oil of lemon eucalyptus, para-menthane-diol, or 2-undecanone.

- When used as directed, these insect repellents are proven safe and effective even for pregnant and breastfeeding women.
  - Always follow the product label instructions.
  - Reapply insect repellent as directed.
  - Do not spray repellent on skin under clothing. Put on clothing first, and then apply repellent to any exposed skin.
  - If you are also using sunscreen, apply sunscreen before applying insect repellent.
- Treat clothing and gear with permethrin or buy permethrin-treated items.
  - Treated clothing can protect after multiple washings.
  - If treating items yourself, follow the product instructions carefully.
  - Do not use permethrin products directly on skin. They are intended to treat clothing.

Even if you do not feel sick, travelers returning from an area with risk of Zika should take steps to prevent mosquito bites for three weeks so they do not pass Zika to mosquitoes that could then spread the virus to other people.

If you have a baby or child:

- Do not use insect repellent on babies younger than two months old.
- Do not use products containing oil of lemon eucalyptus or para-menthane-diol on children younger than three years old.
- Dress your child in clothing that covers arms and legs.
- Cover cribs, strollers, and baby carriers with mosquito netting.
- Do not apply insect repellent onto a child's hands, eyes, mouth, or cut or irritated skin.
- Spray insect repellent onto your hands and then apply to your child's face.

Prevent mosquito bites even after you return from traveling to areas with Zika. If you get infected, even if you do not get sick, Zika virus can be found in your blood and passed to mosquitoes through mosquito bites. Infected mosquitoes can then spread the virus to other people.

Transmission Methods
Through Mosquito Bites

Zika virus is transmitted to people primarily through the bite of an infected Aedes species mosquito (*Ae. aegypti* and *Ae. albopictus*). These are the same mosquitoes that spread dengue and chikungunya viruses.

- These mosquitoes typically lay eggs in or near standing water in things such as buckets, bowls, animal dishes, flower pots, and vases. They prefer to bite people and live indoors and outdoors near people.

- Mosquitoes that spread chikungunya, dengue, and Zika bite during the day and night.

- Mosquitoes become infected when they feed on a person already infected with the virus. Infected mosquitoes can then spread the virus to other people through bites.

From Mother to Child

- A pregnant woman can pass Zika virus to her fetus during pregnancy. Zika is a cause of microcephaly and other severe fetal brain defects. Researchers are studying the full range of other potential health problems that Zika virus infection during pregnancy may cause.

- A pregnant woman already infected with Zika virus can pass the virus to her fetus during the pregnancy or around the time of birth.

- Zika virus has been found in breast milk. Possible Zika virus infections have been identified in breastfeeding babies, but Zika virus transmission through breast milk has not been confirmed. Additionally, researchers do not yet know the long-term effects of Zika virus on young infants infected after birth. Because current evidence suggests that the benefits of breastfeeding outweigh the risk of Zika virus spreading through breast milk, the Centers for Disease Control and Prevention (CDC) continues to encourage mothers to breastfeed, even if they were infected or lived in or traveled to an area with risk of Zika. The CDC continues to study Zika virus and the ways it can spread and will update recommendations as new information becomes available.

Through Sexual Intercourse

- Zika can be passed through sex from a person who has Zika to a partner. Zika can be passed through sex, even if the infected person does not have symptoms at the time.

  - Zika can be passed from a person with Zika before their symptoms start, while they have symptoms, and after their symptoms end.

  - Though not well documented, the virus may also be passed by a person who carries the virus but never develops symptoms.

- Studies are underway to find out how long Zika stays in the semen and vaginal fluids of people who have Zika, and how long it can be passed to sex partners. Researchers know that Zika can remain in semen longer than in other body fluids, including vaginal fluids, urine, and blood.

Through Blood Transfusion

- To date, there have not been any confirmed blood transfusion transmission cases in the United States.

- There have been multiple reports of possible blood transfusion transmission cases in Brazil.

- During the French Polynesian outbreak, 2.8 percent of blood donors tested positive for Zika and in previous outbreaks, the virus has been found in blood donors.

Through Laboratory and Healthcare-Setting Exposure

- There are reports of laboratory-acquired Zika virus infections, although the route of transmission was not clearly established in all cases.

- To date, no cases of Zika virus transmission in healthcare settings have been identified in the United States. Recommendations are available for healthcare providers to help prevent exposure to Zika virus in healthcare settings.

Testing for Zika
How Zika Is Diagnosed

- To diagnose Zika, a doctor or other healthcare provider will ask about any recent travel and any signs and symptoms.

- They may order blood or urine tests to help determine if you have Zika.

Remember to ask for your Zika test results even if you are feeling better.

Need Zika Testing

Zika virus testing is recommended only for certain people. If you have questions or think you should be tested, talk to your healthcare provider.

If you have symptoms:

- Zika testing is recommended if you have symptoms of Zika

  - You live in or traveled to an area with risk of Zika, or

  - You had sex without a condom with a partner who lives in or traveled to an area with risk of Zika

Pregnant Women

Zika testing is recommended for pregnant women who do not have Zika symptoms in certain cases. You should be tested for Zika if you are pregnant and

- You have ongoing exposure to Zika because you live in or frequently travel to an area with risk of Zika, or

- Your doctor sees Zika-associated abnormalities on an ultrasound or you deliver a baby with birth defects that may be related to Zika

Positive for Zika Testing

- If you are pregnant, you can pass Zika to your fetus.

- You can pass Zika to your sex partners.

- You can pass Zika to mosquitoes, which can bite you, get infected with Zika virus, and spread the virus to other people. Learn how you can prevent mosquito bites.

Sexual Transmission and Testing

A blood or urine test can help determine if you have Zika from sexual transmission; however, testing blood, semen, vaginal fluids, or urine is not recommended to determine how likely a person is to pass Zika virus through sex.

Treatment

There is no specific medicine or vaccine for Zika virus.

- Treat the symptoms.

- Get plenty of rest.

- Drink fluids to prevent dehydration.

- Take medicine such as acetaminophen to reduce fever and pain.

- Do not take aspirin and other nonsteroidal anti-inflammatory drugs (NSAIDs) until dengue can be ruled out to reduce the risk of bleeding.

- If you are taking medicine for another medical condition, talk to your healthcare provider before taking additional medication.

Chapter 10

Bacterial Infectious Diseases

Chapter Contents

Section 10.1

Bioterrorism-Related Anthrax

This section includes text excerpted from "Bioterrorism," Centers for Disease Control and Prevention (CDC), September 10, 2018.

Bioterrorism

A biological attack, or bioterrorism, is the intentional release of viruses, bacteria, or other germs that can sicken or kill people, livestock, or crops. *Bacillus anthracis* (*B. anthracis*), the bacteria that causes anthrax, is one of the most likely agents to be used in a biological attack.

The Threat

We do not know if or when another anthrax attack might occur. However, federal agencies have worked for years with health departments across the country to plan and prepare for an anthrax attack. If such an emergency were to occur in the United States, the Centers for Disease Control and Prevention (CDC) and other federal agencies would work closely with local and state partners to coordinate a response.

Why Would Anthrax Be Used as a Weapon?

If a bioterrorist attack were to happen, *Bacillus anthracis*, the bacteria that causes anthrax, would be one of the biological agents most likely to be used. Biological agents are germs that can sicken or kill people, livestock, or crops. Anthrax is one of the most likely agents to be used because:

- Anthrax spores are easily found in nature, can be produced in a lab, and can last for a long time in the environment.

- Anthrax makes a good weapon because it can be released quietly and without anyone knowing. The microscopic spores could be put into powders, sprays, food, and water. Because they are so small, you may not be able to see, smell, or taste them.

- Anthrax has been used as a weapon before.

Anthrax has been used as a weapon around the world for nearly a century. In 2001, powdered anthrax spores were deliberately put into letters that were mailed through the U.S. postal system. Twenty-two people, including 12 mail handlers, got anthrax, and 5 of these 22 people died.

How Dangerous Is Anthrax?

A subset of select agents and toxins has been designated as a Tier 1 agent because these biological agents and toxins present the greatest risk of deliberate misuse with significant potential for mass casualties or a devastating effect on the economy, critical infrastructure, or public confidence, and pose a severe threat to public health and safety. *Bacillus anthracis* is a Tier 1 agent.

B. *anthracis* is a select agent. The possession, use, or transfer of B. *anthracis* is regulated by the Division of Select Agents and Toxins (DSAT), located in the CDC's Office of Public Health Preparedness and Response (OPHPR).

What Might an Anthrax Attack Look Like?

An anthrax attack could take many forms. For example, it could be placed in letters and mailed, as was done in 2001, or it could be put into food or water. Anthrax also could be released into the air from a truck, building, or plane. This type of attack would mean the anthrax spores could easily be blown around by the wind or carried on people's clothes, shoes, and other objects. It only takes a small amount of anthrax to infect a large number of people.

If anthrax spores were released into the air, people could breathe them in and get sick with anthrax. Inhalation anthrax is the most serious form and can kill quickly if not treated immediately. If the attack were not detected by one of the monitoring systems in place in the United States, it might go unnoticed until doctors begin to see unusual patterns of illness among sick people showing up at emergency rooms.

Preparedness

Hopefully, an attack involving anthrax will never happen in the United States. However, there are steps that you and your family can take to help prepare if an anthrax emergency ever did happen. If such an emergency were to occur in the United States, the CDC and other federal agencies would be ready to respond.

What You Can Do to Prepare?
Get a Kit, Make a Plan, Stay Informed

For details about how to put together an emergency kit, develop a family disaster plan, and stay informed about all types of emergencies, go to the CDC's Emergency Preparedness and You website. These basic preparedness steps would be essential during an anthrax emergency.

People in areas where anthrax is released would also need to know how to get antibiotics, how to create a family medical history, and how to recognize the symptoms of anthrax.

Know How You Would Get Antibiotics During an Anthrax Crisis

If an anthrax emergency happened in your area, your community might need to receive large amounts of antibiotics and medical supplies from the federal government. The supplies would be sent to sites that are usually called "points of dispensing" (PODs). PODs would be located in your community in safe, familiar places such as schools or convention centers.

In an anthrax emergency, you would be able to find out where the nearest POD is located and what to bring to the POD by listening to news updates on TV and the radio, visiting your health department's website, and staying alert for messages from community leaders.

PODs are designed to provide medicine to a large number of people in a short period of time, so you could expect to stand in line. While at the POD, you would be asked to fill out a form that includes some basic information about your medical history. Once you complete your form, a POD staff member would review it and determine which antibiotic is best for you.

Keep a Family Medical History

In some cases, you may be able to pick up antibiotics for others in your household. If you live with family members, it is important to keep a medical history for each person in your family, including:

- Medical conditions

- Allergies

- Any medicines they are taking

- Each child's weight

During an emergency, you may be asked to bring this information to a POD to make sure you get the right antibiotics for everyone in your family.

In an anthrax emergency, many lives would be saved if people started taking antibiotics right away. It would be very important to start taking antibiotics as soon as you get them, take them as directed, and keep taking them for as long as you are told to.

The CDC hopes there is never an anthrax emergency that requires PODs to open, but if there is, be assured that the process is in place to get antibiotics to you and your family as quickly as possible.

Be Aware of the Symptoms of Anthrax

During an anthrax emergency, you would need to be able to recognize the symptoms of anthrax, especially inhalation anthrax, and be prepared to get medical care if you have any of these symptoms.

What the Centers for Disease Control and Prevention Is Doing to Prepare

The CDC is working with other federal agencies and health departments across the country to prepare for an anthrax attack. Activities include:

- Providing funds and guidance to help health departments strengthen their abilities to respond to all types of public-health incidents and build more resilient communities

- Providing training in emergency response for the public-health workforce and healthcare providers, as well as leaders in the public and private sector

- Coordinating response activities and providing resources to health departments through the CDC's Emergency Operations Center (EOC)

- Regulating the possession, use, and transfer of biological agents and toxins that could pose a severe threat to public health and safety through the CDC Select Agent Program (SAP)

- Promoting science and practices to strengthen preparedness and response activities

- Ensuring that the United States has enough laboratories that can quickly conduct tests when anthrax is suspected

- Working with hospitals, laboratories, emergency response teams, and healthcare providers to make sure they have the medicine and supplies they would need if an anthrax attack occurred

- Developing guidance to protect the health and safety of workers who would be responding during an anthrax emergency

Section 10.2

Mycobacteria

This section includes text excerpted from "*Mycobacterium abscessus* in Healthcare Settings," Centers for Disease Control and Prevention (CDC), November 24, 2010. Reviewed May 2019.

About Mycobacterium abscessus

Mycobacterium abscessus (also called "*M. abscessus*") is a bacterium distantly related to the ones that cause tuberculosis and Hansen disease (leprosy). It is part of a group of environmental mycobacteria and is found in water, soil, and dust. It has been known to contaminate medications and products, including medical devices.

M. abscessus can cause a variety of infections. Healthcare-associated infections due to this bacterium are usually of the skin and the soft tissues under the skin. It is also a cause of serious lung infections in persons with various chronic lung diseases, such as cystic fibrosis.

People with open wounds or who receive injections without appropriate skin disinfection may be at risk for infection by *M. abscessus*. Rarely, individuals with underlying respiratory conditions or impaired immune systems are at risk of lung infection.

Mycobacterium abscessus is a bacterium distantly related to the ones that cause tuberculosis and leprosy. It is part of a group known as "rapidly growing mycobacteria" and is found in water, soil, and dust. It has been known to contaminate medications and products, including medical devices.

Symptoms of Mycobacterium abscessus

Skin infected with *M. abscessus* is usually red, warm, tender to the touch, swollen, and/or painful. Infected areas can also develop boils or pus-filled vesicles. Other signs of *M. abscessus* infection are fever, chills, muscle aches, and a general feeling of illness. However, for a definite diagnosis, the organism has to be cultured from the infection site or, in severe cases, from a blood culture. A medical provider should evaluate the infection to determine if it may be due to *M. abscessus*.

Diagnosis is made by growing this bacterium in the laboratory from a sample of the pus or biopsy of the infected area. When the infection is severe, the bacterium can be found in the blood and isolated from a blood sample. To make the diagnosis, your healthcare provider will have to take a sample from the infected area and/or blood and send it to a laboratory for identification. It is important that persons who have any evidence of infection at a site where they received procedures, such as surgery or injections, let their doctors know so the appropriate tests can be done.

Transmission of Mycobacterium abscessus

Transmission of *M. abscessus* can occur in several ways. Infection with *M. abscessus* is usually caused by injections of substances contaminated with the bacterium or through invasive medical procedures employing contaminated equipment or material. Infection can also occur after an accidental injury where the wound is contaminated by soil. There is very little risk of transmission from person to person.

Prevention of Mycobacterium abscessus

Anyone who touches or cares for the infected site should wash their hands carefully with soap and water. Patients should follow all instructions given by their healthcare provider following any surgery or medical procedure. Avoid receiving procedures or injections by unlicensed persons.

Treatment of Mycobacterium abscessus

Treatment of infections due to *M. abscessus* consists of draining collections of pus or removing the infected tissue and administering the appropriate combination of antibiotics for a prolonged period of time. Infection with this bacterium usually does not improve with the usual antibiotics used to treat skin infections. Testing the bacteria against different antibiotics is helpful in guiding doctors to the most appropriate treatment for each patient.

Chapter 11

Fungal and Parasitic Infectious Diseases

Chapter Contents

Section 11.1

Cryptococcus gattii *Infection*

This section includes text excerpted from
"*C. gattii* Infection," Centers for Disease Control and
Prevention (CDC), October 18, 2018.

Cryptococcus gattii (*C. gattii*) cryptococcosis is a rare infection caused by *Cryptococcus gattii*, a fungus that lives in soil and in association with certain trees. *C. gattii* primarily lives in tropical and subtropical regions of the world, particularly Australia and Papua New Guinea, but it has also been found in parts of Africa, Asia, Europe, Mexico, and South America. Since 1999, *C. gattii* has been recognized as causing infections in humans and animals on Vancouver Island, British Columbia, and *C. gattii* infections were first recognized the United States Pacific Northwest (Oregon and Washington) in 2004. A small number of people have also gotten *C. gattii* infections in other areas of the United States, particularly in the Southeast, without a history of travel to Oregon or Washington.

People can become infected with *C. gattii* after breathing in the microscopic fungus from the environment. Infection with the fungus Cryptococcus (either *C. gattii* or *C. neoformans*) is called "cryptococcosis." Cryptococcosis usually affects the lungs or the central nervous system (the brain and spinal cord), but it can also affect other parts of the body. Brain infections with the fungus Cryptococcus are called "cryptococcal meningitis."

Sources of Cryptococcus gattii
Where Does Cryptococcus gattii *Live?*

C. gattii lives in the environment, usually near trees and in the soil around trees. The fungus primarily lives in tropical and subtropical areas of the world, particularly Australia and Papua New Guinea, and also in parts of Africa, Asia, Europe, Mexico, and South America. It also lives in mainland British Columbia, Vancouver Island, and the United States Pacific Northwest (Oregon and Washington). *C. gattii* may also live in other areas of the United States, such as California and the Southeastern United States because a few people from these parts of the United States have gotten *C. gattii* infections without traveling outside of these areas.

Life Cycle of **Cryptococcus gattii**

C. gattii infections are not contagious. Humans and animals can become infected with *C. gattii* after inhaling airborne, dried yeast cells or spores from the environment. *C. gattii* travels through the airway and enters the lungs. The body's temperature allows *C. gattii* to transform into its yeast form, and the cells grow thick outer layers to protect themselves. The yeasts then divide and multiply by budding. After infecting the lungs, *C. gattii* can travel through the bloodstream to infect other areas of the body, such as the central nervous system.

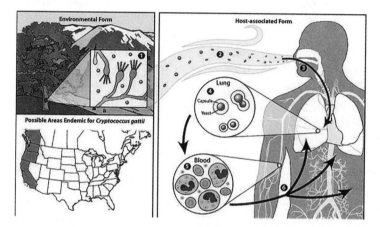

Figure 11.1. *Biology of* Cryptococcus gattii

Cryptococcus gattii *lives in the environment, usually in association with certain trees or soil around trees. Humans and animals can become infected with* C. gattii *after inhaling airborne, dehydrated yeast cells or spores, which travel through the respiratory tract and enter the lungs of the host. The small size of the yeast and/or spores allows them to become lodged deep in the lung tissue. The environment inside the host body signals* C. gattii *to transform into its yeast form and the cells grow thick capsules to protect themselves. The yeasts then divide and multiply by building. After infecting the lungs,* C. gattii *cells can travel through the bloodstream—either on their own or within macrophage cells—to infect other areas of the body, typically the central nervous system.*

I Am Worried That **Cryptococcus gattii** *Is in the Environment near My Home. Can Someone Test the Trees or Soil to Find out If the Fungus Is There?*

No, in this case, testing the environment for *C. gattii* is not likely to be useful. A sample that tests positive for Cryptococcus does not necessarily mean that it is a source of infection, and a sample that tests negative does not necessarily mean that the fungus is not there. Also, there are no commercially-available tests to detect *C. gattii* in the environment. Testing environmental samples for *C. gattii* is currently only done for scientific research.

Species of Cryptococcus and Genetic Types of Cryptococcus gattii

The genus Cryptococcus contains over 30 species, but 2 species, Cryptococcus neoformans and *Cryptococcus gattii*, cause nearly all cryptococcal infections. *Cryptococcus gattii* used to be called "Cryptococcus neoformans var. gattii," but it was determined to be a separate species from *C. neoformans* in 2002. *C. neoformans* and *C. gattii* tend to affect different patient populations. *C. neoformans* most often causes meningitis in people who have HIV infection or who are otherwise immunocompromised. *C. gattii* affects healthy people, as well as people who have weakened immune systems, and it usually infects the lungs, the central nervous system, or both.

There are four known molecular types of *C. gattii*: VGI, VGII, VGIII, and VGIV. Type VGII can be further divided into the molecular subtypes VGIIa, VGIIb, and VGIIc. The different molecular types of *C. gattii* can be found in different parts of the world. Most *C. gattii* infections in British Columbia, Canada, and the United States Pacific Northwest are caused by the molecular type VGII, but VGI is the most common type in Australia and Papua New Guinea. VGII appears to mostly cause lung infections, whereas the other types usually cause meningitis in people who do not have any prior medical problems; however, scientists are still learning about the differences between the types of *C. gattii*.

Symptoms of Cryptococcus gattii *Infection*

C. gattii usually infects the lungs or the central nervous system (the brain and spinal cord), but it can also affect other parts of the body. The symptoms of the infection depend on the parts of the body that are affected.

In the Lungs

A *C. gattii* infection in the lungs can cause a pneumonia-like illness. The symptoms are often similar to those of many other illnesses, and can include:

156

- Cough
- Shortness of breath
- Chest pain
- Fever

In the Brain (Cryptococcal Meningitis)

Cryptococcal meningitis is an infection caused by the fungus Cryptococcus after it spreads from the lungs to the brain. The symptoms of cryptococcal meningitis include:

- Headache
- Fever
- Neck pain
- Nausea and vomiting
- Sensitivity to light
- Confusion or changes in behavior

C. gattii infection can also cause cryptococcomas (fungal growths) to develop in the lungs, skin, brain or other organs, causing symptoms in other parts of the body.

If you have symptoms that you think may be due to a *C. gattii* infection, please contact your healthcare provider.

How Soon Do the Symptoms of Cryptococcus gattii Infection Appear?

The incubation period of *C. gattii* is not well-established. A few studies have shown that symptoms of *C. gattii* infection can appear between 2 to 13 months after breathing in the fungus, with an average of approximately 6 to 7 months. However, for some people, it may take even longer for symptoms to show up after breathing in the fungus; for example, one person did not develop symptoms until 3 years after traveling to an area where the fungus is known to live.

Cryptococcus gattii Infection Risk and Prevention
Who Gets Cryptococcus gattii Infections

Anyone can be infected with *C. gattii* if they have been in an area where the fungus lives in the environment. However, in different parts of the world, different characteristics may make some people more likely to get *C. gattii* infections than others. For example, in Australia and New Zealand, *C. gattii* infections are thought to be more common among people who are otherwise healthy, males, and people of Australian aborigine ethnicity. However, a study of people who got *C. gattii* infections in British Columbia, Canada found that the disease was more likely to occur in people who:

- Have weakened immune systems, for example, by:
  - Human immunodeficiency virus (HIV)/acquired immune deficiency syndrome (AIDS)
  - Cancer treatment
  - Medications that weaken the immune system such as corticosteroids
- Have other lung conditions
- Are 50 years of age or older
- Smoke tobacco

Scientists are still learning about why *C. gattii* appears to affect different groups of people in different areas of the world.

Is **Cryptococcus gattii** Infection *Contagious?*

No. The infection cannot spread between people or between people and animals.

Can Pets Get **Cryptococcus gattii** *Infections?*

Yes. Pets can get *C. gattii* infections, but it is very rare, and the infection cannot spread between animals and people. The symptoms of *C. gattii* infection in pets, such as cats and dogs, are similar to the symptoms in humans. If you are concerned about your pet's risk of getting a *C. gattii* infection, or if you think that your pet has the infection, please talk to a veterinarian.

How Can I Prevent a **Cryptococcus gattii** *Infection?*

There are no formal recommendations to prevent *C. gattii* infection. Most people breathe in small amounts of many fungi every day but never become sick. If you have symptoms that you think may be caused by *C. gattii*, you should see a healthcare provider as soon as possible.

What Are Public Health Agencies Doing about Cryptococcus gattii?

- **Surveillance.** In Oregon and Washington, healthcare providers and laboratories are required to report *C. gattii* cases to public health authorities. Disease reporting helps government officials and healthcare providers monitor trends in the number of *C. gattii* cases.

- **International partnerships.** Medical, public health, and laboratory professionals in Australia, Europe, Canada, and the United States are working together to compare and better understand *C. gattii* infections in different parts of the world.

Diagnosis and Testing for Cryptococcus gattii Infection

How Is a Cryptococcus gattii Infection Diagnosed?

Healthcare providers use your medical and travel history, symptoms, physical examinations, and laboratory tests to diagnose a *C. gattii* infection.

Your healthcare provider will take a sample of tissue or body fluid (such as blood, cerebrospinal fluid, or sputum) and send the sample to a laboratory to be examined under a microscope, tested with an antigen test, or cultured (see Testing for *C. gattii* infection versus *C. neoformans* infection). Your healthcare provider may also perform tests, such as a chest X-ray or CT scan of your lungs, brain, or other parts of the body.

Testing for Cryptococcus gattii Infection versus Cryptococcus neoformans Infection

Testing serum (a component of blood) or cerebrospinal fluid for cryptococcal antigen is useful as a first test for cryptococcal infection, but the test does not tell the difference between *Cryptococcus neoformans* and *Cryptococcus gattii*. Culture is traditionally used to tell if a cryptococcal infection is due to *C. neoformans* or *C. gattii*. On canavanine-glycine-bromthymol blue (CGB) agar, *C. gattii* will turn the culture medium blue, but *C. neoformans* will leave the color of the medium unaffected (yellow to green).

159

Treatment for Cryptococcus gattii *Infection*
How Are Cryptococcus gattii *Infections Treated?*

People who have *C. gattii* infection need to take prescription anti-fungal medication for at least six months, often longer. The type of treatment usually depends on the severity of the infection and the parts of the body that are affected.

- For people who have asymptomatic infections or mild-to-moderate pulmonary infections, the treatment is usually fluconazole.

- For people who have severe lung infections or infections in the central nervous system (brain and spinal cord), the recommended initial treatment is amphotericin B in combination with flucytosine. After that, patients usually need to take fluconazole for an extended time to clear the infection.

The type, dose, and duration of antifungal treatment may differ for certain groups of people, such as pregnant women, children, and people in resource-limited settings. Some people may also need surgery to remove fungal growths (cryptococcomas).

Section 11.2

Cryptosporidium *Disinfection*

This section includes text excerpted from *"Cryptosporidium* (Crypto) and Drinking Water from Private Wells," Centers for Disease Control and Prevention (CDC), July 1, 2015. Reviewed May 2019.

What Is Cryptosporidiosis*?*

Cryptosporidiosis is a diarrheal disease caused by a microscopic parasite, *Cryptosporidium,* that can live in the intestine of humans and animals and is passed in the stool of an infected person or animal. Both the disease and the parasite are commonly known as "Crypto." The parasite is protected by an outer shell that allows it to survive outside the body for long periods of time and makes it very resistant to chlorine-based disinfectants. During the past two decades, Crypto has become recognized as one of the most common causes of water-borne disease (recreational water and drinking water) in humans in the United States. The parasite is found in every region of the United States and throughout the world.

Where and How Does Crypto Get into Drinking Water?

Crypto is found in every part of the United States and throughout the world. Millions of Crypto can be released in a bowel movement from an infected human or animal. Crypto may be found in water sources, such as private wells that have been contaminated with feces from infected humans or animals. Water can be contaminated through sewage overflows, sewage systems that are not working properly, polluted stormwater runoff, and agricultural runoff. Wells may be more vulnerable to such contamination after flooding, particularly if the wells are shallow, have been dug or bored, or have been submerged by floodwater for long periods of time.

How Can I Find Out Whether There Is Cryptosporidium *in My Drinking Water?*

If you suspect a problem and your drinking water comes from a private well, you may contact your state certification officer for a list of laboratories in your area that will perform tests on drinking water for a fee.

How Do I Remove Crypto from My Drinking Water?

To kill or inactivate Crypto, bring your water to a rolling boil for 1 minute (at elevations above 6,500 feet, boil for 3 minutes). Water should then be allowed to cool; stored in a clean, sanitized container with a tight cover; and refrigerated.

An alternative to boiling water is using a point-of-use filter. Not all home water filters remove Crypto. Filters that are designed to remove Crypto should have one of the following labels:

- Reverse osmosis

- Absolute pore size of 1 micron or smaller

161

- Tested and certified to the National Science Foundation (NSF)/ American National Standards Institute (ANSI) Standard 53 or 58 for cyst removal

- Tested and certified to NSF/ANSI Standard 53 for cyst reduction

You may also disinfect your well. However, it is important to note that Crypto is extremely tolerant of chlorination, making chlorination an ineffective intervention. Alternative disinfection processes to consider include systems that utilize ultraviolet (UV) light or ozone. Contact your local health department for recommended procedures. Remember to have your well water tested regularly, at least once a year, after disinfection to make sure the problem does not recur.

Chapter 12

Tick-Borne Diseases

Chapter Contents

Section 12.1

Common Tick-Borne Diseases

This section contains text excerpted from the following
sources: Text in this section begins with excerpts from "Tick-Borne
Diseases," Centers for Disease Control and Prevention (CDC),
September 22, 2011. Reviewed May 2019; Text under the heading
"Tick-Borne Diseases of the United States" is excerpted from
"Tickborne Diseases of the United States," Centers for Disease
Control and Prevention (CDC), January 10, 2019.

Tick-borne pathogens can be passed to humans through the bite of
infected ticks. Ticks can be infected with bacteria, viruses, or parasites.
Some of the most common tick-borne diseases in the United States
include Lyme disease, babesiosis, ehrlichiosis, Rocky Mountain spotted
fever, anaplasmosis, Southern tick-associated rash illness (STARI),
tick-borne relapsing fever, and tularemia. Other tick-borne diseases in
the United States include Colorado tick fever, Powassan encephalitis,
and Q fever. Lyme disease is the most commonly reported tick-borne
disease in the United States. In 2010, more than 22,500 confirmed and
7,500 probable cases of Lyme disease were reported to the Centers for
Disease Control and Prevention (CDC).

Outdoor workers are at risk of exposure to tick-borne diseases if
they work at sites with ticks. Worksites with woods, bushes, high
grass, or leaf litter are likely to have more ticks. Outdoor workers in
most regions of the United States should be extra careful to protect
themselves in the spring, summer, and fall when ticks are most
active. Ticks may be active all year in some regions with warmer
weather.

Tick-Borne Diseases of the United States

In the United States, some ticks carry pathogens that can cause
human disease, including:

- **Anaplasmosis** is transmitted to humans by tick bites primarily
  from the blacklegged tick (Ixodes scapularis) in the northeastern
  and upper midwestern United States and from the western
  blacklegged tick (Ixodes pacificus) along the Pacific coast.

- **Babesiosis** is caused by microscopic parasites that infect red
  blood cells. Most human cases of babesiosis in the United States
  are caused by *Babesia microti*. *Babesia microti* is transmitted by

the blacklegged tick and is found primarily in the northeast and upper Midwest.

- *Borrelia mayonii* infection has recently been described as a cause of illness in the upper midwestern United States. It has been found in blacklegged ticks in Minnesota and Wisconsin. *Borrelia mayonii* is a new species and is the only species besides *B. burgdorferi* known to cause Lyme disease in North America.

- *Borrelia miyamotoi* infection has recently been described as a cause of illness in the United States. It is transmitted by the blacklegged tick and has a range similar to that of Lyme disease.

- **Bourbon virus** infection has been identified in a limited number of patients in the Midwest and southern United States. At this time, it is unknown if the virus might be found in other areas of the United States.

- **Colorado tick fever** is caused by a virus transmitted by the Rocky Mountain wood tick (*Dermacentor andersoni*). It occurs in the Rocky Mountain states at elevations of 4,000 to 10,500 feet.

- **Ehrlichiosis** is transmitted to humans by the lone star tick (Amblyomma americanum), found primarily in the south-central and eastern United States.

- **Heartland virus** cases have been identified in the Midwestern and southern United States. Studies suggest that lone star ticks can transmit the virus. It is unknown if the virus may be found in other areas of the United States.

- **Lyme disease** is transmitted by the blacklegged tick in the northeastern and upper midwestern United States and by the western blacklegged tick (*Ixodes pacificus*) along the Pacific coast.

- **Powassan disease** is transmitted by the blacklegged tick and the groundhog tick (*Ixodes cookei*). Cases have been reported primarily from northeastern states and the Great Lakes region.

- **Rickettsia parkeri rickettsiosis** is transmitted to humans by the Gulf Coast tick (*Amblyomma maculatum*).

- **Rocky Mountain spotted fever (RMSF)** is transmitted by the American dog tick (*Dermacentor variabilis*), Rocky Mountain wood tick, and the brown dog tick (*Rhipicephalus sanguineus*) in the United States. The brown dog tick and other tick species are associated with RMSF in Central and South America.

- **Southern tick-associated rash illness (STARI)** is transmitted via bites from the lone star tick and found in the eastern and southeastern United States.

- **Tick-borne relapsing fever (TBRF)** is transmitted to humans through the bite of infected soft ticks. TBRF has been reported in 15 states: Arizona, California, Colorado, Idaho, Kansas, Montana, Nevada, New Mexico, Ohio, Oklahoma, Oregon, Texas, Utah, Washington, and Wyoming and is associated with sleeping in rustic cabins and vacation homes.

- **Tularemia** is transmitted to humans by the dog tick, the wood tick (Dermacentor andersoni), and the lone star tick. Tularemia occurs throughout the United States.

- **364D rickettsiosis** (Rickettsia phillipi, proposed) is transmitted to humans by the Pacific Coast tick. This is a new disease that has been found in California.

Section 12.2

Lyme Disease

This section includes text excerpted from "Lyme Disease," Centers for Disease Control and Prevention (CDC), December 21, 2018.

What Is Lyme Disease?

Lyme disease is caused by the bacterium *Borrelia burgdorferi* and is transmitted to humans through the bite of infected blacklegged ticks. Typical symptoms include fever, headache, fatigue, and a characteristic skin rash called "erythema migrans." If left untreated, the infection can spread to joints, the heart, and the nervous system. Lyme disease is diagnosed based on symptoms, physical findings (e.g., rash), and the possibility of exposure to infected ticks. Laboratory testing is helpful if used correctly and performed with validated methods. Most cases of Lyme disease can be treated successfully with a few weeks of antibiotics. Steps to prevent Lyme disease include using insect repellent, removing ticks promptly, applying pesticides, and reducing tick habitat. The ticks that transmit Lyme disease can occasionally transmit other tick-borne diseases as well.

Signs and Symptoms of Untreated Lyme Disease

Untreated Lyme disease can produce a wide range of symptoms, depending on the stage of infection. These include fever, rash, facial paralysis, and arthritis. Seek medical attention if you observe any of these symptoms and have had a tick bite, live in an area known for Lyme disease, or have recently traveled to an area where Lyme disease occurs.

Early Signs and Symptoms (3 to 30 Days after Tick Bite)

- Fever, chills, headache, fatigue, muscle and joint aches, and swollen lymph nodes
- Erythema migrans (EM) rash:
  - Occurs in approximately 70 to 80 percent of infected persons
  - Begins at the site of a tick bite after a delay of 3 to 30 days (average is about 7 days)
  - Expands gradually over a period of days, reaching up to 12 inches or more (30 cm) across
  - May feel warm to the touch but is rarely itchy or painful
  - Sometimes clears as it enlarges, resulting in a target or "bullseye" appearance
  - May appear on any area of the body

Later Signs and Symptoms (Days to Months after Tick Bite)

- Severe headaches and neck stiffness
- Additional EM rashes on other areas of the body
- Arthritis with severe joint pain and swelling, particularly of the knees and other large joints

- Facial palsy (loss of muscle tone or droop on one or both sides of the face)

- Intermittent pain in tendons, muscles, joints, and bones

- Heart palpitations or an irregular heartbeat (Lyme carditis)

- Episodes of dizziness or shortness of breath

- Inflammation of the brain and spinal cord

- Nerve pain

- Shooting pains, numbness, or tingling in the hands or feet

- Problems with short-term memory

Diagnosis and Testing

Lyme disease is diagnosed based on:

- Signs and symptoms

- A history of possible exposure to infected blacklegged ticks

Laboratory blood tests are helpful if used correctly and performed with validated methods. Laboratory tests are not recommended for patients who do not have symptoms typical of Lyme disease. Just as it is important to correctly diagnose Lyme disease when a patient has it, it is important to avoid misdiagnosis and treatment of Lyme disease when the true cause of the illness is something else.

Tick Removal and Testing
Removing a Tick

If you find a tick attached to your skin, there is no need to panic—the key is to remove the tick as soon as possible. There are several tick-removal devices on the market, but a plain set of fine-tipped tweezers work very well.

How to Remove a Tick

- Use fine-tipped tweezers to grasp the tick as close to the skin's surface as possible.

- Pull upward with steady, even pressure. Do not twist or jerk the tick; this can cause the mouth parts to break off and remain in the skin. If this happens, remove the mouth parts with tweezers.

If you are unable to remove the mouth easily with clean tweezers, leave it alone and let the skin heal.

- After removing the tick, thoroughly clean the bite area and your hands with rubbing alcohol or soap and water.

- Never crush a tick with your fingers. Dispose of a live tick by putting it in alcohol, placing it in a sealed bag/container, wrapping it tightly in tape, or flushing it down the toilet.

Testing of Ticks

People who have removed a tick sometimes wonder if they should have it tested for evidence of infection. Although some commercial groups offer testing, in general this is not recommended because:

- Laboratories that conduct tick testing are not required to meet the high standards of quality control used by clinical diagnostic laboratories. Results of tick testing should not be used for treatment decisions.

- Positive results showing that the tick contains a disease-causing organism do not necessarily mean that you have been infected.

- Negative results can lead to false assurance. You may have been unknowingly bitten by a different tick that was infected.

- If you have been infected, you will probably develop symptoms before results of the tick test are available. If you do become ill, you should not wait for tick testing results before beginning appropriate treatment.

However, you may want to learn to identify various ticks. Different ticks live in different parts of the country and transmit different diseases.

Preventing Tick Bites

Reducing exposure to ticks is the best defense against Lyme disease, Rocky Mountain spotted fever, and other tick-borne infections. You and your family can take several steps to prevent and control Lyme disease:

Preventing Tick Bites on People

Tick exposure can occur year round, but ticks are most active during warmer months (April to September).

Before You Go Outdoors

- **Know where to expect ticks.** Ticks live in grassy, brushy, or wooded areas, or even on animals. Spending time outside walking your dog, camping, gardening, or hunting could bring you in close contact with ticks. Many people get ticks in their yard or neighborhood.

- **Treat clothing and gear with products containing 0.5 percent permethrin.** Permethrin can be used to treat boots, clothing, and camping gear that remain protective through several washings. Alternatively, you can buy permethrin-treated clothing and gear.

- **Use U.S. Environmental Protection Agency (EPA)-** registered insect repellents containing DEET, picaridin, IR3535, oil of lemon eucalyptus (OLE), para-menthane-diol (PMD), or 2-undecanone. The EPA's helpful online search tool can help you find the product that best suits your needs. Always follow product instructions.

  - Do not use insect repellent on babies younger than two months of age.

  - Do not use products containing OLE or PMD on children under three years of age.

- Avoid contact with ticks.

  - Avoid wooded and bushy areas with high grass and leaf litter.

  - Walk in the center of trails.

After You Come Indoors

Check your clothing for ticks. Ticks may be carried into the house on clothing. Any ticks that are found should be removed. Tumble dry clothes in a dryer on high heat for 10 minutes to kill ticks on dry clothing after you come indoors. If the clothes are damp, additional time may be needed. If the clothes require washing first, hot water is recommended. Cold and medium temperature water will not kill ticks.

Examine gear and pets. Ticks can ride into the home on clothing and pets, then attach to a person later, so carefully examine pets, coats, and daypacks.

Shower soon after being outdoors. Showering within two hours of coming indoors has been shown to reduce your risk of getting Lyme disease and may be effective in reducing the risk of other tick-borne diseases. Showering may help wash off unattached ticks, and it is a good opportunity to do a tick check.

Check your body for ticks after being outdoors. Conduct a full-body check upon returning from potentially tick-infested areas, including your own backyard. Use a handheld or full-length mirror to view all parts of your body. Check these parts of your body and your child's body for ticks:

- Under the arms

- In and around the ears

- Inside the belly button

- Back of the knees

- In and around the hair

- Between the legs

- Around the waist

Transmission

The Lyme disease bacterium *Borrelia burgdorferi* is spread through the bite of infected ticks. The blacklegged tick, or deer tick (Ixodes scapularis), spreads the disease in the northeastern, mid-Atlantic, and north-central United States. The western blacklegged tick (Ixodes pacificus) spreads the disease on the Pacific Coast.

Ticks can attach to any part of the human body but are often found in hard-to-see areas such as the groin, armpits, and scalp. In most cases, the tick must be attached for 36 to 48 hours or more before the Lyme disease bacterium can be transmitted.

Most humans are infected through the bites of immature ticks called "nymphs." Nymphs are tiny (less than 2 mm) and difficult to see; they feed during the spring and summer months. Adult ticks can also transmit Lyme disease bacteria, but they are much larger and are more likely to be discovered and removed before they have had time to transmit the bacteria. Adult Ixodes ticks are most active during the cooler months of the year.

Treatment

People treated with appropriate antibiotics in the early stages of Lyme disease usually recover rapidly and completely. Antibiotics commonly used for oral treatment include doxycycline, amoxicillin, or cefuroxime axetil. People with certain neurological or cardiac forms of illness may require intravenous treatment with antibiotics such as ceftriaxone or penicillin.

Treatment regimens listed in the following table are for localized (early) Lyme disease.

Table 12.1. Treatment Regimens for Lyme Disease*

Age Category	Drug	Dosage	Maximum	Duration, Days
Adults	Doxycycline	100 mg, twice per day orally	N/A	10–21*
	Cefuroxime axetil	500 mg, twice per day orally	N/A	14–21
	Amoxicillin	500 mg, three times per day orally	N/A	14–21
Children	Amoxicillin	50 mg/kg per day orally, divided into 3 doses	500 mg per dose	14–21
	Doxycycline	4 mg/kg per day orally, divided into 2 doses	100 mg per dose	10–21*
	Cefuroxime axetil	30 mg/kg per day orally, divided into 2 doses	500 mg per dose	14–21

* Recent publications suggest the efficacy of shorter courses of treatment for early Lyme disease.

Post-Treatment Lyme Disease Syndrome

Lyme disease is an infection caused by the bacterium *Borrelia burgdorferi*. In the majority of cases, it is successfully treated with oral antibiotics. Physicians sometimes describe patients who have nonspecific symptoms (such as fatigue, pain, and joint and muscle aches) after the treatment of Lyme disease as having post-treatment Lyme disease syndrome (PTLDS) or post-Lyme disease syndrome (PLDS).

Data and Surveillance

Possible cases of Lyme disease are reported to state and local health departments by healthcare providers and laboratories. State health departments classify cases according to standard criteria outlined in the Lyme disease case definition and report confirmed and probable cases to the Centers for Disease Control and Prevention (CDC). The extent of case investigations varies by state. Investigations are often dependent on available resources and staff time. Some states describe their surveillance methods in detail on their health-department website.

Each year, approximately 30,000 cases of Lyme disease are reported to the CDC by state health departments and the District of Columbia. However, this number does not reflect every case of Lyme disease that is diagnosed in the United States every year. Standard national surveillance is only one way that public-health officials can track where the disease is occurring and with what frequency. Estimates using other methods suggest that approximately 300,000 people may get Lyme disease each year in the United States.

Chapter 13

Prion Diseases

Chapter Contents

Section 13.1

Bovine Spongiform Encephalopathy

This section includes text excerpted from "Bovine Spongiform Encephalopathy (BSE), or Mad Cow Disease," Centers for Disease Control and Prevention (CDC), October 9, 2018.

Bovine spongiform encephalopathy (BSE) is a progressive neurological disorder of cattle that results from infection by an unusual transmissible agent called a "prion." The nature of the transmissible agent is not well understood. Currently, the most accepted theory is that the agent is a modified form of a normal protein known as "prion protein." For reasons that are not yet understood, the normal prion protein changes into a pathogenic (harmful) form that then damages the central nervous system of cattle.

Research indicates that the first probable infections of BSE in cows occurred during the 1970s, with two cases of BSE being identified in 1986. BSE possibly originated as a result of feeding cattle meat-and-bone meal that contained BSE-infected products from a spontaneously occurring case of BSE or scrapie-infected sheep products. Scrapie is a prion disease of sheep. There is strong evidence and general agreement that the outbreak was then amplified and spread throughout the United Kingdom cattle industry by feeding rendered, prion-infected, bovine meat-and-bone meal to young calves.

The BSE epizootic in the United Kingdom peaked in January 1993 at almost 1,000 new cases per week. Since then, the annual numbers of BSE cases in the United Kingdom have dropped sharply.

- 2 cases in 2015

- 11 cases in 2010

- 225 cases in 2005

- 1,443 cases in 2000

- 14,562 cases in 1995

Cumulatively, through the end of 2015, more than 184,500 cases of BSE had been confirmed in the United Kingdom alone in more than 35,000 herds. Regularly updated numbers of reported BSE cases, by country, are available on the website of the Office International des Epizooties.

Strong epidemiologic and laboratory evidence exists for a causal association between a new human prion disease called "variant

Creutzfeldt-Jakob disease" (vCJD) that was first reported from the United Kingdom in 1996 and the BSE outbreak in cattle. The interval between the most likely period for the initial extended exposure of the population to potentially BSE-contaminated food (1984–1986) and the onset of initial variant CJD cases (1994–1996) is consistent with known incubation periods for the human forms of prion disease.

Prevalence

Based on World Organization of Animal Health (OIE) standards for BSE surveillance, the reported national prevalence rates of BSE in North American cattle, particularly in animals born in the United States, is very low, and therefore, difficult to measure accurately. In September 2007, the United States Department of Agriculture (USDA) published updated results of the two statistical models used by Harvard University investigators to estimate the prevalence of BSE in Canada. The results incorporated the 11 Canadian-born animals with BSE that had been reported at that time. A key advantage of these models is that they provide statistical confidence limits that measure some of the uncertainty associated with expected estimates.

The model for evaluating national surveillance programs for BSE is most comparable to the observed surveillance data. This model estimated that the true prevalence of BSE in Canada is 90 percent likely to be between 18-fold and 48-fold higher than the previously published best estimate of the prevalence of BSE in the United States (3 to 8 cases per million in Canada compared to a best estimate of 0.167 cases per million in the United States).

The previously published best estimate of Canada's BSE prevalence in 2006 using the BSurveE model was 23-fold higher than that of the United States and is the estimate of the BSE prevalence in Canada that continues to be used in the Harvard Risk Assessments' "worst-case" analyses when evaluating the risk of imported Canadian cattle causing BSE to spread among U.S. animals.

Bovine Spongiform Encephalopathy in North America

Through August 2018, BSE surveillance has identified 26 cases of BSE in North America: 6 BSE cases in the United States and 20 in Canada. Of the 6 cases identified in the United States, one was born in Canada; of the 20 cases identified in Canada, one was imported from the United Kingdom.

Strong evidence indicates that classic BSE has been transmitted to people primarily in the United Kingdom, causing a variant form of Creutzfeldt-Jakob disease. In the United Kingdom, where over 1 million cattle may have been infected with classic BSE, a substantial species barrier appears to protect people from widespread illness. Since vCJD was first reported in 1996, a total of only 231 patients with this disease, including 3 secondary, blood transfusion-related cases, have been reported worldwide. The risk to human health from BSE in the United States is extremely low.

Control Measures

Public health-control measures, such as surveillance, culling sick animals, or banning specified risk materials, have been instituted in many countries, particularly in those with indigenous cases of confirmed BSE, in order to prevent potentially BSE-infected tissues from entering the human food supply.

The most stringent control measures include a United Kingdom program that excludes all animals more than 30 months of age from human food and animal feed supplies. The program appears to be highly effective.

In June 2000, the European Union (EU) Commission on Food Safety and Animal Welfare strengthened the EU's BSE control measures by requiring all member states to remove specified risk materials from animal feed and human food chains as of October 1, 2000; such bans had already been instituted in most member states. Other control measures include banning the use of mechanically recovered meat from the vertebral column of cattle, sheep, and goats for human food and BSE testing of all cattle more than 30 months of age destined for human consumption.

Section 13.2

Chronic Wasting Disease

This section includes text excerpted from "Chronic
Wasting Disease (CWD)," Centers for Disease Control and
Prevention (CDC), February 25, 2019.

Chronic wasting disease (CWD) is a prion disease that affects deer,
elk, reindeer, sika deer, and moose. It has been found in some areas
of North America, including Canada and the United States, and in
Norway and South Korea. It may take over a year before an infected
animal develops symptoms, which can include drastic weight loss
(wasting), stumbling, listlessness, and other neurologic symptoms.
CWD can affect animals of all ages and some infected animals may
die without ever developing the disease. CWD is fatal to animals and
there are no treatments or vaccines.

To date, there have been no reported cases of CWD infection in people. However, some animal studies suggest CWD poses a risk to certain
types of nonhuman primates, such as monkeys, that eat meat from
CWD-infected animals or come in contact with brain or body fluids
from infected deer or elk. These studies raise concerns that there may
also be a risk to people. Since 1997, the World Health Organization
(WHO) has recommended that it is important to keep the agents of all
known prion diseases from entering the human food chain.

Occurrence

As of March 6, 2019, CWD in free-ranging deer, elk, and/or moose
has been reported in at least 24 states in the continental United
States, as well as two provinces in Canada. In addition, CWD has
been reported in reindeer and moose in Norway and Finland, and a
small number of imported cases have been reported in South Korea.
The disease has also been found in farmed deer and elk.

CWD was first identified in captive deer in a Colorado research
facility in the late 1960s, and in wild deer in 1981. By the 1990s, it
had been reported in surrounding areas in northern Colorado and
southern Wyoming. Since 2000, the area known to be affected by CWD
in free-ranging animals has increased to at least 24 states, including
states in the Midwest, Southwest, and limited areas on the East Coast.
It is possible that CWD may also occur in other states without strong
animal surveillance systems, but that cases haven't been detected yet.

Once CWD is established in an area, the risk can remain for a long time in the environment. The affected areas are likely to continue to expand.

Nationwide, the overall occurrence of CWD in free-ranging deer and elk is relatively low. However, in several locations where the disease is established, infection rates may exceed 10 percent (1 in 10), and localized infection rates of more than 25 percent (1 in 4) have been reported. The infection rates among some captive deer can be much higher, with a rate of 79 percent (nearly 4 in 5) reported from at least one captive herd.

Transmission

Scientists believe CWD proteins (prions) likely spread between animals through body fluids like feces, saliva, blood, or urine, either through direct contact or indirectly through environmental contamination of soil, food or water. Once introduced into an area or farm, the CWD protein is contagious within deer and elk populations and can spread quickly. Experts believe CWD prions can remain in the environment for a long time, so other animals can contract CWD from the environment even after an infected deer or elk has died.

The CWD prion has been shown to experimentally infect squirrel monkeys, and also laboratory mice that carry some human genes. An additional study begun in 2009 by Canadian and German scientists, which has not yet been published in the scientific literature, is evaluating whether CWD can be transmitted to macaques—a type of monkey that is genetically closer to people than any other animal that has been infected with CWD previously. On July 10, 2017, the scientists presented a summary of the study's progress, in which they showed that CWD was transmitted to monkeys that were fed infected meat (muscle tissue) or brain tissue from CWD-infected deer and elk. Some of the meat came from asymptomatic deer that had CWD (i.e., deer that appeared healthy and had not begun to show signs of the illness yet). Meat from these asymptomatic deer was also able to infect the monkeys with CWD. CWD was also able to spread to macaques that had the infectious material placed directly into their brains.

This study showed different results than a previous study published in the Journal of Virology in 2018, which had not shown successful transmission of CWD to macaques. The reasons for the different experimental results are unknown. To date, there is no strong evidence for the occurrence of CWD in people, and it is not known if people can get infected with CWD prions. Nevertheless, these experimental studies raise the concern that CWD may pose a risk to people and suggest that it is important to prevent human exposures to CWD.

Additional studies are underway to identify if any prion diseases could be occurring at a higher rate in people who are at increased risk for contact with potentially CWD-infected deer or elk meat. Because of the long time it takes before any symptoms of disease appear, scientists expect the study to take many years before they will determine what the risk, if any, of CWD is to people.

Prevention

If CWD could spread to people, it would most likely be through eating infected deer and elk. In a 2006–2007 CDC survey of U.S. residents, nearly 20 percent of those surveyed said they had hunted deer or elk and more than two-thirds said they had eaten venison or elk meat. However, to date, there is no strong evidence for the occurrence of CWD in people, and it is not known if people can get infected with CWD prions.

Hunters must consider many factors when determining whether to eat meat from deer and elk harvested from areas with CWD, including the level of risk they are willing to accept. Hunters harvesting wild deer and elk from areas with reported CWD should check state wildlife and public-health guidance to see whether testing of animals is recommended or required in a given state or region. In areas where CWD is known to be present, the CDC recommends that hunters strongly consider having those animals tested before eating the meat.

Tests for CWD are monitoring tools that some state wildlife officials use to look at the rates of CWD in certain animal populations. Testing may not be available in every state, and states may use these tests in different ways. A negative test result does not guarantee that an individual animal is not infected with CWD, but it does make it considerably less likely and may reduce your risk of exposure to CWD.

To be as safe as possible and decrease their potential risk of exposure to CWD, hunters should take the following steps when hunting in areas with CWD:

- Do not shoot, handle, or eat meat from deer and elk that look sick, are acting strangely, or are found dead (roadkill).

- When field dressing a deer:

  - Wear latex or rubber gloves when dressing the animal or handling the meat.

- Minimize how much you handle the organs of the animal, particularly the brain or spinal cord tissues.

- Do not use household knives or other kitchen utensils for field dressing.

- Check state wildlife and public-health guidance to see whether testing of animals is recommended or required. Recommendations vary by state, but information about testing is available from many state wildlife agencies.

- Strongly consider having the deer or elk tested for CWD before you eat the meat.

- If you have your deer or elk commercially processed, consider asking that your animal be processed individually to avoid mixing meat from multiple animals.

- If your animal tests positive for CWD, do not eat meat from that animal.

The U.S. Department of Agriculture's Animal and Plant Health Inspection Service regulates commercially farmed deer and elk. The agency operates a national CWD herd certification program. As part of the voluntary program, states and individual herd owners agree to meet requirements meant to decrease the risk of CWD in their herds. Privately owned herds that do not participate in the herd certification program may be at increased risk for CWD.

Section 13.3

Creutzfeldt-Jakob Disease

This section includes text excerpted from "Creutzfeldt-Jakob Disease, Classic (CJD)," Centers for Disease Control and Prevention (CDC), October 9, 2018.

Classic Creutzfeldt-Jakob disease (CJD) is a human prion disease. It is a neurodegenerative disorder with characteristic clinical and diagnostic features. This disease is rapidly progressive and always fatal. Infection with this disease leads to death usually within one year of onset of illness.

Creutzfeldt-Jakob disease is a rapidly progressive, invariably fatal neurodegenerative disorder believed to be caused by an abnormal isoform of a cellular glycoprotein known as the "prion protein." CJD occurs worldwide and the estimated annual incidence in many countries, including the United States, has been reported to be about one case per million.

The vast majority of CJD patients die within one year of illness onset. CJD is classified as a transmissible spongiform encephalopathy (TSE) along with other prion diseases that occur in humans and animals. In about 85 percent of patients, CJD occurs as a sporadic disease with no recognizable pattern of transmission. A smaller proportion of patients (5 to 15%) develop CJD because of inherited mutations of the prion protein gene. These inherited forms include Gerstmann-Straussler-Scheinker syndrome and fatal familial insomnia.

Physicians suspect a diagnosis of CJD on the basis of the typical signs and symptoms and progression of the disease. In most CJD patients, the presence of 14-3-3 protein in the cerebrospinal fluid and/or a typical electroencephalogram (EEG) pattern, both of which are believed to be diagnostic for CJD, have been reported. However, a confirmatory diagnosis of CJD requires neuropathologic and/or immuno-diagnostic testing of brain tissue obtained either at biopsy or autopsy.

Diagnostic Criteria
1. Sporadic Creutzfeldt-Jakob Disease
Definite

Diagnosed by standard neuropathological techniques; and/or immunocytochemically; and/or Western blot- confirmed protease-resistant PrP; and/or presence of scrapie-associated fibrils.

Probable

Neuropsychiatric disorder plus positive RT-QuIC in cerebrospinal fluid (CSF) or other tissues

OR

Rapidly progressive dementia; and at least two out of the following four clinical features:

1. Myoclonus

2. Visual or cerebellar signs

3. Pyramidal/extrapyramidal signs

4. Akinetic mutism

AND a positive result on at least one of the following laboratory tests:

- A typical EEG (periodic sharp wave complexes) during an illness of any duration

- A positive 14-3-3 CSF assay in patients with a disease duration of less than two years

- High signal in caudate/putamen on magnetic resonance imaging (MRI) brain scan or at least two cortical regions (temporal, parietal, occipital) either on diffusion-weighted imaging (DWI) or fluid-attenuated inversion recovery (FLAIR)

AND without routine investigations indicating an alternative diagnosis.

Possible

Progressive dementia; and at least two out of the following four clinical features:

1. Myoclonus

2. Visual or cerebellar signs

3. Pyramidal/extrapyramidal signs

4. Akinetic mutism

AND the absence of a positive result for any of the four tests above that would classify a case as "probable"
AND duration of illness less than two years
AND without routine investigations indicating an alternative diagnosis.

2. Iatrogenic Creutzfeldt-Jakob Disease

Progressive cerebellar syndrome in a recipient of human cadaveric-derived pituitary hormone; or sporadic CJD with a recognized exposure risk, e.g., antecedent neurosurgery with dura mater implantation.

3. Familial Creutzfeldt-Jakob Disease

Definite or probable CJD plus definite or probable CJD in a first-degree relative; and/or neuropsychiatric disorder plus disease-specific PrP gene mutation.

Infection Control
Iatrogenic Transmission of Creutzfeldt-Jakob Disease

Iatrogenic transmission of the CJD agent has been reported in over 250 patients worldwide. These cases have been linked to the use of contaminated human growth hormone, dura mater and corneal grafts, or neurosurgical equipment. Of the six cases linked to the use of contaminated equipment, four were associated with neurosurgical instruments, and two with stereotactic EEG depth electrodes.

All of these equipment-related cases occurred before the routine implementation of sterilization procedures currently used in healthcare facilities. No such cases have been reported since 1976, and no iatrogenic CJD cases associated with exposure to the CJD agent from surfaces such as floors, walls, or countertops have been identified.

Reprocessing Surgical Instruments Used on Suspected or Confirmed Creutzfeldt-Jakob Disease Patients

Inactivation studies have not rigorously evaluated the effectiveness of actual cleaning and reprocessing methods used in healthcare facilities. Recommendations to reprocess instruments potentially contaminated with the CJD agent are primarily derived from in vitro inactivation studies that used either brain tissues or tissue homogenates, both of which pose enormous challenges to any sterilization process.

The World Health Organization (WHO) has developed CJD infection control guidelines that can be a valuable guide to infection-control personnel and other healthcare workers involved in the care of CJD patients. Destruction of heat-resistant surgical instruments that come in contact with high infectivity tissues, albeit the safest and most unambiguous method as described in the WHO guidelines, may not be practical or cost effective.

One of the three most stringent chemical and autoclave sterilization methods outlined in Annex III of the WHO guidelines should be used to reprocess heat-resistant instruments that come in contact with high infectivity tissues (brain, spinal cord, and eyes) and low infectivity tissues (cerebrospinal fluid, kidneys, liver, lungs, lymph nodes, spleen, olfactory epithelium, and placenta) of patients with suspected or confirmed CJD. High and low infectivity tissues were defined on the basis of available experimental data of the WHO guidelines. The stringent sterilization methods described below should be used to reprocess medical instruments that come in contact with high infectivity tissues of persons known to be blood relatives of patients with inheritable forms of TSEs. In addition, instruments should be kept moist and not allowed to air dry throughout the surgical procedure by immersing them in water or disinfectant solution.

Chemical and Autoclave Sterilization Methods Outlined in Annex III of the World Health Organization Infection Control Guidelines for Transmissible Spongiform Encephalopathies

The three most stringent sterilization methods for heat-resistant instruments described in Annex III of the WHO guidelines are listed below; the methods are listed in order of more to less severe treatments. Sodium hypochlorite may be corrosive to some instruments, such as gold-plated instruments. Before instruments are immersed in sodium hypochlorite, the instrument manufacturer should be consulted about the instrument's tolerance of exposure to sodium hypochlorite. Instruments should be decontaminated by a combination of the chemical and recommended autoclaving methods before subjecting them to cleaning in a washer cycle and routine sterilization.

1. Immerse in a pan containing 1N sodium hydroxide (NaOH) and heat in a gravity displacement autoclave at 121°C for 30 min; clean; rinse in water; and subject to routine sterilization. [CDC NOTE: The pan containing sodium hydroxide should be covered, and care should be taken to avoid sodium hydroxide spills in the autoclave. To avoid autoclave exposure to gaseous sodium hydroxide condensing on the lid of the container, the use of containers with a rim and lid designed for condensation to collect and drip back into the pan is recommended. Persons who use this procedure should be cautious in handling hot sodium hydroxide solution (postautoclave) and in avoiding potential exposure to gaseous sodium hydroxide, exercise caution during all sterilization steps, and allow the autoclave, instruments, and solutions to cool down before removal. An experiment conducted by the U.S. Food and Drug Administration (FDA) investigators

indicated that the use of appropriate containment pans and lids prevents escape of sodium hydroxide vapors that may cause damage to the autoclave (Brown and Merritt. Am J Infect Control 2003;31:257–260).]

2. Immerse in 1N NaOH or sodium hypochlorite (20,000 ppm available chlorine) for 1 hour; transfer instruments to water; heat in a gravity displacement autoclave at 121°C for 1 hour; clean; and subject to routine sterilization.

3. Immerse in 1N NaOH or sodium hypochlorite (20,000 ppm available chlorine) for 1 hour; remove and rinse in water, and then transfer to open pan and heat in a gravity displacement (121°C) or porous load (134°C) autoclave for 1 hour; clean; and subject to routine sterilization. [CDC NOTE: Sodium hypochlorite may be corrosive to some instruments.]

FDA investigators evaluated the effects to surgical instruments of the steps involved in the sterilization protocols listed above; some of the protocols they assessed subjected the instruments to harsher conditions than those prescribed above. Their findings indicate that much of the damage from autoclaving in sodium hydroxide was cosmetic and would not affect the performance or cleaning of the instruments. Soaking in sodium hydroxide had the least damaging effect on instruments, but immersion in sodium hypochlorite bleach caused severe damage to some instruments. The article summarizing the findings of this experiment by Brown et al. of the FDA was published in the Journal of Biomedical Materials Research (electronic version published October 2004).

Reprocessing Instruments Used in Patients with No Clear Diagnosis of Creutzfeldt-Jakob Disease at the Time of Their Neurosurgical Procedure

In some patients undergoing neurosurgery, a CJD diagnosis that is not suspected before the procedure may be confirmed after the neurosurgery. For this group of patients, in whom the clinical diagnosis leading to the neurosurgical procedure remains unclear, the instruments should be reprocessed in the same manner as that for instruments used in procedures involving suspected or confirmed CJD patients. Unless a clear nonCJD diagnosis is established, these patients should be considered as potentially suspected CJD patients for all other infection control requirements.

Decontaminating Heat-Sensitive Instruments or Materials That Come in Contact with Suspected or Confirmed Creutzfeldt-Jakob Disease Patients

All disposable instruments, materials, and wastes that come in contact with high infectivity tissues (brain, spinal cord, and eyes) and low infectivity tissues (cerebrospinal fluid, kidneys, liver, lungs, lymph nodes, spleen, and placenta) of suspected or confirmed TSE patients should be disposed of by incineration. Surfaces and heat-sensitive reusable instruments that come in contact with high infectivity and low infectivity tissues should be decontaminated by flooding with or soaking in 2N NaOH or undiluted sodium hypochlorite for one hour and rinsed with water.

Precautions for Embalming the Bodies of Patients with Suspected or Confirmed Creutzfeldt-Jakob Disease

An autopsied or traumatized body of a suspected or confirmed CJD patient can be embalmed, using the precautions outlined in the WHO CJD infection control guidelines. CJD patients who have not been autopsied or whose bodies have not been traumatized can be embalmed using standard Precautions. Family members of CJD patients should be advised to avoid superficial contact (such as touching or kissing the patient's face) with the body of a CJD patient who has been autopsied. However, if the patient has not been autopsied, such contact need not be discouraged.

Occurrence and Transmission

Classic CJD has been recognized since the early 1920s. The most common form of classic CJD is believed to occur sporadically, caused by the spontaneous transformation of normal prion proteins into abnormal prions. This sporadic disease occurs worldwide, including the United States, at a rate of roughly 1 to 1.5 cases per 1 million per year, although rates of up to two cases per million are not unusual. The risk of CJD increases with age; the 1979–2017 average annual rate in the United States was 3.5 cases per million in persons over 50 years of age.

Whereas the majority of cases of CJD (about 85%) occur as sporadic disease, a smaller proportion of patients (5 to 15%) develop CJD because of inherited mutations of the prion protein gene. These inherited forms include Gerstmann-Straussler-Scheinker syndrome and fatal familial insomnia.

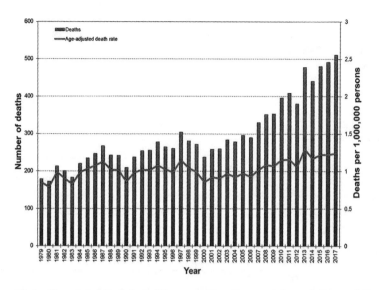

Figure 13.1. *Creutzfeldt-Jakob Disease Deaths and Age-Adjusted Death Rate, United States, 1979–2017**

* Deaths obtained from the multiple cause-of-death data for 1979–1998 are based on ICD-9 codes, and those beginning in 1999 are based on ICD-10 codes with available computerized literal death certificate data. Death information was also obtained from other surveillance mechanisms; data include familial prion diseases. Rates are adjusted to the U.S. standard 2000 projected population.

Table 13.1. Creutzfeldt-Jakob Disease Deaths and Age-Adjusted Death Rate, United States, 1979–2017*

Year	Deaths (Approximate)	Age-Adjusted Death Rate
1979	179	0.85
1980	172	0.787
1981	214	0.988
1982	201	0.901
1983	183	0.825
1984	221	0.985
1985	235	1.033
1986	247	1.073
1987	268	1.129
1988	243	1.02
1989	242	1.011
1990	210	0.859

Table 13.1. Continued

Year	Deaths (Approximate)	Age-Adjusted Death Rate
1991	238	0.982
1992	255	1.018
1993	256	1.012
1994	278	1.079
1995	265	1.023
1996	261	0.984
1997	305	1.152
1998	281	1.038
1999	272	0.99
2000	238	0.853
2001	259	0.917
2002	260	0.904
2003	284	0.967
2004	279	0.921
2005	296	0.972
2006	290	0.925
2007	330	1.019
2008	352	1.086
2009	353	1.067
2010	396	1.149
2011	409	1.16
2012	380	1.053
2013	478	1.299
2014	441	1.167
2015	481	1.225
2016	492	1.223
2017	511	1.241

* Deaths obtained from the multiple cause-of-death data for 1979–1998 are based on ICD-9 codes, and those beginning in 1999 are based on ICD-10 codes with available computerized literal death certificate data. Death information was also obtained from other surveillance mechanisms; data include familial prion diseases. Rates are adjusted to the U.S. standard 2000 projected population.

Treatment

Treatment of prion diseases remains supportive; no specific therapy has been shown to stop the progression of these diseases.

Section 13.4

Variant Creutzfeldt-Jakob Disease

This section includes text excerpted from "Variant
Creutzfeldt-Jakob Disease (vCJD)," Centers for Disease
Control and Prevention (CDC), October 9, 2018.

About Variant Creutzfeldt-Jakob Disease

Variant Creutzfeldt-Jakob disease (vCJD) is a prion disease that
was first described in 1996 in the United Kingdom. There is now strong
scientific evidence that the agent responsible for the outbreak of prion
disease in cows, bovine spongiform encephalopathy (BSE), or "mad
cow" disease, is the same agent responsible for the outbreak of vCJD
in humans.

Variant CJD is not the same disease as classic Creutzfeldt-Jakob
disease (often simply called "CJD"). It has different clinical and patho-
logic characteristics from classic CJD. Each disease also has a particular genetic profile of the prion protein gene. Both disorders are
invariably fatal brain diseases with unusually long incubation periods
measured in years, and are caused by an unconventional transmissible
agent called a "prion."

Diagnostic Criteria
Definite Variant Creutzfeldt-Jakob Disease

Neuropathologic examination of brain tissue is required to confirm
a diagnosis of variant CJD. The following confirmatory features should
be present.

- Numerous widespread kuru-type amyloid plaques surrounded by
  vacuoles in both the cerebellum and cerebrum—florid plaques

- Spongiform change and extensive prion protein deposition
  shown by immunohistochemistry throughout the cerebellum and
  cerebrum

Suspected Variant Creutzfeldt-Jakob Disease

- Current age or age at death <55 years (a brain autopsy is
  recommended, however, for all physician-diagnosed CJD cases)

- Psychiatric symptoms at illness onset and/or persistent painful
  sensory symptoms (frank pain and/or dysesthesia)

- Dementia, and development ≥4 months after illness onset of at least two of the following five neurologic signs: poor coordination, myoclonus, chorea, hyperreflexia, or visual signs. (If persistent painful sensory symptoms exist, ≥4 months delay in the development of the neurologic signs is not required.)

- A normal or an abnormal EEG, but not the diagnostic EEG changes often seen in classic CJD

- Duration of illness of over 6 months

- Routine investigations of the patient do not suggest an alternative, nonCJD diagnosis.

- No history of receipt of cadaveric human pituitary growth hormone or a dura mater graft.

- No history of CJD in a first-degree relative or prion protein gene mutation in the patient.

Surveillance for Variant Creutzfeldt-Jakob Disease

The Centers for Disease Control and Prevention (CDC) monitors the trends and current incidence of CJD in the United States using several surveillance mechanisms. On a routine basis, the CDC reviews the national multiple cause-of-death data taken from death certificates and compiled by the National Center for Health Statistics, CDC. The most systematic method includes analyzing death certificate information from U.S. multiple cause-of-death data, compiled by the National Center for Health Statistics, CDC.

Currently, the CDC works with selected state health departments on various enhanced CJD surveillance projects and education programs regarding the importance of autopsy to both the surveillance and diagnosis of CJD. In addition, CDC collects, reviews, and when indicated, actively investigates specific reports by healthcare personnel or institutions in all states of possible iatrogenic CJD and variant CJD cases. In addition, with the support of the Council of State and Territorial Epidemiologists, the CDC conducts follow-up review of clinical and neuropathology records of CJD decedents aged <55 years who are identified through the national mortality data analysis or reported by healthcare workers. This is the age group in which almost all of the vCJD cases worldwide have occurred to date.

In 1996-97, the CDC established at Case Western Reserve University, in collaboration with the American Association of Neuropathologists, the National Prion Disease Pathology Surveillance Center, which performs special state-of-the-art diagnostic tests for prion diseases, including postmortem tests for vCJD.

These surveillance methods for CJD enhance the ability to identify cases of variant CJD if and when such cases occur in the United States.

A summary of the analysis of multiple cause-of-death data was published in the *Journal of the American Medical Association* (JAMA) on November 8, 2000 (Volume 284, No. 18, pp. 2322–23) and in *Clinics of Laboratory Medicine* in December 2002 (Volume 22, pp. 849–62).

Treatment

Treatment of prion diseases remains supportive; no specific therapy has been shown to stop the progression of these diseases.

Chapter 14

Zoonoses

What Does Zoonoses Mean?

Some animals, even those that look perfectly healthy, can carry harmful organisms that can make people sick. Those organisms that originate in animals can cause diseases in humans. (Sometimes this process works the other way, and organisms from humans can cause diseases in animals). Those diseases are called "zoonotic diseases" or "zoonoses." Zoonoses are common in the United States and around the world. In fact, as many as 60 percent of all communicable diseases and 75 percent of emerging infectious diseases (EID) of people originated with animals. Zoonoses can be caused by bacteria, fungi, mycobacteria, parasites, viruses, and prions.

How Are Zoonotic Disease Agents Transmitted to Humans?

Direct contact: Contact with an animal's body fluids, such as saliva, blood, urine, mucus, or feces, that can occur when petting or touching animals or being bitten or scratched.

This chapter contains text excerpted from the following sources: Text beginning with the heading "What Does Zoonoses Mean?" is excerpted from "Zoonoses—Emerging Infectious Disease Journal," Centers for Disease Control and Prevention (CDC), February 28, 2018; Text beginning with the heading "Who Is at a Higher Risk of Serious Illness from Zoonotic Diseases?" is excerpted from "Zoonotic Diseases," Centers for Disease Control and Prevention (CDC), July 14, 2017.

Foodborne: Eating or drinking something unsafe (such as unpasteurized milk, undercooked meat or eggs, or raw fruits and vegetables) that are contaminated with feces from an infected animal.

Indirect contact: Contact with items in areas where animals live and roam or with objects or surfaces contaminated with germs. Examples include aquarium tank water; pet living areas, food bowls, and water dishes; chicken coops; plants; and soil.

Inhalation: Breathing in airborne organisms or spores.

Vector-borne: Being bitten by an infected tick or an insect (such as a mosquito or flea).

Examples of Zoonoses

Myriad zoonoses are known to exist. Here a few examples:

- Rabies, which you can get from the bite of a rabid infected animal, often a raccoon, skunk, bat, or fox.

- Anthrax, which you can get from contact with an infected animal or animal products (e.g., hides); sources include domestic and wild animals such as cattle, sheep, goats, antelope, and deer.

- Dengue, malaria, Zika virus infection, and Lyme disease, which you can get from the bite of an infected mosquito in areas where those diseases are common.

- Salmonella infection, which you can get after handling an infected baby chick, chicken, duck, turtle, or snake, or by eating contaminated food.

- *Escherichia coli* infection, which you can catch by touching surfaces in areas such as petting zoos or dairy farms where some of the animals may be infected, or by eating contaminated food.

Why Are Zoonoses a Public-Health Concern?

Zoonoses are a threat to public health for a number of reasons.

- The number and types of zoonotic diseases are increasing as people, animals, and vectors can travel the globe in less time than it takes for disease symptoms to develop after exposure (incubation period).

- Human manipulation of the environment (e.g., climate change) is helping some zoonotic disease vectors thrive.

- Overuse of antibiotics has made some of these diseases harder to treat (antibiotic resistance).

- Some organisms that cause zoonoses could be used for bioterrorism.

- Vaccines are not available to protect humans against many zoonoses.

- Treatments may not exist or be readily available for people infected with some zoonoses.

- Some zoonoses may take a different, or more deadly, form in people than in animals.

Who Is at a Higher Risk of Serious Illness from Zoonotic Diseases?

Anyone can become sick from a zoonotic disease, including healthy people. However, some people may be more at risk than others and should take steps to protect themselves or family members. These people are more likely than others to get really sick, and even die, from infection with certain diseases. These groups of people include:

- Children younger than 5 years of age

- Adults older than 65 years of age

- People with weakened immune systems

What Can You Do to Protect Yourself and Your Family from Zoonotic Diseases?

People can come into contact with animals in many places. This includes at home and away from home, in places such as petting zoos, fairs, schools, stores, and parks. Insects, such as mosquitoes and fleas, and ticks bite people and animals day and night. Thankfully, there are things you can do to protect yourself and your family from zoonotic diseases.

- Keep your hands clean. Washing your hands right after being around animals, even if you did not touch any animals, is one of the most important steps you can take to avoid getting sick and spreading germs to others.

- Always wash your hands after being around animals, even if you did not touch the animals.

- Many germs are spread by not washing hands with soap and clean, running water.

- If clean, running water is not accessible, use soap and available water.

- If soap and water are unavailable, use an alcohol-based hand sanitizer that contains at least 60 percent alcohol to clean hands. Because hand sanitizers do not eliminate all types of germs, it is important to wash your hands as soon as soap and water are available.

- Know the simple things you can do to stay safe around your pets.

- Prevent bites from mosquitoes, ticks, and fleas.

- Learn more about ways to handle food safely—whether it is for yourself or your family, your pet, or other animals.

- Be aware of zoonotic diseases both at home, away from home (such as at petting zoos or other animal exhibits), in child care settings or schools, and when you travel.

- Avoid bites and scratches from animals.

Part Three

Emerging Infectious Diseases Risk due to Climate Change

Chapter 15

Climate Change and Human Health

Human health has always been influenced by climate and weather. Changes in climate and climate variability, particularly changes in weather extremes, affect the environment that provides us with clean air, food, water, shelter, and security. Climate change, together with other natural and human-made health stressors, threatens human health and well-being in numerous ways. Some of these health impacts are already being experienced in the United States.

Given that the impacts of climate change are projected to increase over the next century, certain existing health threats will intensify, and new health threats may emerge. Connecting our understanding of how climate is changing with an understanding of how those changes may affect human health can inform decisions about mitigating (reducing) the amount of future climate change, suggest priorities for protecting public health, and help identify research needs.

Our Changing Climate
Observed Climate Change

The fact that the Earth has warmed over the last century is unequivocal. Multiple observations of air and ocean temperatures, sea level,

This chapter includes text excerpted from "Climate Change and Human Health," GlobalChange.gov, U.S. Global Change Research Program (USGCRP), April 4, 2016.

and snow and ice have shown these changes to be unprecedented over decades to millennia. Human influence has been the dominant cause of this observed warming. The 2014 U.S. National Climate Assessment (NCA) found that rising temperatures, the resulting increases in the frequency or intensity of some extreme weather events, rising sea levels, and melting snow and ice are already disrupting people's lives and damaging some sectors of the U.S. economy.

The concepts of climate and weather are often confused. Weather is the state of the atmosphere at any given time and place. Weather patterns vary greatly from year to year and from region to region. Familiar aspects of weather include temperature, precipitation, clouds, and wind that people experience throughout the course of a day. Severe weather conditions include hurricanes, tornadoes, blizzards, and droughts. Climate is the average weather conditions that persist over multiple decades or longer. While the weather can change in minutes or hours, identifying a change in climate has required observations over a time period of decades to centuries or longer. Climate change encompasses both increases and decreases in temperature, as well as shifts in precipitation, changing risks of certain types of severe weather events, and changes to other features of the climate system.

Some climate and weather changes already observed in the United States include:

- The U.S. average temperature has increased by 1.3°F to 1.9°F since record keeping began in 1895; most of this increase has occurred since about 1970. The first decade of the 2000s (2000–2009) was the warmest on record throughout the United States.

- Average U.S. precipitation has increased since 1900, but some areas have experienced increases greater than the national average, and some areas have experienced decreases.

- Heavy downpours are increasing nationally, especially over the last three to five decades. The largest increases are in the Midwest and Northeast, where floods have also been increasing.

- Drought has increased in the west. Over the last decade, the Southwest has experienced the most persistent droughts since record-keeping began in 1895. Changes in precipitation and runoff, combined with changes in consumption and withdrawal, have reduced surface and groundwater supplies in many areas.

- There have been changes in some other types of extreme weather events over the last several decades. Heat waves have become more frequent and intense, especially in the west. Cold waves have become less frequent and intense across the nation.

- The intensity, frequency, and duration of North Atlantic hurricanes, as well as the frequency of the strongest (category 4 and 5) hurricanes, have all increased since the early 1980s. The relative contributions of human and natural causes to these increases remain uncertain.

Projected Climate Change

Projections of future climate conditions are based on results from climate models—sophisticated computer programs that simulate the behavior of the Earth's climate system. These climate models are used to project how the climate system is expected to change under different possible scenarios. These scenarios describe future changes in atmospheric greenhouse gas concentrations, land use, other human influences on climate, and natural factors. The most recent set of coordinated climate model simulations use a set of scenarios called Representative Concentration Pathways (RCPs), which describe four possible trajectories in greenhouse gas concentrations. Actual future greenhouse gas concentrations, and the resulting amount of future climate change, will still largely be determined by choices society makes about emissions.

Some of the projected changes in climate in the United States as described in the 2014 National Climate Assessment (NCA) are listed below:

- Temperatures in the United States are expected to continue to rise. This temperature rise has not been, and will not be, uniform across the country or over time.

- Increases are also projected for extreme temperature conditions. The temperature of both the hottest day and coldest night of the year are projected to increase.

- More winter and spring precipitation is projected for the northern United States, and less for the Southwest, over this century.

- Increases in the frequency and intensity of extreme precipitation events are projected for all the United States areas.

- Short-term (seasonal or shorter) droughts are expected to intensify in most U.S. regions. Longer-term droughts are expected to intensify in large areas of the Southwest, the southern Great Plains, and the Southeast. Trends in reduced surface and groundwater supplies in many areas are expected to continue, increasing the likelihood of water shortages for many uses.

- Heat waves are projected to become more intense, and cold waves less intense, everywhere in the United States.

- Hurricane-associated storm intensity and rainfall rates are projected to increase as the climate continues to warm.

How Does Climate Change Affect Health?

The influences of weather and climate on human health are significant and varied. They range from the clear threats of temperature extremes and severe storms to connections that may seem less obvious. For example, weather and climate affect the survival, distribution, and behavior of mosquitoes, ticks, and rodents that carry diseases, such as West Nile virus or Lyme disease. Climate and weather can also affect water and food quality in particular areas, with implications for human health. In addition, the effects of global climate change on mental health and well-being are integral parts of the overall climate-related human health impact.

A useful approach to understand how climate change affects health is to consider specific exposure pathways and how they can lead to human disease. The concept of exposure pathways is adapted from its use in chemical risk assessment, and in this context describes the main routes by which climate change affects health (see Figure 15.1). Exposure pathways differ over time and in different locations, and climate-change related exposures can affect different people and different communities to different degrees. While often assessed individually, exposure to multiple climate change threats can occur simultaneously, resulting in compounding or cascading health impacts. Climate change threats may also accumulate over time, leading to longer-term changes in resilience and health.

Whether or not a person is exposed to a health threat or suffers illness or other adverse health outcomes from that exposure depends on a complex set of vulnerability factors. Vulnerability is the tendency or predisposition to be adversely affected by climate-related health effects, and encompasses three elements: exposure, sensitivity, or susceptibility to harm, and the capacity to adapt or to cope. Because multiple disciplines use these terms differently and multiple definitions exist in the literature, the distinctions between them are not always clear. All three of these elements can change over time and are place- and system-specific.

Vulnerability, and the three components of vulnerability, are factors that operate at multiple levels, from the individual and community to the country level, and affect all people to some degree. For an individual, these factors include human behavioral choices and the degree to which that person is vulnerable based on her or his level of exposure, sensitivity, and adaptive capacity. Vulnerability is also influenced by social determinants of health, including those that affect a person's adaptive capacity, such as social capital and social cohesion (for example, the strength of interpersonal networks and social patterns in a community).

At a larger community or societal scale, health outcomes are strongly influenced by adaptive capacity factors, including those related to the natural and built environments (for example, the state of infrastructure), governance and management (health-protective surveillance programs, regulations and enforcement, or community health programs), and institutions (organizations operating at all levels to form a national public health system). For example, water resource, public health, and environmental agencies in the United States provide many public health safeguards, such as monitoring water quality and issuing advisories to reduce the risk of exposure and illness if water becomes contaminated. Some aspects of climate change health impacts in the United States may, therefore, be mediated by factors, such as strong social capital, fully functional governance/management, and institutions that maintain the nation's generally high level of adaptive capacity. On the other hand, the evidence base regarding the effectiveness of public health interventions in a climate change context is still relatively weak. Current levels of adaptive capacity may not be sufficient to address multiple impacts that occur simultaneously or in close succession, or impacts of climate change that result in unprecedented damages.

The three components of vulnerability (exposure, sensitivity, and adaptive capacity) are associated with social and demographic factors, including level of wealth and education, as well as other characteristics of people and places, such as the condition of infrastructure and extent of ecosystem degradation. For example, poverty can leave people more exposed to climate and weather threats, increase sensitivity because of associations with higher rates of illness and nutritional deficits, and limit people's adaptive capacity. As another example, people living in a city with degraded coastal ecosystems and inadequate water and wastewater infrastructure may be at greater risk of health consequences from severe storms. Figure 15.1 demonstrates the interactions among climate drivers, health impacts, and other factors that influence people's vulnerability to health impacts.

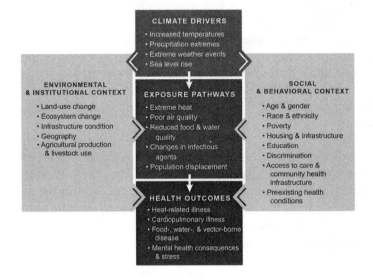

Figure 15.1. *Climate Change and Health*

Conceptual diagram illustrating the exposure pathways by which climate change affects human health. Exposure pathways exist within the context of other factors that positively or negatively influence health outcomes. Key factors that influence vulnerability for individuals are shown in the right box and include social determinants of health and behavioral choices. Key factors that influence vulnerability at larger scales, such as natural and built environments, governance and management, and institutions, are shown in the left box. All of these influencing factors can affect an individual's or a community's vulnerability through changes in exposure, sensitivity, and adaptive capacity and may also be affected by climate change.

We are already experiencing changes in the frequency, severity, and even the location of some weather and climate phenomena, including extreme temperatures, heavy rains and droughts, and some other kinds of severe weather, and these changes are projected to continue. This means that areas already experiencing health-threatening weather and climate phenomena, such as severe heat or hurricanes, are likely to experience worsening impacts, such as even higher temperatures and increased storm intensity, rainfall rates, and storm surge. It also means that some areas will experience new climate-related health threats. For example, areas previously unaffected by toxic algal blooms or waterborne diseases because of cooler water temperatures may face these hazards in the future as increasing water temperatures allow the organisms that cause these health risks to thrive. Even areas that currently experience these health threats may see a shift in the timing of the seasons that pose the greatest risk to human health.

Climate change can, therefore, affect human health in two main ways: first, by changing the severity or frequency of health problems that are already affected by climate or weather factors; and second, by creating unprecedented or unanticipated health problems or health threats in places where they have not previously occurred.

Our Changing Health

In order to understand how climate change creates or exacerbates health problems, assessments of climate change health impacts must start with what is known about the current state and observed trends in a wide array of health conditions. In addition, because preexisting health conditions, socioeconomic status, and life stage all contribute to vulnerability to climate-related and weather-related health effects, assessments of climate change health impacts should be informed by projected changes in these factors. In cases where people's health or socioeconomic status is getting worse, climate change may accentuate the health burdens associated with those worsening trends. Conversely, in cases where people's health or socioeconomic status is improving, the effect of climate change may be to slow or reduce that improvement. Where the state of scientific understanding allows, the inclusion of projected trends in health and socioeconomic conditions into models of climate change impacts on health can provide useful insights into these interactions between nonclimate factors and climate change effects.

Demographic and Socioeconomic Trends

The United States is in the midst of several significant demographic changes: the population is aging, growing in number, becoming more ethnically diverse, and demonstrating greater disparities between the wealthy and the poor. Immigration is having a major influence on both the size and age distribution of the population. Each of these demographic trends has implications for climate-change related human health impacts. Some of these trends and projections are summarized below:

Trends in Population Growth

- The total U.S. population has more than doubled since 1950, from 151,325,798 persons in 1950 to 308,745,538 in 2010.

- The Census Bureau projects that the U.S. population will grow to almost 400 million by 2050 (from estimates of about 320 million in 2014).

Trends in the Elderly Population

- The nation's older adult population (65 years of age and older) will nearly double in number from 2015 through 2050, from approximately 48 million to 88 million. Of those 88 million older adults, a little under 19 million will be 85 years of age and older.

Trends in Racial and Ethnic Diversity

- As the United States becomes more diverse, the aggregate minority population is projected to become the majority by 2042. The non-Hispanic or non-Latino White population will increase but more slowly than other racial groups. Non-Hispanic Whites are projected to become a minority by 2050.

- Projections for 2050 suggest that nearly 19 percent of the population will be immigrants, compared with 12 percent in 2005.

- The Hispanic population is projected to nearly double from 12.5 percent of the U.S. population in 2000 to 24.6 percent in 2050.

Trends in Economic Disparity

- Income inequality rose and then stabilized during the last 30 years and is projected to resume rising over the next 20 years, though at a somewhat slower overall rate that declines to near 0 by 2035. For example, the Gini coefficient, a measure of income inequality, is estimated to have risen by 18 percent between 1984 and 2000, and is projected to rise by an additional 17 percent for all workers between 2009 and 2035.

- America's communities of color have disproportionately higher poverty rates and lower income levels. While racial disparities in household wealth were higher in the late 1980s than now, trends in more recent years have been toward greater inequality. The ratio of the median net household worth of White, non-Hispanic versus non-White or Hispanic households increased from 6.0 to 7.8 between 2007 and 2013. In 2009, 25.8 percent of non-Hispanic Blacks and 25.3 percent of Hispanics had incomes below the poverty level as compared to 9.4 percent of non-Hispanic Whites and 12.5 percent of Asian Americans. In 2014, the median income level for a non-Hispanic Black household was approximately $35,000, $25,000 lower than a non-Hispanic White household.

Population growth and migration in the United States may place more people at risk of the health impacts of climate change, especially as more people are located in and around vulnerable areas, such as coastal, low-lying, or flood-prone zones; densely populated urban areas; and drought-stricken or wildfire-prone regions. Increases in racial and ethnic diversity and in the number of persons living near the poverty line may increase the risk of health impacts from climate change. Economic disparity can make it difficult for some populations to respond to dangerous weather conditions, especially when evacuation is necessary or when the aftermath requires rebuilding of homes and businesses not covered by home or property insurance.

Trends in Health Status

As a nation, trends in the population's health are mixed. Some major indicators of health, such as life expectancy, are consistently improving, while others, such as rate and number of diabetes deaths, are getting worse. Changes in these metrics may differ across populations and over time. For example, though rates of obesity have increased in both children and adults over the last 30 years or more, rates over just the last decade have remained steady for adults but increased among children.

Climate change impacts to human health will act on top of these underlying trends. Some of these underlying health conditions can increase sensitivity to climate change effects, such as heat waves and worsening air quality. Understanding the trends in these conditions is, therefore, important in considering how many people are likely to experience illness when exposed to these climate change effects. Potential climate-change related health impacts may reduce the improvements that would otherwise be expected in some indicators of health status and accentuate trends towards poorer health in other health indicators.

Examples of health indicators that have been improving between 2000 and 2013 include the following:

- Life expectancy at birth increased from 76.8 to 78.8 years.

- Death rates per 100,000 people from heart disease and cancer decreased from 257.6 to 169.8 and from 199.6 to 163.2, respectively.

- The percent of people over the age of 18 who say they smoke decreased from 23.2 to 17.8 percent.

At the same time, some health trends related to the prevalence of chronic diseases, self-reported ill health, and disease risk factors have been getting worse. For example:

- The percentage of adult (18 years of age and older) Americans describing their health as "poor" or "fair" increased from 8.9 percent in 2000 to 10.3 percent in 2012.

- Prevalence of physician-diagnosed diabetes among adults 20 years of age and older increased from 5.2 percent in 1988–1994 to 8.4 percent in 2009–2012.

- The prevalence of obesity among adults (between the ages of 20 and 74) increased by almost three-fold from 1960–1962 (13.4% of adults classified as obese) to 2009–2010 (36.1% of adults classified as obese).

- In the past 30 years, obesity has more than doubled in children and quadrupled in adolescents in the United States. The percentage of children between the ages of 6 and 11 who were obese increased from 7 percent in 1980 to nearly 18 percent in 2012. Similarly, the percentage of adolescents between the ages of 12 and 19s who were obese increased from 5 percent to nearly 21 percent over the same period. In 2012, approximately one-third of American children and adolescents were overweight or obese.

Table 15.1 shows some examples of underlying health conditions that are associated with increased vulnerability to health effects from climate-change related exposures and provides information on current status and future trends.

Health status is often associated with demographics and socio-economic status. Changes in the overall size of the population, racial and ethnic composition, and age distribution affect the health status of the population. Poverty, educational attainment, access to care, and discrimination all contribute to disparities in the incidence and prevalence of a variety of medical conditions. Some examples of these interactions include:

- Older adults. In 2013, the percentage of adults 75 years of age and older described as persons in fair or poor health totaled 27.6 percent, as compared to 6.2 percent for adults between the ages of 18 and 44. Among adults 65 years of age and older, the number in nursing homes or other residential care facilities totaled 1.8 million in 2012, with more than 1 million utilizing home healthcare.

- Children. Approximately 9.0 percent of children in the United States have asthma. Between 2011 and 2013, rates for Black (15.3%) and Hispanic (8.6%) children were higher than the rate for White (7.8%) children. Rates of asthma were also higher in poor children who live below 100% of the poverty level (12.4%).

- Non-Hispanic Blacks. In 2014, the percentage of non-Hispanic Blacks of all ages who were described as persons in fair or poor health totaled 14.3 percent as compared to 8.7 percent for Whites. Health risk factors for this population include high rates of smoking, obesity, and hypertension in adults, as well as high infant death rates.

- Hispanics. The percentage of Hispanics of all ages who were described as persons in fair or poor health totaled 12.7 percent in 2014. Health disparities for Hispanics include moderately higher rates of smoking in adults, low birth weights, and infant deaths.

The impacts of climate change may worsen these health disparities by exacerbating some of the underlying conditions they create. For example, disparities in life expectancy may be exacerbated by the effects of climate-change related heat and air pollution on minority populations that have higher rates of hypertension, smoking, and diabetes. Conversely, public health measures that reduce disparities and overall rates of illness in populations would lessen vulnerability to worsening of health status from climate change effects.

211

Table 15.1. Current Estimates and Future Trends in Chronic Health Conditions That Interact with the Health Risks Associated with Climate Change

Health Conditions	Current Estimates	Future Trends	Possible Influences of Climate Change
Alzheimer Disease	Approximately 5 million Americans over 65 had Alzheimer's disease in 2013.	Prevalence of Alzheimer is expected to triple to 13.8 million by 2050.	Persons with cognitive impairments are vulnerable to extreme weather events that require evacuation or other emergency responses.
Asthma	Average asthma prevalence in the U.S. was higher in children (9% in 2014) than in adults (7% in 2013).35 Since the 1980s, asthma prevalence increased, but rates of asthma deaths and hospital admissions declined.,	Stable incidence and increasing prevalence of asthma is projected in the U.S. in coming decades.	Asthma is exacerbated by changes in pollen season and allergenicity and in exposures to air pollutants affected by changes in temperature, humidity, and wind.
Chronic Obstructive Pulmonary Disease (COPD)	In 2012, approximately 6.3% of adults had COPD. Deaths from chronic lung diseases increased by 50% from 1980 to 2010.	Chronic respiratory diseases are the third leading cause of death and are expected to become some of the most costly illnesses in coming decades.	COPD patients are more sensitive than the general population to changes in ambient air quality associated with climate change.
Diabetes	In 2012, approximately 9% of the total U.S. population had diabetes. Approximately 18,400 people younger than age 20 were newly diagnosed with type 1 diabetes in 2008–2009; an additional 5,000 were diagnosed with type 2.	New diabetes cases are projected to increase from about 8 cases per 1,000 in 2008 to about 15 per 1,000 in 2050. If recent increases continue, prevalence is projected to increase to 33% of Americans by 2050.	Diabetes increases sensitivity to heat stress; medication and dietary needs may increase vulnerability during and after extreme weather events.

Table 15.1. Continued

Health Conditions	Current Estimates	Future Trends	Possible Influences of Climate Change
Cardiovascular disease	Cardiovascular disease (CVD) is the leading cause of death in the U.S.	By 2030, approximately 41% of the U.S. population is projected to have some form of CVD.	Cardiovascular disease increases sensitivity to heat stress.
Mental Illness	Depression is one of the most common types of mental illness, with approximately 7% of adults reporting a major episode in the past year. Lifetime prevalence is approximately twice as high for women as for men. Lifetime prevalence is more than 15% for anxiety disorders and nearly 4% for bipolar disorder.	By 2050, the total number of U.S. adults with depressive disorder is projected to increase by 35%, from 33.9 million to 45.8 million, with those over age 65 having a 117% increase.	Mental illness may impair responses to extreme events; certain medications increase sensitivity to heat stress.
Obesity	In 2009–2010, approximately 35% of American adults were obese. In 2012, approximately 32% of youth (aged 2–19) were overweight or obese.	By 2030, 51% of the U.S. population is expected to be obese. Projections suggest a 33% increase in obesity and a 130% increase in severe obesity.	Obesity increases sensitivity to high ambient temperatures.
Disability	Approximately 18.7% of the U.S. population has a disability. In 2010, the percent of American adults with a disability was approximately 16.6% for those age 21–64 and 49.8% for persons 65 and older.	The number of older adults with activity limitations is expected to grow from 22 million in 2005 to 38 million in 2030.	Persons with disabilities may find it hard to respond when evacuation is required and when there is no available means of transportation or easy exit from residences.

Quantifying Health Impacts

For some changes in exposures to health risks related to climate change, the future rate of a health impact associated with any given environmental exposure can be estimated by multiplying three values: 1. the baseline rate of the health impact, 2. the expected change in exposure, and 3. the exposure–response function. An exposure–response function is an estimate of how the risk of a health impact changes with changes in exposures and is related to sensitivity, one of the three components of vulnerability. For example, an exposure–response function for extreme heat might be used to quantify the increase in heat-related deaths in a region (the change in health impact) for every 1°F increase in daily ambient temperature (the change in exposure).

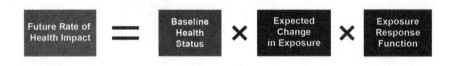

Figure 15.2. *Quantifying Health Impacts*

The ability to quantify many types of health impacts is dependent on the availability of data on the baseline incidence or prevalence of the health impact, the ability to characterize the future changes in the types of exposures relevant to that health impact, and how well the relationship between these exposures and health impacts is understood. Health impacts with many intervening factors, such as infectious diseases, may require different and more complex modeling approaches. Where our understanding of these relationships is strong, some health impacts, even those occurring in unprecedented places or times of the year, may in fact be predictable. Where there is a lack of data or these relationships are poorly understood, health impacts are harder to project.

Data on the incidence and prevalence of health conditions are obtained through a complicated system of state- and city-level surveillance programs, national health surveys, and national collection of data on hospitalizations, emergency room visits, and deaths. For example, data on the incidence of a number of infectious diseases are captured through the National Notifiable Diseases Surveillance System. This system relies first on the mandatory reporting of specific diseases by healthcare providers to state, local, territorial, and tribal health departments. These reporting jurisdictions then have the option of voluntarily providing the Centers for Disease Control and Prevention (CDC) with data on a set of nationally notifiable diseases. Because of challenges with getting healthcare providers to confirm and report specific diagnoses of reportable diseases in their patients, and the lack of requirements for reporting a consistent set of diseases and forwarding data to the CDC, incidence of infectious disease is generally believed to be underreported, and actual rates are uncertain.

Characterizing certain types of climate-change related exposures can be a challenge. Exposures can consist of temperature changes and other weather conditions, inhaling air pollutants and pollens, consuming unsafe food supplies or contaminated water, or experiencing trauma or other mental-health consequences from weather disasters. For some health impacts, the ability to understand the relationships between climate-related exposures and health impacts is limited by these difficulties in characterizing exposures or in obtaining accurate data on the occurrence of illnesses. For these health impacts, scientists may not have the capability to project changes in a health outcome (such as the incidence of diseases) and can only estimate how risks of exposure will change. For example, modeling capabilities allow projections of the impact of rising water temperatures on the concentration of Vibrio bacteria, which provides an understanding of geographic changes in exposure but does not capture how people may be exposed and how many will actually become sick. Nonetheless, the ability to project changes in exposure or in intermediate determinants of health impacts may improve understanding of the change in health risks, even if modeling quantitative changes in health impacts is not possible. For example, seasonal temperature and precipitation projections may be combined to assess future changes in ambient pollen concentrations (the exposure that creates risk), even though the potential associated increase in respiratory and allergic diseases (the health impacts) cannot be directly modeled.

Modeling Approaches Used in This Report

Adverse health effects attributed to climate change can have many economic and social consequences, including direct medical costs, work loss, increased caregiving, and other limitations on everyday activities. Though economic impacts are a crucial component to understanding risk from climate change and may have important direct and secondary impacts on human health and well-being by reducing resources available for other preventative health measures, economic valuation of the health impacts was not reported in this assessment.

Uncertainty in Health Impact Assessments

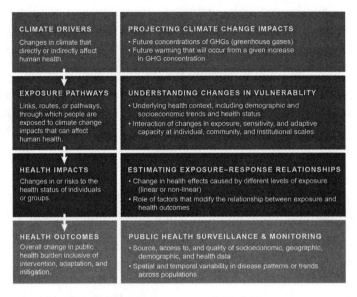

Figure 15.3. *Sources of Uncertainty*

Examples of sources of uncertainty in projecting impacts of climate change on human health. The left column illustrates the exposure pathway through which climate change can affect human health. The right column lists examples of key sources of uncertainty surrounding effects of climate change at each stage along the exposure pathway.

Two of the key uncertainties in projecting future global temperatures are 1) uncertainty about future concentrations of greenhouse gases and 2) uncertainty about how much warming will occur for a given increase in greenhouse gas concentrations. The Intergovernmental Panel on Climate Change's Fifth Assessment Report found that the most likely response of the climate system to a doubling of carbon dioxide concentrations lie between a 1.5 percent and 4.5 percent (2.7°F to 8.1°F) increase in global average temperature. Future concentrations depend on both future emissions and how long these emissions remain in the atmosphere (which can vary depending on how natural systems process those emissions). To capture these uncertainties, climate modelers often use multiple models, analyze multiple scenarios, and conduct sensitivity analyses to assess the significance of these uncertainties.

Uncertainty in current and future estimates of health or socioeconomic status is related to several factors. In general, estimates are more uncertain for less-prevalent health conditions (such as rare cancers versus cardiovascular disease), smaller subpopulations (such as Hispanic subpopulations versus White adults), smaller geographic areas (census tracts versus state or national scale), and time periods further into the future (decades versus seasons or years). Most current estimates of disease prevalence or socioeconomic status have uncertainty expressed as standard errors or confidence intervals that are derived from sampling methods and sample sizes. When modeling health impacts using data on health prevalence or socioeconomic status, these measures of uncertainty are typically included in the analysis to help establish a range of plausible results. Expert judgment is typically used to assess the overall effects of uncertainty from estimates of health or socioeconomic status when assessing the scientific literature.

The factors related to uncertainty in exposure–response functions are similar to those for the projections of health or socioeconomic status. Estimates are more uncertain for smaller subpopulations, less-prevalent health conditions, and smaller geographic areas. Because these estimates are based on observations of real populations, their validity when applied to populations in the future is more uncertain the further into the future the application occurs. Uncertainty in the estimates of the exposure–outcome relationship also comes from factors related to the scientific quality of relevant studies, including appropriateness of methods, source of data, and size of study populations. Expert judgment is used to evaluate the validity of an individual study, as well as the collected group of relevant studies in assessing uncertainty in estimates of exposure–outcome relationships.

Approach to Reporting Uncertainty in Key Findings

Despite the sources of uncertainty described above, the current state of the science allows an examination of the likely direction of and trends in the health impacts of climate change. Over the past 10 years, the models used for climate and health assessments have become more useful and more accurate. This assessment builds on that improved capability.

Two kinds of language are used when describing the uncertainty associated with specific statements in this report: confidence language and likelihood language. Confidence in the validity of a finding is expressed qualitatively and is based on the type, amount, quality, strength, and consistency of evidence and the degree of expert agreement on the finding. Likelihood, or the projected probability of an impact occurring, is based on quantitative estimates or measures of

217

uncertainty expressed probabilistically (in other words, based on statistical analysis of observations or model results, or on expert judgment). Whether a key finding has a confidence level associated with it or, where findings can be quantified, both a confidence and likelihood level associated with it, involves the expert assessment and consensus of the chapter author teams.

Table 15.2. Likelihood and Confidence Level

Likelihood				
Very Likely ≥9 in 10	Likely ≥2 in 3	As Likely as Not ≈ 1 in 2	Unlikely ≤ 1 in 3	Very Unlikely ≤1 in 10
Confidence Level				
Very High Strong evidence (established theory, multiple sources, consistent results, well documented and accepted methods, etc.), high consensus	**High** Moderate evidence (several sources, some consistency, methods vary and/or documentation limited, etc.), medium consensus	**Medium** Suggestive evidence (a few sources, limited consistency, models incomplete, methods emerging, etc.), competing schools of thought	**Low** Inconclusive evidence (limited sources, extrapolations, inconsistent findings, poor documentation and/or methods not tested, etc.), disagreement or lack of opinions among experts	

Chapter 16

Populations of Concern

Climate change is already causing and is expected to continue to cause a range of health impacts that vary across different population groups in the United States. The vulnerability of any given group is a function of its sensitivity to climate-change related health risks, its exposure to those risks, and its capacity for responding to or coping with climate variability and change. Vulnerable groups of people, described here as populations of concern, include those with low income, some communities of color, immigrant groups (including those with limited English proficiency), Indigenous peoples, children and pregnant women, older adults, vulnerable occupational groups, persons with disabilities, and persons with preexisting or chronic medical conditions. Planners and public health officials, politicians and physicians, scientists, and social service providers are tasked with understanding and responding to the health impacts of climate change. Collectively, their characterization of vulnerability should consider how populations of concern experience disproportionate, multiple, and complex risks to their health and well-being in response to climate change.

Some groups face a number of stressors related to both climate and nonclimate factors. For example, people living in impoverished urban or isolated rural areas, floodplains, coastlines, and other at-risk locations are more vulnerable not only to extreme weather and persistent climate change but also to social and economic stressors. Many of these stressors can occur simultaneously or consecutively. Over time,

This chapter includes text excerpted from "Populations of Concern," Global-Change.gov, U.S. Global Change Research Program (USGCRP), April 4, 2016.

this accumulation of multiple, complex stressors is expected to become more evident as climate impacts interact with stressors associated with existing mental- and physical-health conditions and with other socioeconomic and demographic factors.

A Framework for Understanding Vulnerability

Some populations of concern demonstrate relatively greater vulnerability to the health impacts of climate change. The definitions of the following key concepts are important to understand how some people or communities are disproportionately affected by climate-related health risks. Definitions are adapted from the Intergovernmental Panel on Climate Change (IPCC) and the National Research Council (NRC).

- **Vulnerability** is the tendency or predisposition to be adversely affected by climate-related health effects and encompasses three elements: exposure, sensitivity or susceptibility to harm, and the capacity to adapt to or to cope with change. Exposure is contact between a person and one or more biological, chemical, or physical stressors, including stressors affected by climate change. Contact may occur in a single instance or repeatedly over time, and may occur in one location or over a wider geographic area. Sensitivity is the degree to which people or communities are affected, either adversely or beneficially, by climate variability and change. Adaptive capacity is the ability of communities, institutions, or people to adjust to potential hazards, to take advantage of opportunities, or to respond to consequences. A related term, "resilience," is the ability to prepare and plan for, absorb, recover from, and more successfully adapt to adverse events. People and communities with strong adaptive capacity have greater resilience.

- **Risk** is the potential for consequences to develop where something of value (such as human health) is at stake and where the outcome is uncertain. Risk is often represented as the probability of the occurrence of a hazardous event multiplied by the expected severity of the impacts of that event.

- **Stressors** are events or trends, whether related to climate change or other factors, that increase vulnerability to health effects.

People or communities can have greater or lesser vulnerability to health risks depending on social, political, and economic factors that are collectively known as "social determinants of health." Some groups are disproportionately disadvantaged by social determinants of health that limit resources and opportunities for health promoting behaviors and conditions of daily life, such as living/working circumstances and access to healthcare services. In disadvantaged groups, social determinants of health interact with the three elements of vulnerability by contributing to increased exposure, increased sensitivity, and reduced adaptive capacity (see Figure 16.1).

Health risks and vulnerability may increase in locations or instances where combinations of social determinants of health that amplify health threats occur simultaneously or close in time or space. For example, people with limited economic resources living in areas with deteriorating infrastructure are more likely to experience disproportionate impacts and are less able to recover following extreme events, increasing their vulnerability to climate-related health effects. Understanding the role of social determinants of health can help characterize

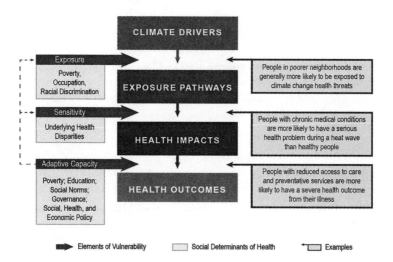

Figure 16.1. *Intersection of Social Determinants of Health and Vulnerability*

Social determinants of health interact with the three elements of vulnerability. The left side boxes provide examples of social determinants of health associated with each of the elements of vulnerability. Increased exposure, increased sensitivity and reduced adaptive capacity all affect vulnerability at different points in the causal chain from climate drivers to health outcomes (middle boxes). Adaptive capacity can influence exposure and sensitivity and also can influence the resilience of individuals or populations experiencing health impacts by influencing access to care and preventive services. The right side boxes provide illustrative examples of the implications of social determinants on increased exposure, increased sensitivity, and reduced adaptive capacity.

climate change impacts and identify public health interventions or actions to reduce or prevent exposures in populations of concern.

Factors That Contribute to Exposure

Exposures to climate-related variability and change are determined by a range of factors that individually and collectively shape the nature and extent of exposures. These factors include:

- **Occupation:** Certain occupations have a greater risk of exposure to climate impacts. People working outdoors or performing duties that expose them to extreme weather, such as emergency responders, utility repair crews, farm workers, construction workers, and other outdoor laborers, are at particular risk.

- **Time spent in risk-prone locations:** Where a person lives, goes to school, works, or spends leisure time will contribute to exposure. Locations with greater health threats include urban areas (due to, for example, the heat island effect or air quality concerns), areas where airborne allergens and other air pollutants occur at levels that aggravate respiratory illnesses, communities experiencing depleted water supplies or vulnerable energy and transportation infrastructure, coastal and other flood-prone areas, and locations affected by drought and wildfire.

- **Responses to extreme events:** A person's ability or, in some cases, their choice whether to evacuate or shelter-in-place in response to an extreme event such as a hurricane, flood, or wildfire affects their exposure to health threats. Low-income populations are generally less likely to evacuate in response to a warning.

- **Socioeconomic status:** Persons living in poverty are more likely to be exposed to extreme heat and air pollution. Poverty also determines, at least in part, how people perceive the risks to which they are exposed, how they respond to evacuation orders and other emergency warnings, and their ability to evacuate or relocate to a less risk-prone location.

- **Infrastructure condition and access:** Older buildings may expose occupants to increased indoor air pollutants and mold, stagnant airflow, or high indoor temperatures. Persons preparing for or responding to flooding, wildfires, or other weather-related emergencies may be hampered by disruption to transportation, utilities, medical, or communication infrastructure. Lack of access to these resources, in either urban or rural settings, can increase a person's vulnerability.

- **Compromised mobility, cognitive function, and other mental or behavioral factors:** These factors can lead to increased exposure to climate-related health impacts if people are not aware of health threats or are unable to take actions to avoid, limit, or respond to risks. People with access and functional needs may be particularly at risk if these factors interfere with their ability to access or receive medical care before, during, or after a disaster or emergency.

Characterizing Biological Sensitivity

The sensitivity of human communities and individuals to climate-change stressors is determined, at least in part, by biological traits. Among those traits are the overall health status, age, and life stage. From fetus, to infant, to toddler, to child, to adolescent, to adult, to the elderly, persons at every life stage have varying sensitivity to climate change impacts. For instance, the relatively immature immune systems of very young children make them more sensitive to aeroallergen exposure (such as airborne pollens). In addition to life stage, people experiencing long-term chronic medical and/or psychological conditions are more sensitive to climate stressors. Persons with asthma or chronic obstructive pulmonary disease (COPD) are more sensitive to exposures to wildfire smoke and other respiratory irritants. Social and economic factors also affect disparities in the prevalence of chronic medical conditions that aggravate biological sensitivity.

Adaptive Capacity and Response to Climate Change

Many of the same factors that contribute to exposure or sensitivity also influence the ability of both individuals and communities to adapt to climate variability and change. Socioeconomic status (SES), the condition and accessibility of infrastructure, the accessibility of healthcare, certain demographic characteristics, human and social capital (the skills, knowledge, experience, and social cohesion of a community), and other institutional resources all contribute to the timeliness and effectiveness of adaptive capacity.

Concerned Population
Communities of Color, Low Income, Immigrants, and Limited English Proficiency Groups

In the United States, some communities of color, low-income groups, people with limited English proficiency (LEP), and certain immigrant groups (especially those who are undocumented) live with many of the factors that contribute to their vulnerability to the health impacts of climate change. These populations are at increased risk of exposure given their higher likelihood of living in risk-prone areas (such as urban heat islands, isolated rural areas, or coastal and other flood-prone areas), areas with older or poorly maintained infrastructure, or areas with an increased burden of air pollution. These groups of people also experience relatively greater incidence of chronic medical conditions, such as cardiovascular and kidney disease, diabetes, asthma, and COPD, which can be exacerbated by climate-related health impacts. Socioeconomic and educational factors, limited transportation, limited access to health education, and social isolation related to language deficiencies collectively impede their ability to prepare for, respond to, and cope with climate-related health risks. These populations also may have limited access to medical care and may not be able to afford medications or other treatments. For LEP and undocumented persons, high poverty rates, language and cultural barriers, and citizenship status limit access to and use of healthcare and other social services and make these groups more hesitant to seek out help that might compromise their immigration status in the United States.

The number of people of color in the United States who may be affected by heightened vulnerability to climate-related health risks will continue to grow. Currently, Hispanics or Latinos, Blacks or African Americans, American Indians and Alaska Natives, Asian Americans, and Native Hawaiians and Pacific Islanders represent 37 percent of the total U.S. population. By 2042, they are projected to become the majority. People of color already constitute the majority in 4 states (California, Hawaii, New Mexico, and Texas) and in many cities. Numbers of LEP and undocumented immigrant populations have also increased. In 2011, LEP groups comprised approximately 9 percent (25.3 million individuals) of the U.S. population five years of age and older. In 2010, approximately 11.2 million people in the United States were undocumented.

Vulnerability to Climate-Related Health Stressors

Key climate impacts for some communities of color and low-income, LEP, and immigrant populations include heat waves, other extreme weather events, poor air quality, food safety, infectious diseases, and psychological stressors.

Race is an important factor in vulnerability to climate-related stress, but it can be difficult to isolate the role of race from other related socioeconomic and geographic factors. Some racial minorities are also members of low-income groups, immigrants, and people with limited English proficiency, and it is their socioeconomic status (SES) that contributes most directly to their vulnerability to climate-change related stressors. SES is a measure of a person's economic and social status, often defined by income, education, and occupation. Additional factors such as age, gender, preexisting medical conditions, psychosocial factors, and physical and mental stress are also associated with vulnerability to climate change. Because many of these variables are highly related to one another, statistical models must account for these factors in order to accurately measure the relative importance of various risk factors. For instance, minority race and low SES are jointly linked to increased prevalence of underlying health conditions that may affect sensitivity to climate change. When adjusted for age, gender, and level of education, the number of potential life years (LY) lost from all causes of death was found to be 35 percent greater for Blacks than for Whites in the United States, indicating an independent effect of race.

Extreme heat events. Some communities of color and some low-income, homeless, and immigrant populations are more exposed to heat waves, as these groups often reside in urban areas affected by heat island effects. In addition, these populations are likely to have limited adaptive capacity due to a lack of adequately insulated housing; inability to afford or to use air conditioning; inadequate access to public shelters, such as cooling centers; and inadequate access to both routine and emergency healthcare. These social, economic, and health risk factors give rise to the observed increase in deaths and disease from extreme heat in some immigrant and impoverished communities. Elevated risks for mortality associated with exposures to high ambient temperatures are also reported for Blacks as compared to Whites, a finding that persists once air conditioning use is accounted for.

Other weather extremes. As observed during and after Hurricane Katrina and Hurricane/Post-Tropical Cyclone Sandy, some communities of color and low-income people experienced increased illness or injury, death, or displacement due to poor quality housing, lack of access to emergency communications, lack of access to transportation, inadequate access to healthcare services and medications, limited postdisaster employment, and limited or no health and property insurance. Following a 2006 flood in El Paso, Texas, Hispanic ethnicity was identified as a significant risk factor for adverse health effects after controlling for other important socioeconomic factors (for example, age and housing quality). Adaptation measures to address these risk factors—such as providing transportation during evacuations or targeted employment assistance during the recovery phase—may help reduce or eliminate these health impact disparities, but they may not be readily available or affordable.

Degraded air quality. Climate change impacts on outdoor air quality will increase exposure in urban areas where large proportions of minority, low-income, homeless, and immigrant populations reside. Fine particulate matter and ozone levels already exceed the U.S. National Ambient Air Quality Standards (NAAQS) in many urban areas. Given the relatively higher rates of cardiovascular and respiratory diseases in low-income urban populations, these populations are more sensitive to degraded air quality, resulting in increases in illness, hospitalization, and premature death. In addition, climate change can contribute to increases in aeroallergens, which exacerbate asthma, an illness that is relatively more common among some communities of color and low-income groups. People of color are especially impacted by air pollution due to both disproportionate exposures for persons living in urban areas, as well as higher prevalence of underlying diseases, such as asthma and COPD, which increase their inherent sensitivity. In 2000, the prevalence of asthma was 122 per 1,000 Black persons and 104 per 1,000 White persons in the United States. At that time, asthma mortality was approximately 3 times higher among Blacks as compared to Whites.

Waterborne and vector-borne diseases. Climate change is expected to increase exposure to waterborne pathogens that cause a variety of illnesses—most commonly gastrointestinal illness and diarrhea. Health risks increase in crowded shelter conditions following floods or hurricanes, which suggests that some low-income groups living in crowded housing (particularly prevalent among foreign-born or Hispanic populations) may face increased exposure risk. Substandard or deteriorating water infrastructure (including sewerage, drainage, and stormwater systems, and drinking water systems) in both urban and rural low-income areas also contribute to increased risk of exposure to waterborne pathogens. Low-income populations in some regions may also be more vulnerable to the changes in the distribution of some vector-borne diseases that are expected to result from climate change. For example, higher incidence of West Nile virus disease has been linked to poverty and to urban location in the southeastern and northeastern United States, respectively.

Food safety and security. Climate change affects food safety and is projected to reduce the nutrient and protein content of some crops, such as wheat and rice. Some communities of color and low-income populations are more likely to be affected because they spend a relatively larger portion of their household income on food compared to more affluent households. These groups often suffer from poor-quality diets and limited access to full-service grocery stores that offer healthy and affordable dietary choices.

Psychological stress. Some communities of color, low-income populations, immigrants, and LEP groups are more likely to experience stress-related mental-health impacts, particularly during and after extreme events. Other contributing factors include barriers in accessing and affording mental healthcare, such as counseling in native languages, and the availability and affordability of appropriate medications.

Indigenous Peoples in the United States

A number of health risks are higher among Indigenous populations, such as poor mental health related to historical or personal trauma, alcohol abuse, suicide, infant/child mortality, environmental exposures from pollutants or toxic substances, and diabetes caused by inadequate or improper diets. Because of existing vulnerabilities, Indigenous people, especially those who are dependent on the environment for sustenance or who live in geographically isolated or impoverished communities, are likely to experience greater exposure and lower resilience to climate-related health effects. Indigenous Arctic communities have already experienced difficulty adapting to climate change effects, such as reductions in sea ice thickness, thawing permafrost, increases in coastal erosion, and landslide frequency, alterations in the ranges of some fish, increased weather unpredictability, and northward advance of the tree line. These climate changes have disrupted traditional hunting and subsistence practices and may threaten infrastructure, such as the condition of housing, transportation, and pipelines, which ultimately may force relocation of villages.

Food safety and security. Examples of how climate changes can affect the health of Indigenous peoples include changes in the abundance and nutrient content of certain foodstuffs, such as berries for Alaska Native communities; declining moose populations in Minnesota, which are significant to many Ojibwe peoples and an important source of dietary protein; rising temperatures and lack of available water for farming among Navajo people; and declines in traditional rice harvests among the Ojibwe in the upper Great Lakes region. Traditional foods and livelihoods are embedded in Indigenous cultural beliefs and subsistence practices. Climate impacts on traditional foods may result in poor nutrition and increased obesity and diabetes.

Changes in aquatic habitats and species also affect subsistence fishing. Rising temperatures affect water quality and availability. Lower oxygen levels in freshwater and seawater degrade water quality and promote the growth of disease-causing bacteria, viruses, and parasites. Warming can exacerbate shellfish disease and make mercury more readily absorbed in fish tissue. Elevated sea surface temperatures, consistent with projected trends in climate warming, have been associated with increased accumulation of methylmercury in fish and increased human exposure. Mercury is a neurotoxin that adversely affects people at all life stages, particularly during the prenatal stage. In addition, oceans are becoming more acidic as they absorb some of the carbon dioxide (CO_2) added to the atmosphere by fossil fuel burning and other sources, and this change in acidity can lower shellfish survival. This affects Indigenous peoples on the West and Gulf Coasts and Alaska Natives whose livelihoods depend on shellfish harvests. Rising sea levels will also destroy fresh- and saltwater habitats that some Indigenous peoples located along the Gulf Coast rely upon for subsistence food.

Water security. Indigenous peoples may lack access to water resources and to adequate infrastructure for water treatment and supply. A significant number of Indigenous persons living on remote reservations lack indoor plumbing and rely on unregulated water supplies that are vulnerable to drought, changes in water quality, and contamination of water in local systems. Existing infrastructure may be poorly maintained or in need of significant and costly upgrades. Heavy rainfall events and warm temperatures have been linked to diarrheal outbreaks and bacterial contamination of drinking water sources. Acute diarrheal disease has been shown to disproportionately affect children on the Fort Apache reservation in Arizona and result in higher overall hospitalization rates for American Indian/

Alaska Native infants. Increased extreme precipitation and potential increases in cyanobacterial blooms are also expected to stress existing water infrastructure on tribal lands and increase exposure to water-borne pathogens.

Loss of cultural identity. Climate change threatens sacred ceremonial and cultural practices through changing the availability of culturally relevant plant and animal species. Climate-related threats may compound historical impacts associated with colonialism, as well as current effects on tribal culture as more young people leave reservations for education and employment opportunities. Loss of tribal territory and disruption of cultural resources and traditional ways of life, lead to loss of cultural identity. The loss of medicinal plants due to climate change may leave ceremonial and traditional practitioners without the resources they need to practice traditional healing. The relocation of young people may reduce interactions across generations and undermine the sharing of traditional knowledge, tribal lore, and oral history.

Degraded infrastructure and other impacts. Rising temperatures may damage transportation infrastructure on tribal lands. Changing ice or thawing permafrost, flooding, and drought-related dust storms may block roads and cut off communities from access to evacuation routes and emergency medical care or social services. Poor air quality from blowing dust affects southwestern Indigenous communities, particularly in Arizona and New Mexico, and is likely to worsen with drought conditions. Exposure to impaired air quality also affects Indigenous communities, especially those downwind from urban areas or industrial complexes.

Children and Pregnant Women

Children are vulnerable to adverse health effects associated with environmental exposures due to factors related to their immature physiology and metabolism, their unique exposure pathways, their biological sensitivities, and limits to their adaptive capacity. Children pass through a series of windows of vulnerability that begin in the womb and continue through their second decade of life. Children have a proportionately higher intake of air, food, and water relative to their body weight when compared to adults. They also share unique behaviors and interactions with their environment that may increase their exposure to environmental contaminants. For example, small children often play indoors on the floor or outdoors on the ground and place hands and other objects in their mouths, increasing their exposure to dust and other contaminants, such as pesticides, mold spores, and allergens. There is, however, large variation in vulnerability among children at different life stages due to differing physiology and behaviors (see Figure 16.2). Climate change—interacting with factors such as economic status, diet, living situation, and stage of development—will increase children's exposure to health threats. The impact of poverty on children's health is a critical factor to consider in ascertaining how climate change will be manifest in children. Poor and low-income households have difficulty accessing healthcare and meeting the basic needs that are crucial for healthy child development. In addition, children in poverty are less likely to have access to air conditioning to mitigate the effects of extreme heat. Children living in poverty are also less likely to be able to respond to or escape from extreme weather events.

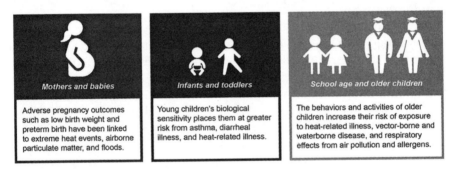

Figure 16.2. *Vulnerability to the Health Impacts of Climate Change at Different Life Stages*

Children's vulnerability to climate change results from distinct exposures, biological sensitivities (developing bodies and immune systems), and limitations to adaptive capacity (dependency on caregivers) at different life stages.

Vulnerability to Climate-Related Health Stressors

Extreme heat events. An increase in the frequency and intensity of extreme heat events will affect children who spend time outdoors or in nonclimate controlled indoor settings. Student athletes and other children who are susceptible to heat-related illnesses when they exercise or play outdoors in hot and humid weather may be poorly acclimated to physical exertion in the heat. Some 9,000 high-school athletes in the United States are treated for exertional heat illness (such as heat stroke and muscle cramps) each year, with the greatest risk among high-school football players. This appears to be a worsening trend. Between 1997 and 2006, emergency department visits for all heat-related illness increased 133 percent, and youth made up almost 50 percent of those cases. From 2000 through 2013, the number of deaths due to heat stroke doubled among U.S. high-school and college football players. Other data show effects of extreme heat on children of all ages, including increases in heat illness, fluid and electrolyte imbalances, and asthma. Children in homes or schools without air conditioning are also more vulnerable during heat events.

Other weather extremes. Climate change is likely to affect the mental health and well-being of children, primarily by increasing exposure to traumatic weather events that result in injury, death, or displacement. In 2003, more than 10 percent of U.S. children from infancy to 18 years of age reported experiencing a disaster (fire, tornado, flood, hurricane, earthquake, etc.) during their lifetimes. Exposures to traumatic events can impact children's capacity to regulate emotions, undermine cognitive development and academic performance, and contribute to posttraumatic stress disorder (PTSD) and other psychiatric disorders (such as depression, anxiety, phobia, and panic). Children's ability to cope with disasters is affected by factors such as socioeconomic status, available support systems, and timeliness of treatment. Negative mental-health effects in children, if untreated, can extend into adulthood.

Degraded air quality. Several factors make children more sensitive to the effects of respiratory hazards, including lung development that continues through adolescence, the size of the child's airways, their level of physical activity, and body weight. Climate change has the potential to affect future ground-level ozone concentrations, particulate matter concentrations, and levels of some aeroallergens. Ground-level ozone and particulate matter are associated with increases in asthma episodes and other adverse respiratory effects in children. Nearly 7 million, or about 9 percent, of children in the United States, suffer from asthma. Asthma accounts for 10 million missed school days each year. Particulate matter, such as dust and emissions from coal-fired electricity generation plants, is also associated with decreases in lung maturation in children.

Changes in climate also contribute to longer, more severe pollen seasons that may be associated with increases in childhood asthma episodes and other allergic illnesses. Children may also be exposed

231

to indoor air pollutants, including both particulate matter originating outdoors and indoor sources, such as tobacco smoke and mold. In addition, high outdoor temperatures may increase the amount of time children spend indoors. Homes, childcare centers, and schools—places where children spend large amounts of their time—are all settings where indoor air quality issues may affect children's health. In communities where these buildings are insufficiently supplied with screens, air conditioning, humidity controls, or pest control, children's health may be at risk.

Waterborne illnesses. Climate change induced increases in heavy rainfall, flooding, and coastal storm events are expected to increase children's risk of gastrointestinal illness from ingestion of or contact with contaminated water. An increased association between heavy rainfall and increased acute gastrointestinal illness has already been observed in children in the United States. Children may be especially vulnerable to recreational exposures to waterborne pathogens, in part because they swallow roughly twice as much water as adults while swimming. In addition, children comprised 40 percent of swimming-related eye and ear infections from the waterborne bacteria *Vibrio alginolyticus* during the period 1997–2006 and 66 percent (between the ages of 1 and 19) of those seeking treatment for illness associated with harmful algal bloom toxins in 2009–2010.

Vector-borne and other infectious diseases. The changes in the distribution of infectious diseases that are expected to result from climate change may introduce new exposures to children. Due to physiological vulnerability or changes in their body's immune system, fetuses, pregnant women, and children are at increased risk of acquiring or having complications from certain infectious diseases, such as listeriosis, dengue fever, and influenza. Children spend more time outdoors than adults, increasing their exposure to mosquito and tick bites that can cause vector-borne diseases that disproportionately affect children, such as La Crosse encephalitis or Lyme disease. Lyme disease is most frequently reported among male children between five and nine years of age, and a disproportionate increasing trend was observed in all children from 1992 to 2006.

Food safety and security. Climate change, including rising levels of atmospheric CO_2, significantly reduces food quality and threatens availability and access for children. Because of the importance of nutrition during certain stages of physical and mental growth and development, the direct effect of the continued rise of CO_2 on reducing food quality will be an increasingly significant issue for children globally. For the United States, disruptions in food production or distribution due to extreme events, such as drought, can increase costs and limit availability or access, particularly for food-insecure households, which include nearly 16 percent of households with children in the United States. Children are also more susceptible to severe infection or complications from *Escherichia coli* infections, such as hemolytic uremic syndrome (HUS).

Vulnerability Related to Life Stage

Prenatal and pregnancy outcomes for mothers and babies. Climate-related exposures may lead to adverse pregnancy and newborn health outcomes, including spontaneous abortion, low birth weight (less than 5.5 pounds), preterm birth (birth before 37 weeks of pregnancy), increased neonatal death, dehydration and associated renal failure, malnutrition, diarrhea, and respiratory disease. Other risk factors that may influence maternal and newborn health include water scarcity, poverty, and population displacement. The rate of preterm births is relatively high in the United States (1 of every 9 infants born), where they contribute substantially to neonatal death and illness. Of the 1.2 million preterm births estimated to occur annually in high-income countries, more than 500 thousand (42% of the total) occur in the United States. Extreme heat events have been associated with adverse birth outcomes, such as low birth weight, preterm birth, and infant mortality, as well as congenital cataracts. Newborns are especially sensitive to ambient temperatures that are too high or too low because their capacity for regulating body temperature is limited.

In addition, exposure of pregnant women to inhaled particulate matter is associated with negative birth outcomes. Incidences of diarrheal diseases and dehydration may increase in extent and severity, which can be associated with adverse effects on pregnancy outcomes and the health of newborns. Floods are associated with an increased risk of maternal exposure to environmental toxins and mold, reduced access to safe food and water, psychological stress, and disrupted healthcare. Other flood-related health outcomes for mothers and babies include maternal risk of anemia (a condition associated with low red blood cell (RBC) counts sometimes caused by low iron intake), eclampsia (a condition that can cause seizures in pregnant women), and spontaneous abortion.

Infants and toddlers. Infants and toddlers are particularly sensitive to air pollutants, extreme heat, and microbial water contamination, which are all affected by climate change. Ozone exposure in young children and exposure to air pollutants and toxins in wildfire smoke are associated with increased asthma risk and other respiratory illnesses. Young children and infants are particularly vulnerable to heat-related illness and death, as their bodies are less able to adapt to heat than are adults. Children under four years of age experience higher hospital admissions for respiratory illnesses during heat waves. Rates of diarrheal illness have been shown to be higher in children under the age of five in the United States, and climate change is expected to increase children's risk of gastrointestinal illness from ingestion or contact with contaminated water.

Older Adults

Older adults (generally defined as persons 65 years of age and older) are vulnerable to the health impacts associated with climate change and weather extremes. The number of older adults in the United States is projected to grow substantially in the coming decades. The nation's older adult population (65 years of age and older) will nearly double in number from 2015 through 2050, from approximately 48 million to 88 million. Of those 88 million older adults, a little under 19 million will be 85 years of age and older. This projected population growth is largely due to the aging of the Baby Boomer generation (an estimated 76 million people born in the United States between 1946 and 1964), along with increases in lifespan and survivorship. Older adults in the United States are not uniform with regard to their climate-related vulnerabilities, but are a diverse group with distinct subpopulations that can be identified not only by age but also by race, educational attainment, socioeconomic status, social support networks, overall physical and mental health, and disability status.

Vulnerability to Climate-Related Health Stressors

The potential climate-change related health impacts for older adults include rising temperatures and heat waves; increased risk of more intense hurricanes (Categories IV and V), floods, droughts, and wildfires; degraded air quality; exposure to infectious diseases; and other climate-related hazards.

Extreme heat events. Older adults exposed to extreme heat can experience multiple adverse effects. In the coming decades, extreme heat events are projected to become more frequent, more intense, and of longer duration, especially in higher latitudes and large metropolitan areas. Between 1979 and 2004, 5,279 deaths were reported in the United States related to heat exposure, with those deaths reported most commonly among adults aged 65 and older. Disease incidence among older adults is expected to increase even in regions with relatively modest temperature changes (as demonstrated by case studies of a 2006 California heat wave). In New York City, extreme high temperatures were associated with an increase in hospital admissions for cardiovascular and respiratory disorders, with the elderly among the most affected. Hospital admissions for respiratory illness were greatest for the elderly, with a 4.7 percent increase per degree Centigrade increase. Future climate-related increases in summertime temperatures may increase the risk of death in older people with chronic conditions, particularly those suffering from congestive heart failure and diabetes. The percentage of older adults with diabetes, which puts individuals at higher risk for heat-related illness and death, has increased from 9.1 percent in 1980 to 19.9 percent in 2009.

Other weather extremes. Hurricanes and other severe weather events lead to physical, mental, or emotional trauma before, during, and after the event. The need to evacuate an area can pose increased health and safety risks for older adults, especially those who are poor or reside in nursing or assisted living facilities (ALF). Moving patients to a sheltering facility is complicated, costly, and time-consuming and requires concurrent transfer of medical records, medications, and medical equipment.

Degraded air quality. Climate change can affect air quality by increasing ground-level ozone, fine particulate matter, aeroallergens, wildfire smoke, and dust. Exposure to ground-level ozone varies with age and can affect lung function and increase emergency department visits and hospital admissions, even for healthy adults. Air pollution can also exacerbate asthma and chronic obstructive pulmonary disease (COPD) and can increase the risk of heart attack in older adults, especially those who are also diabetic or obese.

Vector-borne and waterborne diseases. The changes in the distribution of disease vectors like ticks and mosquitoes that are expected to result from climate change may increase exposures to pathogens in older adult populations. Some vector-borne diseases, notably mosquito-borne West Nile and St. Louis encephalitis viruses, pose a greater health risk among sensitive older adults with already compromised

235

immune systems. Climate change is also expected to increase exposure risk to waterborne pathogens in sources of drinking water and recreational water. Older adults have a higher risk of contracting gastrointestinal illnesses from contaminated drinking and recreational water and suffering severe health outcomes and death.

Interactions with Nonclimate Stressors

Older adults are particularly vulnerable to climate-change related health effects depending on their geographic location and characteristics of their homes, such as the quality of construction and amenities. More than half of the elderly U.S. adult population is concentrated in 170 countries (5% of all U.S. counties), and approximately 20 percent of older Americans live in a county in which a hurricane or tropical storm made landfall over the last decade. For example, Florida is a traditional retirement destination with an older adult population accounting for 16.8 percent of the total in 2010, nearly 4 percentage points higher than the national average. The increasing severity of tropical storms may pose particular risks for older adults in coastal zones. Other geographic risk factors common to older adults are the urban heat island effect, urban sprawl (which affects mobility), characteristics of the built environment, and perceptions of neighborhood safety.

In neighborhoods where safety and crime are a concern, older residents may fear venturing out of their homes, thus increasing their social isolation and risk of health impacts during events such as heat waves. Degraded infrastructure, including the condition of housing and public transportation, is associated with higher numbers of heat-related deaths in older adults. In multistory residential buildings in which residents rely on elevators, electricity loss makes it difficult, if not impossible, for elderly residents and those with disabilities to leave the building to obtain food, medicine, and other needed services. Also, older adults who own air-conditioning units may not utilize them during heat waves due to high operating costs.

Vulnerability related to physiological factors. Older adults are more sensitive to weather-related events due to age-related physiological factors. Elevated risks for cardiovascular deaths related to exposure to extreme heat have been observed in older adults. Generally, poorer physical health conditions, such as long-term chronic illnesses, are exacerbated by climate change. In addition, aging can impair the mechanisms that regulate body temperature, particularly for those taking medications that interfere with regulation of body temperature, including psychotropic medications used to treat a variety of mental illnesses, such as depression, anxiety, and psychosis. Respiratory impairments already experienced by older adults will be exacerbated by increased exposure to outdoor air pollutants (especially ozone and fine particulate matter), aeroallergens, and wildfire smoke—all of which may be exacerbated by climate change.

Vulnerability related to disabilities. Some functional limitations and mobility impairments increase older adults' sensitivity to climate change, particularly extreme events. In 2010, 49.8 percent of older adults (over the age of 65) were reported to have a disability, compared to 16.6 percent of people between the ages of 21 and 64. Dementia occurs at a rate of 5 percent of the U.S. population between the ages of 71 and 79, with an increase to more than 37 percent at the age of 90 and older. Older adults with mobility or cognitive impairments are likely to experience greater vulnerability to health risks due to difficulty responding to, evacuating, and recovering from extreme events.

Occupational Groups

Climate change may increase the prevalence and severity of known occupational hazards and exposures, as well as the emergence of new ones. Outdoor workers are often among the first to be exposed to the effects of climate change. Climate change is expected to affect the health of outdoor workers through increases in ambient temperature, degraded air quality, extreme weather, vector-borne diseases, industrial exposures, and changes in the built environment. Workers affected by climate change include farmers, ranchers, and other agricultural workers; commercial fishermen; construction workers; paramedics, firefighters, and other first responders; and transportation workers. Also, laborers exposed to hot indoor work environments (such as steel mills, dry cleaners, manufacturing facilities, warehouses, and other areas that lack air conditioning) are at risk for extreme heat exposure.

For some groups, such as migrant workers and day laborers, the health effects of climate change can be cumulative, with occupational exposures exacerbated by exposures associated with poorly insulated housing and lack of air conditioning. Workers may also be exposed to adverse occupational and climate-related conditions that the general public may altogether avoid, such as direct exposure to wildfires.

Extreme heat events. Higher temperatures or longer, more frequent periods of heat may result in more cases of heat-related illnesses (for example, heat stroke and heat exhaustion) and fatigue among workers, especially among more physically demanding occupations. Heat stress and fatigue can also result in reduced vigilance, safety lapses, reduced work capacity, and increased risk of injury. Elevated temperatures can increase levels of air pollution, including ground level ozone, resulting in increased worker exposure and subsequent risk of respiratory illness.

Other weather extremes. Some extreme weather events and natural disasters, such as floods, storms, droughts, and wildfires, are becoming more frequent and intense. An increased need for complex emergency responses will expose rescue and recovery workers to physical and psychological hazards. The safety of workers and their ability to recognize and avoid workplace hazards may be impaired by damage to infrastructure and disrupted communication.

From 2000 to 2013, almost 300 U.S. wildfire firefighters were killed while on duty. With the frequency and severity of wildfires projected to increase, more firefighters will be exposed. Common workplace hazards faced on the fire line include being overrun by fire (as happened during the Yarnell Hill Fire in Arizona in 2013, killing 19 firefighters); heat-related illnesses and injuries; smoke inhalation; vehicle-related injuries (including aircraft); slips, trips, and falls; and exposure to particulate matter and other air pollutants in wildfire smoke. In addition, wildland firefighters are at risk of rhabdomyolysis (a breakdown of muscle tissue) that is associated with prolonged and intense physical exertion.

Other workplace exposures to outdoor health hazards. Other climate-related health threats for outdoor workers include increased waterborne and foodborne pathogens, increased duration of aeroallergen exposure with longer pollen seasons, and expanded habitat ranges of disease-carrying vectors that may influence the risk of human exposure to diseases, such as West Nile virus or Lyme disease.

Persons with Disabilities

Disability refers to any condition or impairment of the body or mind that limits a person's ability to do certain activities or restricts a person's participation in normal life activities, such as school, work, or recreation. The term "disability" covers a wide variety and range of functional limitations related to expressive and receptive communication (hearing and speech), vision, cognition, and mobility. These factors, if not anticipated and accommodated before, during, and after extreme events, can result in illness and death. The extent of disability, or its severity, is reflected in the affected person's need for environmental accessibility and accommodations for their impairment(s).

Disability can occur at any age and is not uniformly distributed across populations. Disability varies by gender, race, ethnicity, and geographic location. Approximately 18.7 percent of the U.S. population has a disability. In 2010, the percent of American adults with a disability was approximately 16.6 percent for those between the ages of 18 and 64 and 49.8 percent for persons 65 years of age and older. In 2014, working-age adults with disabilities were substantially less likely to participate in the labor force (30.2%) than people without disabilities (76.2%) and experience more than twice the rate of unemployment (13.9% and 6.0%, respectively).

People with disabilities experience disproportionately higher rates of social risk factors, such as poverty and lower educational attainment, that contribute to poorer health outcomes during extreme events or climate-related emergencies. These factors compound the risks posed by functional impairments and disrupt planning and emergency response. Of the climate-related health risks experienced by people with disabilities, perhaps the most fundamental is their "invisibility" to decision-makers and planners. There has been relatively limited empirical research documenting how people with disabilities fare during or after an extreme event.

An increase in extreme weather can be expected to disproportionately affect populations with disabilities unless emergency planners make provisions to address their functional needs in preparing emergency response plans. In 2005, Hurricane Katrina had a significant and disproportionate impact on people with disabilities. Of the 986 deaths in Louisiana directly attributable to the storm, 103 occurred among individuals in nursing homes, presumably with a disability. Strong social capital and societal connectedness to other people, especially through faith-based organizations, family networks, and work connections, were considered to be key enabling factors that helped people with disabilities to cope before, during, and after the storm. In the aftermath of Hurricane Sandy, the City of New York lost a lawsuit filed by the Brooklyn Center for Independence of the Disabled, with the finding that the city had not adequately prepared to accommodate the social and medical support needs of New York residents with disabilities.

Risk communication is not always designed or delivered in an accessible format or media for individuals who are deaf or have hearing loss, who are blind or have low vision, or those with diminished cognitive skills. Emergency communication and other important notifications (such as a warning to boil contaminated water) simply may not reach persons with disabilities. In addition, persons with disabilities often rely on medical equipment (such as portable oxygen) that requires an uninterrupted source of electricity. Portable oxygen supplies must be evacuated with the patient.

Persons with Chronic Medical Conditions

Preexisting medical conditions present risk factors for increased illness and death associated with climate-related stressors, especially exposure to extreme heat. In some cases, risks are mediated by the physiology of specific medical conditions that may impair responses to heat exposure. In other cases, the risks are related to unintended side effects of medical treatment that may impair body temperature, fluid, or electrolyte balance and thereby increase risks. In general, the prevalence of common chronic medical conditions, including cardiovascular disease, respiratory disease, diabetes, asthma, and obesity, is anticipated to increase over the coming decades, resulting in larger populations at risk of medical complications from climate-change related exposures.

Excess heat exposure has been shown to increase the risk of disease exacerbation or death for people with various medical conditions. Hospital admissions and emergency room visits increase during heat waves for people with diabetes, cardiovascular diseases, respiratory diseases, and psychiatric illnesses. Medical conditions such as Alzheimer disease or mental illnesses can impair judgment and behavioral responses in crisis situations, which can place people with those conditions at greater risk.

Medications used to treat chronic medical conditions are associated with an increased risk of hospitalization, emergency room admission, and in some cases, death from extreme heat. These medicines include drugs used to treat neurologic or psychiatric conditions, such as antipsychotic drugs, anticholinergic agents, anxiolytics (anti-anxiety medicines), and some antidepressants. In addition, drugs used to treat cardiovascular diseases (CVDs), such as diuretics and beta-blockers, may impair resilience to heat stress.

People with chronic medical conditions also can be more vulnerable to interruption in treatment. For example, interrupting treatment for

240

patients with addiction to drugs or alcohol may lead to withdrawal syndromes. Treatment for chronic medical conditions represents a significant proportion of postdisaster medical demands. Communities that are both medically underserved and have a high prevalence of chronic medical conditions can be especially at risk. While most studies have assessed adults, and especially the elderly, with chronic medical conditions, children with medical conditions such as allergic and respiratory diseases are also at greater risk of symptom exacerbation and hospital admission during heat waves.

Measures of Vulnerability and Mapping

Vulnerability associated with exposures to climate-related hazards is closely tied to place. While an understanding of the individual-level factors associated with vulnerability is essential to assessing population risks and considering possible protective measures, understanding how potential exposures overlap with the geographic location of populations of concern is critical for designing and implementing appropriate adaptations. Analytic capabilities provided by mapping tools allow public health and emergency response workers to consider multiple types of vulnerability and how they interact with place. The development of indices that combine different elements of vulnerability and allow visualization of areas and populations experiencing the highest risks is related to improved geographic information systems (GIS) capabilities.

Approaches to Assessing Vulnerability

There are multiple approaches for developing vulnerability indices to identify populations of concern across large areas, such as state or multistate regions, or small areas, such as households within a county or several counties within a state. The Social Vulnerability Index (SVI) developed by the Centers for Disease Control and Prevention (CDC) aggregates U.S. census data to estimate the social vulnerability of census tracts. The SVI provides a measure of overall social vulnerability, in addition to measures of elements that comprise social vulnerability (including socioeconomic status, household composition, race or ethnicity, native language, and infrastructure conditions). Each census tract receives a separate ranking for overall vulnerability and for each of the four elements, which are available at the census-tract level for the entire United States. A similar methodology has been used to develop a vulnerability index for climate-sensitive health outcomes which, in

241

addition to socioeconomic data, incorporates data on climate-related exposures and adaptive capacity.

Application of Vulnerability Indices

GIS—data management systems used to capture, store, manage, retrieve, analyze, and display geographic information—can be used to quantify and visualize factors that contribute to climate-related health risks. By linking together census data, data on the determinants of health (social, environmental, preexisting health conditions), measures of adaptive capacity (such as healthcare access), and climate data, GIS mapping helps identify and position resources for at-risk populations. For instance, heat-related illnesses have been associated with social isolation in older adults, which can be mapped by combining data for persons living alone (determinants of health data), distribution of people 65 years of age and older (census data), and frequency and severity of heat waves (climate data).

Vulnerability mapping can also enhance emergency and disaster risk management. Vulnerability mapping conducted at finer spatial resolution (for example, census tracts or census blocks) allows public health departments to target vulnerable communities for emergency preparedness, response, recovery, and mitigation. Geographic characteristics of vulnerability can be used to determine where to position emergency medical and social response resources that are most needed before, during, and after climate-change related events.

Emergency response agencies can apply lessons learned by mapping prior events. For example, vulnerability mapping has been used to assess how social disparities affected the geography of recovery in New Orleans following Hurricane Katrina. Maps displaying the intersection of social vulnerability (low, medium, high scores) and flood inundation (none, low, medium, high levels) showed that while the physical manifestation of the disaster had few race or class distinctions, the social vulnerability of communities influenced both pre-impact responses, such as evacuation and postevent recovery. As climate change increases the probability of more frequent or more severe extreme weather events, vulnerability mapping is an important tool for preparing for and responding to health threats.

Chapter 17

Vector-Borne Diseases

Vector-borne diseases are illnesses that are transmitted by vectors, which include mosquitoes, ticks, and fleas. These vectors can carry infectious pathogens, such as viruses, bacteria, and protozoa, which can be transferred from one host (carrier) to another. In the United States, there are currently 14 vector-borne diseases that are of national public health concern. These diseases account for a significant number of human illnesses and deaths each year and are required to be reported to the National Notifiable Diseases Surveillance System (NNDSS) at the Centers for Disease Control and Prevention (CDC). In 2013, state and local health departments reported 51,258 vector-borne disease cases to the CDC (see Table 17.1).

Table 17.1. Summary of Reported Case Counts of Notifiable Vector-Borne Diseases in the United States.

Diseases	2013 Reported Cases	Median (range) 2004–2013 (b)
Tick-Borne		
Lyme disease	36,307	30,495 (19,804–38,468)
Spotted Fever Rickettsia	3,359	2,255 (1,713–4,470)
Anaplasmosis/Ehrlichiosis	4,551	2,187 (875–4,551)
Babesiosis (b)	1,792	1,128 (940–1,792)
Tularemia	203	136 (93–203)

This chapter includes text excerpted from "Vector-Borne Diseases," GlobalChange.gov, U.S. Global Change Research Program (USGCRP), April 4, 2016.

Table 17.1. Continued

Diseases	2013 Reported Cases	Median (range) 2004–2013 (b)
Powassan	15	7 (1–16)
Mosquito-Borne		
West Nile virus	2,469	1,913 (712–5,673)
Malaria	1,594	1,484 (1,255–1,773)
Dengue (b,c)	843	624 (254–843)
California serogroup viruses	112	78 (55–137)
Eastern equine encephalitis	8	7 (4–21)
St. Louis encephalitis	1	10 (1–13)
Flea-Borne		
Plague	4	4 (2–17)

a) State Health Departments are required by law to report regular, frequent, and timely information about individual cases to the CDC in order to assist in the prevention and control of diseases. Case counts are summarized based on annual reports of nationally notifiable infectious diseases.

b) Babesiosis and dengue were added to the list of nationally notifiable diseases in 2011 and 2009, respectively. Median and range values encompass cases reported from 2011 to 2013 for babesiosis and from 2010 to 2013 for dengue.

c) Primarily acquired outside of the United States and based on travel-related exposures.

The seasonality, distribution, and prevalence of vector-borne diseases are influenced significantly by climate factors, primarily high and low temperature extremes and precipitation patterns. Climate change can result in modified weather patterns and an increase in extreme events that can affect disease outbreaks by altering biological variables, such as vector population size and density, vector survival rates, the relative abundance of disease-carrying animal (zoonotic) reservoir hosts, and pathogen reproduction rates. Collectively, these changes may contribute to an increase in the risk of the pathogen being carried to humans.

Climate change is likely to have both short- and long-term effects on vector-borne disease transmission and infection patterns, affecting both seasonal risk and broad geographic changes in disease occurrence over decades. However, models for predicting the effects of climate change on vector-borne diseases are subject to a high degree of uncertainty, largely due to two factors: 1. Vector-borne diseases are maintained in nature in complex transmission cycles that involve vectors, other intermediate zoonotic hosts, and humans; and 2. There are a number of other significant social and environmental drivers of vector-borne disease transmission in addition to climate change. For example, while climate variability and climate change both alter the transmission of vector-borne diseases, they will likely interact with many other factors, including how pathogens adapt and change, the availability of hosts, changing ecosystems and land use, demographics, human behavior, and adaptive capacity. These complex interactions make it difficult to predict the effects of climate change on vector-borne diseases.

The risk of introducing exotic pathogens and vectors not currently present in the United States, while likely to occur, is similarly difficult to project quantitatively. In recent years, several important vector-borne pathogens have been introduced or reintroduced into the United States. These include West Nile virus (WNV), dengue virus, and chikungunya virus. In the case of the 2009 dengue outbreak in southern Florida, climate change was not responsible for the reintroduction of the virus in this area, which arrived via infected travelers from disease-endemic regions of the Caribbean. In fact, vector populations capable of transmitting dengue have been present for many years throughout much of the southern United States, including Florida. Climate change has the potential to increase human exposure risk or disease transmission following shifts in extended spring and summer seasons as dengue becomes more established in the United States. Climate change effects, however, are difficult to quantify due to the adaptive capacity of a population that may reduce exposure to vector-borne pathogens through such means as air conditioning, screens on windows, vector control, and public health practices.

This chapter presents case studies of Lyme disease and West Nile virus infection in relation to weather and climate. Although ticks and mosquitoes transmit multiple infectious pathogens to humans in the United States, Lyme disease and West Nile virus infection are the most commonly reported tick-borne and mosquito-borne diseases in this country (see above Table 17.1). In addition, a substantial number of studies have been conducted to elucidate the role of climate in the transmission of these infectious pathogens. These broad findings, together with the areas of uncertainty from these case studies, are generalizable to other vector-borne diseases.

245

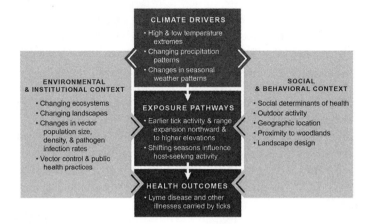

Figure 17.1. *Climate Change and Health—Lyme Disease*

This conceptual diagram illustrates the key pathways by which climate change influences human exposure to Lyme disease and the potential resulting health outcomes (center boxes). These exposure pathways exist within the context of other factors that positively or negatively influence health outcomes. Key factors that influence vulnerability for individuals are shown in the right box, and include social determinants of health and behavioral choices. Key factors that influence vulnerability at larger scales, such as natural and built environments, governance and management, and institutions, are shown in the left box. All of these influencing factors can affect an individual's or a community's vulnerability through changes in exposure, sensitivity, and adaptive capacity and may also be affected by climate change.

Lyme Disease
State of the Science

Lyme disease is a tick-borne bacterial disease that is endemic (commonly found) in parts of North America, Europe, and Asia. In the United States, Lyme disease is caused by the bacterium *Borrelia burgdorferi* sensu stricto (*B. burgdorferi*; one of the spiral-shaped bacteria known as "spirochetes") and is the most commonly reported vector-borne illness. It is primarily transmitted to humans in the eastern United States by the tick species Ixodes scapularis (formerly I. dammini), known as "blacklegged ticks" or "deer ticks," and in the far western United States by I. pacificus, commonly known as "western blacklegged ticks." Illness in humans typically presents with fever, headache, fatigue, and a characteristic skin rash called "erythema migrans." If left untreated, infection can spread to joints, the heart, and the nervous system. Since 1991, when standardized surveillance and reporting of Lyme disease began in the United States, case counts have increased steadily. Since 2007, more than 25,000 Lyme disease cases have been reported annually. The geographic distribution of the disease is limited to specific regions in the United States, transmission occurs seasonally, and year-to-year variation in case counts and in seasonal onset is considerable. Each of these observations suggest that geographic location and seasonal climate variability may play a significant role in determining when and where Lyme disease cases are most likely to occur.

Although the reported incidence of Lyme disease is greater in the eastern United States compared with the westernmost United States, in both geographical regions, nymphs (small immature ticks) are believed to be the life stage that is most significant in pathogen transmission from infected hosts (primarily rodents) to humans. Throughout the United States, the majority of human cases report onset of clinical signs of infection during the months of June, July, and August. The summer is a period of parallel increased activity for both blacklegged and western blacklegged ticks in the nymphal life stage (the more infectious stage) and for human recreational activity outdoors.

Infection rates in humans vary significantly from year to year. From 1992 to 2006, variation in case counts of Lyme disease was as high as 57 percent from one year to the next. Likewise, the precise week of onset of Lyme disease cases across states in the eastern United States, where Lyme disease is endemic, differed by as much as 10 weeks from 1992 to 2007. Much of this variation in timing of disease onset can be explained by geographic region (cases occurred earlier in warmer states in the mid-Atlantic region when compared with cooler states in the North); however, the annual variation of disease onset within regions was notable and linked to winter and spring climate variability.

The geographic and seasonal distributions of Lyme disease case occurrence are driven, in part, by the life cycle of vector ticks. Humans are only exposed to Lyme disease spirochetes (*B. burgdorferi*) in locations where both the vector tick populations and the infection-causing spirochetes are present. Within these locations, the potential for contracting Lyme disease depends on three key factors: 1. Tick vector abundance (the density of host-seeking nymphs being particularly important), 2. Prevalence of *B. burgdorferi* infection in ticks (the prevalence in nymphs being particularly important), and 3. Contact frequency between infected ticks and humans. To varying degrees, climate change can affect all three of these factors.

Aside from short periods of time when they are feeding on hosts (less than three weeks of their two- to three-year life cycle), ticks spend most of their lives off of hosts in various natural landscapes (such as woodlands or grasslands) where weather factors, including temperature, precipitation, and humidity, affect their survival and host-seeking behavior. In general, both low and high temperatures increase tick mortality rates, although increasing humidity can increase their ability to tolerate higher temperatures. Within areas where tick vector populations are present, some studies have demonstrated an association among temperature, humidity, and tick abundance. Factors that are less immediately dependent on climate (for example, landscape and the relative proportions within a community of zoonotic hosts that carry or do not carry Lyme disease-causing bacteria) may be more important in smaller geographic areas. Temperature and humidity also influence the timing of host-seeking activity and which seasons are of highest risk to the public.

In summary, weather-related variables can determine geographic distributions of ticks and seasonal activity patterns. However, the importance of these weather variables in Lyme disease transmission to humans compared with other important predictors is likely scale-dependent. In general, across the entire country, climate-related variables often play a significant role in determining the occurrence of tick vectors and Lyme disease incidence in the United States (for example, Lyme disease vectors are absent in the arid Intermountain West where climate conditions are not suitable for tick survival). However, within areas where conditions are suitable for tick survival, other variables (for example, landscape and the relative proportions within a community of zoonotic hosts that carry or do not carry Lyme disease-causing bacteria) are more important for determining tick abundance, infection rates in ticks, and ultimately human infection rates.

Observed Trends and Measures of Human Risk
Geographic Distribution of Ticks

Because the presence of tick vectors is required for _B. burgdorferi_ transmission to humans, information on where vector tick species live provides basic information on where Lyme disease risk occurs. Minimum temperature appears to be a key variable in defining the geographic distribution of blacklegged ticks. Low minimum temperatures in winter may lead to environmental conditions that are unsuitable for tick population survival. The probability of a given geographic area being suitable for tick populations increases as minimum temperature rises. In the case of the observed northward range expansion of blacklegged ticks into Canada, higher temperatures appear to be a key factor affecting where, and how fast, ticks are colonizing new localities.

Maximum temperatures also significantly affect where blacklegged ticks live. Higher temperatures increase tick development and hatching rates, but reduce tick survival and egg-laying (reproduction) success.

Declines in rainfall amount and humidity are also important in limiting the geographic distribution of blacklegged ticks. Ticks are more likely to reside in moisture areas because increased humidity can increase tick survival.

Geographic Distribution of Infected Ticks

Climate variables have been shown to be strong predictors of geographic locations in which blacklegged ticks reside, but they are less important for determining how many nymphs live in a given area or what proportion of those ticks is infected. The presence of uninfected nymphs and infected nymphs can vary widely over small geographic areas experiencing similar temperature and humidity conditions, which supports the hypothesis that factors other than weather play a significant role in determining nymph survival and infection rates. Additional studies that modeled nymphal density within small portions of the blacklegged tick range (north-central states and Hudson River Valley, NY) and studies that included climate and other nonbiological variables indicate only a weak relationship to nymphal density. Nonetheless, climate variables can be used to model nymphal density in some instances. For example, in a single county in northern coastal California with strong climate gradients, warmer areas with less variation between maximum and minimum monthly water vapor in the air were characteristic of areas with elevated concentrations of infected nymphs. However, it is likely that differences in animal host community structure, which vary with climatic conditions (for example, relative abundances of hosts that carry or do not carry Lyme disease-causing bacteria), influenced the concentration of infected nymphs.

Geographic Distribution of Lyme Disease

Though there are links between climate and tick distribution, studies that look for links between weather and geographical differences in human infection rates do not show a clear or consistent link between temperature and Lyme disease incidence.

Annual and Seasonal Variation in Lyme Disease

Temperature and precipitation both influence the host-seeking activity of ticks, which may result in year-to-year variation in the number of new Lyme disease cases and the timing of the season in which Lyme disease infections occur. However, identified associations between precipitation and Lyme disease incidence, or temperature and Lyme disease incidence, are limited or weak. Overall, the association between summer moisture and Lyme disease infection rates in humans remains inconsistent across studies.

The peak period when ticks are seeking hosts starts earlier in the warmer, more southern, states than in northern states. Correspondingly, the onset of human Lyme disease cases occurs earlier as the growing degree days (a measurement of temperature thresholds that must be met for biological processes to occur) increases, yet, the timing of the end of the Lyme disease season does not appear to be determined by weather-related variables. Rather, the number of potential carriers (for example, deer, birds, and humans) likely influences the timing of the end of the Lyme disease season.

The effects of temperature and humidity or precipitation on the seasonal activity patterns of nymphal western blacklegged ticks are more certain than the impacts of these factors on the timing of Lyme disease case occurrence. Peak nymphal activity is generally reached earlier in hotter and drier areas but lasts for shorter durations. Host-seeking activity ceases earlier in the season in cooler and more humid conditions. The density of nymphal western blacklegged ticks in north-coastal California consistently begins to decline when average daily maximum temperatures are between 70°F (21°C) and 73.5°F (23°C), and when average maximum daily relative humidity decreases below 83 to 85 percent.

Projected Impacts

Warmer winter and spring temperatures are projected to lead to earlier annual onset of Lyme disease cases in the eastern United States and in an earlier onset of nymphal host-seeking behavior. Limited research shows that the geographic distribution of blacklegged ticks is expected to expand to higher latitudes and elevations in the future and retract in the southern United States. Declines in subfreezing temperatures at higher latitudes may be responsible for improved survival of ticks. In many woodlands, ticks can find refuge from far-subzero winter air temperatures in the surface layers of the soil. However, a possibly important impact of climate change will be acceleration of the tick life cycles due to higher temperatures during the spring, summer, and autumn, which would increase the likelihood that ticks survive to reproduce. This prediction is consistent with recent observations of the spread of I. scapularis in Canada.

To accurately project the changes in Lyme disease risk in humans based on climate variability, long-term data collection on tick vector abundance and human infection case counts are needed to better understand the relationships between changing climate conditions, tick vector abundance, and Lyme disease case occurrence.

West Nile Virus
State of the Science

West Nile virus is the leading cause of mosquito-borne disease in the United States. From 1999 to 2013, a total of 39,557 cases of WNV disease were reported in the United States. Annual variation is substantial, both in terms of case counts and the geographic distribution of cases of human infection. Since the late summer of 1999, when an outbreak of WNV first occurred in New York City, human WNV cases have occurred in the United States every year. After the introduction of the virus to the United States, WNV spread westward, and by 2004, WNV activity was reported throughout the contiguous United States. Annual human WNV incidence remained stable through 2007, decreased substantially through 2011, and increased again in 2012, raising questions about the factors driving year-to-year variation in disease transmission. The locations of annual WNV outbreaks vary, but several states have reported consistently high rates of disease over the years, including Arizona, California, Colorado, Idaho, Illinois, Louisiana, New York, North Dakota, South Dakota, and Texas.

The majority (70 to 80%) of people infected with WNV do not show symptoms of the disease. Of those infected, 20 to 30 percent develop acute systemic febrile illness, which may include headache, myalgias (muscle pains), rash, or gastrointestinal symptoms; fewer than 1 percent experience neuroinvasive disease, which may include meningitis (inflammation around the brain and spinal cord), encephalitis (inflammation of the brain), or myelitis (inflammation of the spinal cord). Because most infected persons are asymptomatic (showing no symptoms), there is significant under-reporting of cases. More than three million people were estimated to be infected with WNV in the United States from 1999 to 2010, resulting in about 780,000 illnesses. However, only about 30,700 cases were reported during the same time span.

West Nile virus is maintained in transmission cycles between birds (the natural hosts of the virus) and mosquitoes (see Figure 17.2). The number of birds and mosquitoes infected with WNV increases as mosquitoes pass the virus from bird to bird, starting in late winter or spring. Human infections can occur from a bite of a mosquito that has previously bitten an infected bird. Humans do not pass on the virus to biting mosquitoes because they do not have sufficient concentrations of the virus in their bloodstreams. In rare instances, WNV can be transmitted through blood transfusions or organ transplants. Peak transmission of WNV to humans in the United States typically occurs between June and September, coinciding with the summer season when mosquitoes are most active and temperatures are highest.

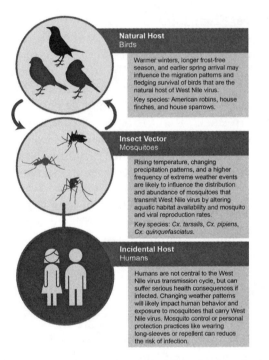

Figure 17.2. *Climate Impacts on West Nile Virus Transmission*

Observed Impacts and Indicators

Mosquito vectors and bird hosts are required for WNV to persist, and the dynamics of both are strongly affected by climate in a number of ways. Geographical variation in average climate constrains the ranges of both vectors and hosts, while shorter-term climate variability affects many aspects of vector and host population dynamics. Unlike ticks, mosquitoes have short life cycles and respond more quickly to climate drivers over relatively short timescales of days to weeks. Impacts on bird abundance are often realized over longer timescales of months to years due to impacts on annual reproduction and migration cycles.

West Nile virus has been detected in 65 mosquito species and more than 300 bird species in the United States; although, only a relatively small number of these species contribute substantially to human infections. Three Culex (Cx.) mosquito species are the primary vectors of the virus in different regions of the continental United States, and differences in their preferred breeding habitats mean that climate change will likely impact human WNV disease risk differently across these regions. Bird species that contribute to WNV transmission include those that develop sufficient viral concentrations in their blood to transmit the virus to feeding mosquitoes. As with mosquitoes, the bird species involved in the transmission cycle are likely to respond differently to climate change, increasing the complexity of projecting future WNV risk.

Impacts of Climate and Weather

Climate, or the long-term average weather, is important for defining WNV's transmission range limits because extreme conditions—too cold, hot, wet, or dry—can alter mosquito and bird habitat availability, increase mortality in mosquitoes or birds, and/or disrupt viral transmission. WNV is an invasive pathogen that was first detected in the United States just over 15 years ago, which is long enough to observe responses of WNV to key weather variables but not long enough to observe responses to climate change trends.

Climate change may influence mosquito survival rates through changes in season length, although mosquitoes are also able to adapt to changing conditions. For example, mosquitoes that transmit WNV are limited to latitudes and altitudes where winters are short enough for them to survive. However, newly emerged adult female mosquitoes have some ability to survive cold temperatures by entering a reproductive arrest called "diapause" as temperatures begin to cool and days grow shorter in late summer. These females will not seek a blood meal until temperatures begin to warm the following year. Even during diapause, very harsh winters may reduce mosquito populations, as temperatures near freezing have been shown to kill diapausing Cx. tarsalis.

During the warmer parts of the year, Culex mosquitoes must have an aquatic habitat available on a nearly continuous basis because their eggs hatch within a few days after they are laid and need moisture to remain viable. The breeding habitats of WNV vectors vary by species, ranging from fresh, sunlit water found in irrigated crops and wetlands preferred by Cx. tarsalis to stagnant, organically enriched water sources, such as urban storm drains, unmaintained swimming pools, or backyard containers, used by Cx. pipiens and Cx. quinquefasciatus.

West Nile virus has become endemic within a wide range of climates in the United States, but there is substantial geographic variation in the intensity of virus transmission. Part of this geographic variation can be attributed to the abundance and distributions of suitable bird hosts. Important hosts, such as robins, migrate annually between summer breeding grounds and winter foraging areas. Migrating birds have shown potential as a vehicle for long-range virus movement. Although the timing of migration is driven by climate, the impact of climate change-driven migration changes on WNV transmission have not yet been documented by scientists. Climate change has already begun to cause shifts in bird breeding and migration patterns, but it is unknown how these changes may affect WNV transmission.

Temperature is the most studied climate driver of the dynamics of WNV transmission. It is clear that warm temperatures accelerate virtually all of the biological processes that affect transmission: accelerating the mosquito life cycle, increasing the mosquito biting rates that determine the frequency of contact between mosquitoes and hosts, and increasing viral replication rates inside the mosquito that decrease the time needed for a blood-fed mosquito to be able to pass on the virus. These relationships between increasing temperatures and the biological processes that affect WNV transmission suggest a subsequent increase in risk of human disease. However, results from models have suggested that extreme high temperatures combined with decreased precipitation may decrease mosquito populations.

Precipitation can create aquatic breeding sites for WNV vectors, and in some areas, snowpack increases the amount of stored water available for urban or agricultural systems, which provide important habitat for WNV vectors; although, effects depend on human water management decisions and vary spatially. Droughts have been associated with increased WNV activity, but the association between decreased precipitation and WNV depends on location and the particular sequence of drought and wetting that precedes the WNV transmission season.

The impact of year-to-year changes in precipitation on mosquito populations varies among the regions of the United States and is affected by the typical climate of the area, as well as other nonclimate factors, such as land use or water infrastructure and management practices. In the northern Great Plains—a hotspot for WNV activity—increased precipitation has been shown to lead to higher Cx. tarsalis abundance a few weeks later. In contrast, in the typically wet Pacific Northwest, weekly precipitation was found to be unrelated to subsequent mosquito abundance. In urban areas, larvae (aquatic immature mosquitoes) may be washed out of their underground breeding habitats by heavy rainfall events, making drier conditions more favorable for WNV transmission. In rural areas or drier regions, increased precipitation or agricultural irrigation may provide the moisture necessary for the development of breeding habitats.

Impacts of Long-Term Climate Trends

The relatively short period of WNV's transmission in the United States prevents direct observation of the impacts of long-term climate trends on WNV incidence. However, despite the short history of WNV in the United States, there are some lessons to be learned from other mosquito-borne diseases with longer histories in the United States.

Western equine encephalomyelitis virus (WEEV) and St. Louis encephalitis virus (SLEV) were first identified in the 1930s and have been circulating in the United States since that time. As with WNV, both viruses are transmitted primarily by Culex mosquitoes and are climate-sensitive. WEEV outbreaks were associated with wet springs followed by warm summers. Outbreaks of SLEV were associated with hot, dry periods when urban mosquito production increased due to stagnation of water in underground systems or when cycles of drought and wetting set up more complex transmission dynamics.

Despite climatic warming that would be expected to favor increased WEEV and SLEV transmission, both viruses have had sharply diminished incidence during the past 30 to 40 years. Although the exact reason for this decline is unknown, it is likely a result of nonclimate factors, such as changes in human behavior or undetected aspects of viral evolution. Several other mosquito-borne pathogens, such as chikungunya and dengue, have grown in importance as global health threats during recent decades; however, a link to climate-change induced disease expansion in the United States has not yet been confirmed. These examples demonstrate the variable impact that climate change can have on different mosquito-borne diseases and help to explain why the direction of future trends in risk for WNV remain unclear.

Projected Impacts

Given West Nile virus' relatively short history in the United States, the described geographic variation in climate responses, and the complexity of transmission cycles, projecting the future distribution of WNV under climate change remains a challenge. Despite the growing body of work examining the connections between WNV and weather, climate-based seasonal forecasts of WNV outbreak risk are not yet available at a national scale. Forecasting the annual presence of WNV disease on the basis of climate and other ecological factors has been attempted for U.S. counties, with general agreement between modeled expectations and observed data, but more quantitative predictions of disease incidence or the risk for human exposure are needed.

Longer-term projections of WNV under climate change scenarios are also rare. WNV is projected to increase in much of the northern and southeastern United States due to rising temperatures and declining precipitation, respectively, with the potential for decreased occurrence across the central United States. Future projections show that the season when mosquitoes are most abundant will begin earlier and end later, possibly resulting in fewer mosquitoes in mid-summer in southern locations where extreme heat is predicted to coincide with decreased summer precipitation.

Populations of Concern

Climate change will influence human vulnerability to vector-borne disease by influencing the seasonality and the location of exposures to pathogens and vectors. These impacts may influence future disease patterns; certain vector-borne diseases may emerge in areas where they had previously not been observed and other diseases may become less common in areas where they had previously been very common. As such, some segments of the U.S. population may be disproportionately affected by, or exposed to, vector-borne diseases in response to climate change.

In addition to climate factors, multiple nonclimate factors also influence human exposure to vector-borne pathogens. Some of these include factors from an environmental or institutional context (see Figure 17.1), such as pathogen adaptation and change, changes in vector and host population and composition, changes in pathogen infection rates, and vector control or other public health practices (pesticide applications, integrated vector management, vaccines, and other disease interventions). Other nonclimate factors that influence vulnerability to vector-borne disease include those from a social and behavioral context, such as outdoor activity, occupation, landscape design, proximity to vector habitat, and personal protective behaviors (applying repellents before spending time in tick habitat, performing tick checks, and bathing after being outdoors). For Lyme disease, behavioral factors, especially the number of hours spent working or playing outdoors in tick habitat, as well as proximity to dense shrubbery, can increase exposure to the ticks that transmit the bacteria that causes Lyme disease. For example, outdoor workers in the northeastern United States are at higher risk for contact with blacklegged ticks and, therefore, are at a greater risk for contracting Lyme disease. If outdoor workers are working in areas where there are infected mosquitoes, occupational exposures can also occur for WNV.

Individual characteristics, such as age, gender, and immune function, may also affect vulnerability by influencing susceptibility to infection. Lyme disease is more frequently reported in children between 5 and 9 years of age and in adults between the ages of 55 and 59, and advanced age and being male contribute to a higher risk for severe WNV infections.

The impacts of climate change on human vulnerability to vector-borne disease may be minimized by individual- or community-level adaptive capacity, or the ability to reduce the potential exposures that may be caused by climate change. For example, socioeconomic status and domestic protective barriers, such as screens on windows and doors, can limit exposures to vector-borne pathogens. From 1980 to 1999, the infected mosquito counts in Laredo, Texas, were significantly higher than in 3 adjoining Mexican states—yet, while there were only 64 cases of dengue fever reported in Texas, more than 62,000 dengue fever cases were reported in the Mexican states. In Texas, socioeconomic factors and adaptive measures, including houses with air conditioning and intact screens, contributed to the significantly lower dengue incidence by reducing human–mosquito contact. The adaptive capacity of a population may augment or limit the impacts of climate change to human vulnerability for vector-borne disease.

Climate factors are useful benchmarks to indicate seasonal risk and broad geographic changes in disease occurrence over decades. However, human vulnerability to vector-borne disease is more holistically evaluated by examining climate factors with nonclimate factors (environmental or institutional context, social and behavioral context, and individual characteristics). Ultimately, a community's capacity to adapt to both the climate and nonclimate factors will affect population vulnerability to vector-borne disease.

Emerging Issues

Some vector-borne diseases may be introduced or become reestablished in the United States by a variety of mechanisms. In conjunction

257

with trade and travel, climate change may contribute by creating habitats suitable for the establishment of disease-carrying vectors or for locally sustained transmission of vector-borne pathogens. Examples of emerging vector-borne diseases in the United States include the West Nile virus, recent outbreaks of locally acquired dengue in Florida and southern Texas, and chikungunya cases in the Caribbean and southern Florida, all of which have raised public health concern about emergence and reemergence of these mosquito-borne diseases in the United States. Collecting data on the spread of disease-causing insect vectors and the viruses that cause dengue and chikungunya is critical to understanding and predicting the threat of emergence or reemergence of these diseases. Understanding the role of climate change in disease emergence and reemergence would also require additional research.

Chapter 18

Water-Related Illness

Across most of the United States, climate change is expected to affect fresh and marine water resources in ways that will increase people's exposure to water-related contaminants that cause illness. Water-related illnesses include waterborne diseases caused by pathogens, such as bacteria, viruses, and protozoa. Water-related illnesses are also caused by toxins produced by certain harmful algae and cyanobacteria (also known as "blue-green algae") and by chemicals introduced into the environment by human activities. Exposure occurs through ingestion, inhalation, or direct contact with contaminated drinking or recreational water and through consumption of fish and shellfish.

Factors related to climate change—including temperature, precipitation and related runoff, hurricanes, and storm surge—affect the growth, survival, spread, and virulence or toxicity of agents (causes) of water-related illness. Heavy downpours are already on the rise and increases in the frequency and intensity of extreme precipitation events are projected for all U.S. regions. Projections of temperature; precipitation; extreme events, such as flooding and drought; and other climate factors vary by region of the United States, and thus, the extent of climate-health impacts will also vary by region.

Waterborne pathogens are estimated to cause 8.5 to 12 percent of acute gastrointestinal illness cases in the United States, affecting

This chapter includes text excerpted from "Water-Related Illness," GlobalChange.gov, U.S. Global Change Research Program (USGCRP), April 4, 2016.

between 12 and 19 million people annually. 8 pathogens, which are all affected to some degree by climate, account for approximately 97 percent of all suspected waterborne illnesses in the United States: the enteric viruses norovirus, rotavirus, and adenovirus; the bacteria *Campylobacter jejuni*, *Escherichia coli* O157: H7 and *Salmonella enterica*; and the protozoa *Cryptosporidium* and *Giardia*.

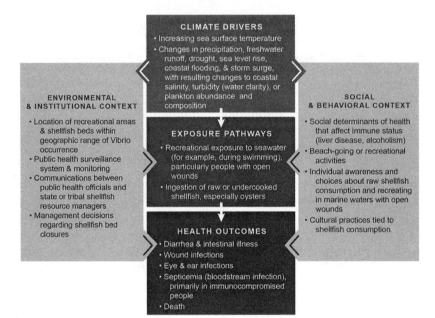

Figure 18.1. *Climate Change and Health–Vibrio*

This conceptual diagram for an example of infection by Vibrio species (V. vulnificus, V. parahaemolyticus, or V. alginolyticus) illustrates the key pathways by which humans are exposed to health threats from climate drivers. These climate drivers create more favorable growing conditions for these naturally occurring pathogens in coastal environments through their effects on coastal salinity, turbidity (water clarity), or plankton abundance and composition. Longer seasons for growth and expanding geographic range of occurrence increase the risk of exposure to Vibrio, which can result in various potential health outcomes (center boxes). These exposure pathways exist within the context of other factors that positively or negatively influence health outcomes (gray side boxes). Key factors that influence vulnerability for individuals are shown in the right box and include social determinants of health and behavioral choices. Key factors that influence vulnerability at larger scales, such as natural and built environments, governance and management, and institutions, are shown in the left box. All of these influencing factors can affect an individual's or a community's vulnerability through changes in exposure, sensitivity, and adaptive capacity and may also be affected by climate change.

Specific health outcomes are determined by different exposure pathways and multiple other social and behavioral factors, some of which are also affected by climate (see Figure 18.1). Most research to date has focused on understanding how climate drivers affect physical and ecological processes that act as key exposure pathways for pathogens and toxins, as shown by the arrow moving from the top to the middle box in figure 18.1. There is currently less information and fewer methods with which to measure actual human exposure and incidence of illness based on those physical and ecological metrics (arrow moving from middle to bottom box in Figure 18.1). Thus, it is often not possible to quantitatively project future health outcomes from water-related illnesses under climate change (bottom box in Figure 18.1).

This chapter covers health risks associated with changes in natural marine, coastal, and freshwater systems and water infrastructure for drinking water, wastewater, and stormwater. This chapter also includes fish and shellfish illnesses associated with the waters in which they grow and which are affected by the same climate factors that affect drinking and recreational waters. The framing of this chapter addresses sources of contaminations, exposure pathways, and health outcomes when available. Based on the available data and research, many of the examples are regionally focused and make evident that the impact of climate change on water-related illness is inherently regional. Table 18.1 lists various health outcomes that can result from exposure to agents of water-related illness as well as key climate-related changes affecting their occurrence.

Whether or not illness result from exposure to contaminated water, fish, or shellfish is dependent on a complex set of factors, including human behavior and social determinants of health that may affect a person's exposure, sensitivity, and adaptive capacity (Figure 18.1). Water resource, public health, and environmental agencies in the United States provide many public health safeguards to reduce the risk of exposure and illness even if water becomes contaminated. These include water quality monitoring, drinking water treatment standards and practices, beach closures, and issuing advisories for boiling drinking water and harvesting shellfish.

Many water-related illnesses are either undiagnosed or unreported, and therefore, the total incidence of waterborne disease is underestimated. On average, illnesses from pathogens associated with water are thought to be underestimated by as much as 43-fold and may be underestimated by up to 143 times for certain Vibrio species.

Table 18.1. Climate Sensitive Agents of Water-Related Illness

Pathogen or Toxin Producer	Exposure Pathway	Selected Health Outcomes and Symptoms	Major Climate Correlation or Driver (Strongest Drivers Listed First)
Algae: Toxigenic marine species of *Alexandrium*, *Pseudo-nitzschia*, *Dinophysis*, *Gambierdiscus*; *Karenia brevis*	Shellfish Fish Recreational waters (aerosolized toxins)	Gastrointestinal and neurologic illness caused by shellfish poisoning (paralytic, amnesic, diarrhetic, neurotoxic) or fish poisoning (ciguatera). Asthma exacerbations, eye irritations caused by contact with aerosolized toxins (K. brevis).	Temperature (increased water temperature), ocean surface currents, ocean acidification, hurricanes (*Gambierdiscus spp.* and *K. brevis*)
Cyanobacteria (multiple freshwater species producing toxins including microcystin)	Drinking water Recreational waters	Liver and kidney damage, gastroenteritis (diarrhea and vomiting), neurological disorders, and respiratory arrest.	Temperature, precipitation patterns
Enteric bacteria and protozoan parasites: *Salmonella enterica*; *Campylobacter* species; Toxigenic *Escherichia coli*; *Cryptosporidium*; *Giardia*	Drinking water Recreational waters Shellfish	Enteric pathogens generally cause gastroenteritis. Some cases may be severe and may be associated with long-term and recurring effects.	Temperature (air and water; both increase and decrease), heavy precipitation, and flooding
Enteric viruses: enteroviruses; rotaviruses; noroviruses; hepatitis A and E	Drinking water Recreational waters Shellfish	Most cases result in gastrointestinal illness. Severe outcomes may include paralysis and infection of the heart or other organs.	Heavy precipitation, flooding, and temperature (air and water; both increase and decrease)

Table 18.1. Continued

Pathogen or Toxin Producer	Exposure Pathway	Selected Health Outcomes and Symptoms	Major Climate Correlation or Driver (Strongest Drivers Listed First)
Leptospira and *Leptonemabacteria*	Recreational waters	Mild to severe flu-like illness (with or without fever) to severe cases of meningitis, kidney, and liver failure.	Flooding, temperature (increased water temperature), heavy precipitation
Vibrio bacteria species	Recreational waters Shellfish	Varies by species but include gastroenteritis (*V. parahaemolyticus*, *V. cholerae*), septicemia (bloodstream infection) through ingestion or wounds (*V. vulnificus*), skin, eye, and ear infections (*V. alginolyticus*).	Temperature (increased water temperature), sea level rise, precipitation patterns (as it affects coastal salinity)

Sources of Water-Related Contaminants

The primary sources of water contamination are human and animal waste and agricultural activities, including the use of fertilizers. Runoff and flooding resulting from expected increases in extreme precipitation, hurricane rainfall, and storm surge may increase risks of contamination. Contamination occurs when agents of water-related illness and nutrients, such as nitrogen and phosphorus, are carried from urban, residential, and agricultural areas into surface waters, groundwater, and coastal waters. The nutrient loading can promote the growth of naturally occurring pathogens and algae. Human exposure occurs via contamination of drinking water sources, recreational waters, and fish and shellfish.

Water contamination by human waste is tied to the failure of local urban or rural water infrastructure, including municipal wastewater, septic, and stormwater conveyance systems. Failure can occur either when rainfall and subsequent runoff overwhelm the capacity of these systems—causing, for example, sewer overflows, basement backups, or localized flooding—or when extreme events, such as flooding and storm surge, damage water conveyance or treatment infrastructure and result in reduction or loss of performance and functionality. Many older cities in the Northeast and around the Great Lakes region of the United States have combined sewer systems (with stormwater and sewage sharing the same pipes), which are prone to discharging raw sewage directly into surface waters after moderate to heavy rainfall. The amount of rain that causes combined sewer overflows is highly variable between cities because of differences in infrastructure capacity and design, and ranges from 5 mm (about 0.2 inches) to 2.5 cm (about 1 inch). Overall, combined sewer overflows are expected to increase, but the site-specific analysis is needed to predict the extent of these increases. Extreme precipitation events will exacerbate existing problems with inadequate, aging, or deteriorating wastewater infrastructure throughout the country. These problems include broken or leaking sewer pipes and failing septic systems that leach sewage into the ground. Runoff or contaminated groundwater discharge also carries pathogens and nutrients into surface water, including freshwater and marine coastal areas and beaches.

Water contamination from agricultural activities is related to the release of microbial pathogens or nutrients in livestock manure and inorganic fertilizers that can stimulate rapid and excessive growth or blooms of harmful algae. Agricultural land covers about 900 million acres across the United States, comprising over 2 million farms, with livestock sectors concentrated in certain regions of the United States. Depending on the type and number of animals, a large livestock operation can produce between 2,800 and 1,600,000 tons of manure each year. With the projected increases in heavy precipitation for all U.S. regions, agricultural sources of contamination can affect water quality across the nation. Runoff from lands where manure has been used as fertilizer or where flooding has caused wastewater lagoons to overflow can carry contamination agents directly from the land into water bodies.

Management practices and technologies, such as better timing of manure application and improved animal feeds, help reduce or eliminate the risks of manure-borne contaminant transport to public water supplies and shellfish harvesting waters, and reduce nutrients that stimulate harmful algal blooms. Drinking water treatment and monitoring practices also help to decrease or eliminate exposure to waterborne illness agents originating from agricultural environments.

Water contamination from wildlife (for example, rodents, birds, deer, and wild pigs) occurs via feces and urine of infected animals, which are reservoirs of enteric and other pathogens. Warmer winters and earlier springs are expected to increase animal activity and alter the ecology and habitat of animals that may carry pathogens. This may lengthen the exposure period for humans and expand the geographic ranges in which pathogens are transmitted.

Exposure Pathways and Health Risks

Humans are exposed to agents of water-related illness through several pathways, including drinking water (treated and untreated), recreational waters (freshwater, coastal, and marine), and fish and shellfish.

Drinking Water

Although the United States has one of the safest municipal drinking water supplies in the world, water-related outbreaks (more than 1 illness case linked to the same source) still occur. Public drinking water systems provide treated water to approximately 90 percent of Americans at their places of residence, work, or schools. However, about 15 percent of the population relies fully or in part on untreated private wells or other private sources for their drinking water. These private sources are not regulated under the Safe Drinking Water Act (SDWA). The majority of drinking water outbreaks in the United States are

265

associated with untreated or inadequately treated groundwater and distribution system deficiencies.

Pathogen and Algal Toxin Contamination

Between 1948 and 1994, 68 percent of waterborne disease outbreaks in the United States were preceded by extreme precipitation events, and heavy rainfall and flooding continue to be cited as contributing factors in more recent outbreaks in multiple regions of the United States. Extreme precipitation events have been statistically linked to increased levels of pathogens in treated drinking water supplies and to an increased incidence of gastrointestinal illness in children. This established relationship suggests that extreme precipitation is a key climate factor for waterborne disease. The Milwaukee *Cryptosporidium* outbreak in 1993—the largest documented waterborne disease outbreak in U.S. history, causing an estimated 403,000 illnesses and more than 50 deaths—was preceded by the heaviest rainfall event in 50 years in the adjacent watersheds. Various treatment plant operational problems were also key contributing factors. Observations in England and Wales also show waterborne disease outbreaks were preceded by weeks of low cumulative rainfall and then heavy precipitation events, suggesting that drought or periods of low rainfall may also be important climate-related factors.

Small community or private groundwater wells or other drinking water systems where water is untreated or minimally treated are especially susceptible to contamination following extreme precipitation events. For example, in May 2000, following heavy rains, livestock waste containing *E. coli* O157: H7 and *Campylobacter* was carried in the runoff to a well that served as the primary drinking water source for the town of Walkerton, Ontario, Canada, resulting in 2,300 illnesses and 7 deaths. High rainfall amounts were an important catalyst for the outbreak, although nonclimate factors, such as well infrastructure, operational and maintenance problems, and lack of communication between public utilities staff and local health officials, were also key factors.

Likewise, extreme precipitation events and subsequent increases in runoff are key climate factors that increase nutrient loading in drinking water sources, which increases the likelihood of harmful cyanobacterial blooms that produce algal toxins. The U.S. Environmental Protection Agency (EPA) has established health advisories for 2 algal toxins (microcystins and cylindrospermopsin) in drinking water. Lakes and reservoirs that serve as sources of drinking water for between 30 and 48 million Americans may be periodically contaminated by algal toxins. Certain drinking water treatment processes can remove cyanobacterial toxins; however, the efficacy of the treatment processes may vary from 60 to 99.9 percent. Ineffective treatment could compromise water quality and may lead to severe treatment disruption or treatment plant shutdown. Such an event occurred in Toledo, Ohio, in August 2014, when nearly 500,000 residents of the state's fourth largest city lost access to their drinking water after tests revealed the presence of toxins from a cyanobacterial bloom in Lake Erie near the water plant's intake.

Water Supply

Climate-related hydrologic changes, such as those related to flooding, drought, runoff, snowpack and snowmelt, and saltwater intrusion (the movement of ocean water into fresh groundwater), have implications for freshwater management and supply. Adequate freshwater supply is essential to many aspects of public health, including the provision of drinking water and proper sanitation, and personal hygiene. For example, following floods or storms, short-term loss of access to potable water has been linked to increased incidence of illnesses, including gastroenteritis and respiratory tract and skin infections. Changes in precipitation and runoff, combined with changes in consumption and withdrawal, have reduced surface and groundwater supplies in many areas, primarily in the Western United States. These trends are expected to continue under future climate change, increasing the likelihood of water shortages for many uses.

Future climate-related water shortages may result in more municipalities and individuals relying on alternative sources for drinking water, including reclaimed water and roof-harvested rainwater. Water reclamation refers to the treatment of stormwater, industrial wastewater, and municipal wastewater for beneficial reuse. States such as California, Arizona, New Mexico, Texas, and Florida are already implementing wastewater reclamation and reuse practices as a means of conserving and adding to freshwater supplies. However, no federal regulations or criteria for public health protection have been developed or proposed specifically for potable water reuse in the United States. Increasing household rainwater collection has also been seen in some areas of the country (primarily Arizona, Colorado, and Texas); although, in some cases, exposure to untreated rainwater has been found to pose health risks from bacterial or protozoan pathogens, such as *Salmonella enterica* and *Giardia lamblia*.

Projected Changes

Runoff from more frequent and intense extreme precipitation events will contribute to contamination of drinking water sources with pathogens and algal toxins, and place additional stresses on the capacity of drinking water treatment facilities and distribution systems. Contamination of drinking water sources may be exacerbated or insufficiently addressed by treatment processes at the treatment plant or by breaches in the distribution system, such as during water main breaks or low-pressure events. Untreated groundwater drawn from municipal and private wells is of particular concern.

Climate change is not expected to substantially increase the risk of contracting illness from drinking water for those people who are served by treated drinking water systems if appropriate treatment and distribution is maintained. However, projections of more frequent or severe extreme precipitation events, flooding, and storm surge suggest that drinking water infrastructure may be at greater risk of disruption or failure due to damage or exceedance of system capacity. Aging drinking water infrastructure is one longstanding limitation in controlling waterborne disease and may be especially susceptible to failure. For example, there are more than 50,000 systems providing treated drinking water to communities in the United States, and most water distribution pipes in these systems are already failing or will reach their expected lifespan and require replacement within 30 years. Breakdowns in drinking water treatment and distribution systems, compounded by aging infrastructure, could lead to more serious and frequent health consequences than those we experience now.

Recreational Waters

Humans are exposed to agents of water-related illness through recreation (such as swimming, fishing, and boating) in freshwater and marine or coastal waters. Exposure may occur directly (ingestion and contact with water) or incidentally (inhalation of aerosolized water droplets).

Pathogen and Algal Toxin Contamination

Enteric viruses, especially noroviruses, from human waste are a primary cause of gastrointestinal illness from exposure to contaminated recreational fresh and marine water (see Table 18.1). Although there are comparatively few reported illnesses and outbreaks of gastrointestinal illness from recreating in marine waters compared to freshwater, marine contamination still presents a significant health risk. Illnesses from marine sources are less likely to be reported than those from freshwater beaches in part because the geographical residences of beachgoers are more widely distributed (for example, tourists may travel to marine beaches for vacation), and illnesses are less often attributed to marine exposure as a common source.

Key climate factors associated with risks of exposure to enteric pathogens in both freshwater and marine recreational waters include extreme precipitation events, flooding, and temperature. For example, *Salmonella* and *Campylobacter* concentrations in freshwater streams in the Southeastern United States increased significantly in the summer months and followed heavy rainfall. In the Great Lakes—a freshwater system—changes in rainfall, higher lake temperatures, and low lake levels have been linked to increases in fecal bacteria levels. The zoonotic bacteria Leptospira are introduced into the water from the urine of animals, and increased illness rates in humans are linked to warm temperatures and flooding events.

In marine waters, recreational exposure to naturally occurring bacterial pathogens (such as Vibrio species) may result in eye, ear, and wound infections; diarrheal illness; or death (see Table 18.1). Reported rates of illness for all Vibrio infections have tripled since 1996, with *V. alginolyticus* infections having increased by 40-fold. Vibrio growth rates are highly responsive to rising sea surface temperatures, particularly in coastal waters, which generally have high levels of the dissolved organic carbon required for Vibrio growth. The distribution of species changes with salinity patterns related to sea level rise and to changes in the delivery of freshwater to coastal waters, which is affected by flooding and drought. For instance, *V. parahaemolyticus* and *V. alginolyticus* favor higher salinities while *V. vulnificus* favors more moderate salinities.

Harmful algal blooms caused by cyanobacteria were responsible for nearly half of all reported outbreaks in untreated recreational freshwater in 2009 and 2010, resulting in approximately 61 illnesses (health effects included dermatologic, gastrointestinal, respiratory, and neurologic symptoms), primarily reported in children/young adults between the ages of 1 and 19. Cyanobacterial blooms are strongly influenced by rising temperatures, altered precipitation patterns, and changes in freshwater discharge or flushing rates of water bodies (see Table 18.1). Higher temperatures (77°F and greater) favor surface-bloom-forming cyanobacteria over less harmful types of algae. In marine water, the toxins associated with harmful "red tide" blooms of Karenia brevis can aerosolize in water droplets through wind and wave action, and cause acute respiratory illness and eye irritation in recreational beachgoers. People with preexisting respiratory diseases, specifically asthma, are at increased risk of illness. Prevailing winds and storms are important climate factors influencing the accumulation of K. brevis cells in the water. For example, in 1996, Tropical Storm Josephine transported a Florida panhandle bloom as far west as Louisiana, the first documented occurrence of K. brevis in that state.

Projected Changes

Overall, climate change will contribute to contamination of recreational waters and increased exposure to agents of water-related illness. Increases in flooding, coastal inundation, and nuisance flooding (linked to sea level rise and storm surge from changing patterns of coastal storms and hurricanes) will negatively affect coastal infrastructure and increase chances for pathogen contamination, especially in populated areas. In areas where increasing temperatures lengthen the seasons for recreational swimming and other water activities, exposure risks are expected to increase.

As average temperatures rise, the seasonal and geographic range of suitable habitat for cyanobacterial species is projected to expand. For example, tropical and subtropical species, such as Cylindrospermopsis raciborskii, Anabaena spp., and Aphanizomenon spp., have already shown poleward expansion into mid-latitudes of Europe, North America, and South America. Increasing variability in precipitation patterns and more frequent and intense extreme precipitation events (which will increase nutrient loading) will also affect cyanobacterial communities. If such events are followed by extended drought periods, the stagnant, low-flow conditions accompanying droughts will favor cyanobacterial dominance and bloom formation.

In recreational waters, projected increases in sea surface temperatures are expected to lengthen the seasonal window of growth and expand the geographic range of Vibrio species, although the certainty of regional projections is affected by the underlying model structure. While the specific response of Vibrio and degree of growth may vary by species and locale, in general, longer seasons and expansion of Vibrio into areas where it had not previously been will increase the likelihood of exposure to Vibrio in recreational waters. Regional climate changes that affect coastal salinity (such as flooding, drought, and sea level rise) can also affect the population dynamics of these agents, with implications for human exposure risk. Increases in hurricane intensity and rainfall are projected as the climate continues to warm. Such increases may redistribute toxic blooms of K. brevis ("red tide" blooms) into new geographic locations, which would change human exposure risk in newly affected areas.

Fish and Shellfish

Water-related contaminants, as well as naturally occurring harmful bacteria and algae, can be accumulated by fish or shellfish, providing a route of human exposure through consumption. Shellfish, including oysters, are often consumed raw or very lightly cooked, which increases the potential for ingestion of an infectious pathogen.

Pathogens Associated with Fish and Shellfish

Enteric viruses (for example, noroviruses and hepatitis A virus) found in sewage are the primary causes of gastrointestinal illness due to shellfish consumption. Rainfall increases the load of contaminants associated with sewage delivered to shellfish harvesting waters and may also temporarily reduce salinity, which can increase the persistence of many enteric bacteria and viruses. Many enteric viruses also exhibit seasonal patterns in infection rates and detection rates in the environment, which may be related to temperature.

Among naturally occurring water-related pathogens, *Vibrio vulnificus* and *V. parahaemolyticus* are the species most often implicated in foodborne illness in the United States, accounting for more than 50 percent of reported shellfish-related illnesses annually. Cases have increased significantly since 1996. Rising sea surface temperatures have contributed to an expanded geographic and seasonal range in outbreaks associated with shellfish.

Precipitation is expected to be the primary climate driver affecting enteric-pathogen loading to shellfish harvesting areas, although temperature also affects bioaccumulation rates of enteric viruses in shellfish. There are currently no national projections for the associated risk of illness from shellfish consumption. Many local and state agencies have developed plans for closing shellfish beds in the event of threshold-exceeding rain events that lead to the loading of these contaminants and deterioration of water quality.

Increases in sea surface temperatures, changes in precipitation and freshwater delivery to coastal waters, and sea level rise will continue to affect Vibrio growth and are expected to increase human exposure risk. Regional models project increased abundance and extended seasonal windows of growth of Vibrio pathogens. The magnitude of health

271

impacts depends on the use of intervention strategies and on public and physician awareness.

Harmful Algal Toxins

Harmful algal blooms (HABs) that contaminate seafood with toxins are becoming increasingly frequent and persistent in coastal marine waters, and some have expanded into new geographic locations. Attribution of this trend has been complicated for some species, with evidence to suggest that human-induced changes (such as ballast water exchange, aquaculture, nutrient loading to coastal waters, and climate change) have contributed to this expansion.

Among harmful algal blooms associated with seafood, ciguatera fish poisoning (CFP) is most strongly influenced by climate. CFP is caused by toxins produced by the benthic algae Gambierdiscus (see Table 18.1) and is the most frequently reported fish poisoning in humans. There is a well-established link between warm sea surface temperatures and increased occurrences of CFP, and in some cases, increases have also been linked to El Niño–Southern Oscillation events. The frequency of tropical cyclones in the United States has also been associated with CFP, but with an 18-month lag period associated with the time required for a new Gambierdiscus habitat to develop.

Paralytic shellfish poisoning (PSP) is the most globally widespread shellfish poisoning associated with algal toxins, and records of PSP toxins in shellfish tissues (an indicator of toxin-producing species of Alexandrium) provide the longest time series in the United States for evaluating climate impacts. Warm phases of the naturally occurring climate pattern known as the "Pacific Decadal Oscillation" co-occur with increased PSP toxins in Puget Sound shellfish on decadal timescales. Further, it is very likely that the 20th-century warming trend also contributed to the observed increase in shellfish toxicity since the 1950s. Warm spring temperatures also contributed to a bloom of Alexandrium in a coastal New York estuary in 2008. Decadal patterns in PSP toxins in the Gulf of Maine shellfish show no clear relationships with long-term trends in climate, but ocean-climate interactions and changing oceanographic conditions are important factors for understanding Alexandrium bloom dynamics in this region.

There is less agreement on the extent of climate impacts on other marine HAB-related diseases in the United States. Increased abundances of Pseudo-nitzschia species, which can cause amnesic shellfish poisoning, have been attributed to nutrient enrichment in the Gulf of Mexico. On the U.S. West Coast, increased abundances of at least some species of Pseudo-nitzschia occur during warm phases associated with El Niño events. For Dinophysis species that can cause diarrhetic shellfish poisoning, data records are too short to evaluate potential relationships with the climate in the United States, but studies in Sweden have found relationships with natural climate oscillations.

The projected impacts of climate change on toxic marine harmful algae include geographic range changes in both warm- and cold-water species, changes in abundance and toxicity, and changes in the timing of the seasonal window of growth. These impacts will likely result from climate change-related impacts on one or more of water temperatures, salinities, enhanced surface stratification, nutrient availability and supply to coastal waters (upwelling and freshwater runoff), and altered winds and ocean currents.

Limited understanding of the interactions among climate and nonclimate stressors and, in some cases, limitations in the design of experiments for investigating decadal- or century-scale trends in phytoplankton communities makes forecasting the direction and magnitude of change in toxic marine HABs challenging. Still, changes to the community composition of marine microalgae, including harmful species, will occur. Conditions for the growth of dinoflagellates—the algal group containing numerous toxic species—could potentially be increasingly favorable with climate change because these species possess certain physiological characteristics that allow them to take advantage of climatically-driven changes in the structure of the ocean (for example, stronger vertical stratification and reduced turbulence).

Climate change, especially continued warming, will dramatically increase the burden of some marine HAB-related diseases in some parts of the United States, with strong implications for disease surveillance and public health preparedness. For example, the projected 4.5°F to 6.3°F increase in sea surface temperature in the Caribbean over the coming century is expected to increase the incidence of ciguatera fish poisoning by 200 to 400 percent. In Puget Sound, warming is projected to increase the seasonal window of growth for Alexandrium by approximately 30 days by 2040, allowing blooms to begin earlier in the year and persist for longer.

Populations of Concern

Climate change impacts on the drinking water exposure pathway will act as an additional stressor on top of existing exposure disparities in the United States. Lack of consistent access to potable drinking water and inequities in exposure to contaminated water disproportionately

273

affects the following populations: tribes and Alaska Natives, especially those in remote reservations or villages; residents of low-income rural subdivisions known as "colonias" along the United States-Mexico border; migrant farm workers; the homeless; and low-income communities not served by public water utilities—which can be urban, suburban, or rural, and some of which are predominately Hispanic or Latino and Black or African American communities in certain regions of the country. In general, the heightened vulnerability of these populations primarily results from unequal access to adequate water and sewer infrastructure, and various environmental, political, economic, and social factors jointly create these disparities.

Children, older adults (primarily those 65 years of age and older), pregnant women, and immunocompromised individuals have a higher risk of gastrointestinal illness and severe health outcomes from contact with contaminated water. Pregnant women who develop severe gastrointestinal illness are at high risk for adverse pregnancy outcomes (pregnancy loss and preterm birth). Because children swallow roughly twice as much water as adults while swimming, they have higher recreational exposure risk for both pathogens and freshwater HABs. Recent cryptosporidiosis and giardiasis cases have frequently been reported in children between the ages of 1 and 9, with the onset of illness peaking during the summer months. In addition, 40 percent of the swimming-related eye and ear infections from *Vibrio alginolyticus* during the period 1997 to 2006 were reported in children (median age of 15).

Traditional tribal consumption of fish and shellfish in the Pacific Northwest and Alaska can be on average 3 to 10 times higher than that of average U.S. consumers or even up to 20 times higher. Climate change will contribute to increased seafood contamination by toxins and potentially by chemical contaminants, with potential health risks and cultural implications for tribal communities. Those who continue to consume traditional diets may face increased health risks from contamination. Alternatively, replacing these traditional nutrition sources may involve consuming less nutritious processed foods and the loss of cultural practices tied to fish and shellfish harvest.

Emerging Issues

A key emerging issue is the impact of climate on new and reemerging pathogens. While cases of nearly-always-fatal primary amoebic meningoencephalitis due to the amoeba *Naegleria fowleri* and other related species remain relatively uncommon, a northward expansion of cases has been observed in the last five years. Evidence suggests that in addition to detection in source water (ground and surface waters), these amoebae may be harbored in biofilms associated with water distribution systems, where increased temperatures decrease efficacy of chlorine disinfection and support survival and potentially growth.

Climate change may also alter the patterns or magnitude of chemical contamination of seafood, leading to altered effects on human health—most of which are chronic conditions. Rising temperatures and reduced ice cover are already linked to increasing burdens of mercury and organohalogens in arctic fish, a sign of increasing contamination of the Arctic food chain. Changes in hydrology resulting from climate change are expected to alter releases of chemical contaminants into the nation's surface waters, with as-yet-unknown effects on seafood contamination.

Chapter 19

Foodborne Infections

A safe and nutritious food supply is a vital component of food security. Food security, in a public health context, can be summarized as permanent access to a sufficient, safe, and nutritious food supply needed to maintain an active and healthy lifestyle.

The impacts of climate change on food production, prices, and trade for the United States and globally have been widely examined, including in the U.S. Global Change Research Program (USGCRP) report, "Climate Change, Global Food Security, and the U.S. Food System;" in the most recent Intergovernmental Panel on Climate Change report; and elsewhere. An overall finding of the USGCRP report was that "climate change is very likely to affect global, regional, and local food security by disrupting food availability, decreasing access to food, and making utilization more difficult."

This chapter focuses on some of the less reported aspects of food security, specifically, the impacts of climate change on food safety, nutrition, and distribution in the context of human health in the United States.

Systems and processes related to food safety, nutrition, and production are inextricably linked to their physical and biological environment. Although production is important, for most developed countries, such as the United States, food shortages are uncommon; rather, nutritional quality and food safety are the primary health concerns.

This chapter includes text excerpted from "Food Safety, Nutrition, and Distribution," GlobalChange.gov, U.S. Global Change Research Program (USGCRP), April 4, 2016.

277

Certain populations, such as the poor, children, and Indigenous populations, may be more vulnerable to climate impacts on food safety, nutrition, and distribution.

There are two overarching means by which increasing carbon dioxide (CO_2) and climate change alter safety, nutrition, and distribution of food. The first is associated with rising global temperatures and the subsequent changes in weather patterns and extreme climate events. Current and anticipated changes in climate and the physical environment have consequences for contamination, spoilage, and the disruption of food distribution.

The second pathway is through the direct CO_2 "fertilization" effect on plant photosynthesis. Higher concentrations of CO_2 stimulate carbohydrate production and plant growth, but can lower the levels of protein and essential minerals in a number of widely consumed crops, including wheat, rice, and potatoes, with potentially negative implications for human nutrition.

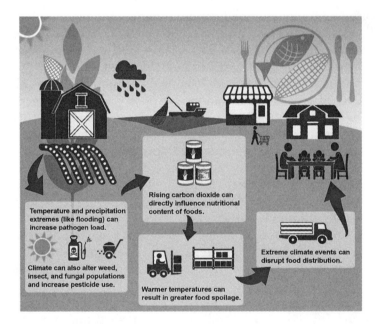

Figure 19.1. *Farm to Table: The Potential Interactions of Rising CO_2 and Climate Change on Food Safety and Nutrition*

The food system involves a network of interactions with our physical and biological environments as food moves from production to consumption, or from "farm to table." Rising CO_2 and climate change will affect the quality and distribution of food, with subsequent effects on food safety and nutrition.

278

Food Safety

Although the United States has one of the safest food supplies in the world, food safety remains an important public health issue. In the United States, the Centers for Disease Control and Prevention (CDC) estimate that there are 48 million cases of foodborne illnesses per year, with approximately 3,000 deaths. As climate change drives changes in environmental variables, such as ambient temperature, precipitation, and weather extremes (particularly flooding and drought), increases in foodborne illnesses are expected.

Most acute illnesses are caused by foodborne viruses (specifically noroviruses), followed by bacterial pathogens. Of the common foodborne illnesses in the United States, most deaths are caused by Salmonella, followed by the parasite *Toxoplasma gondii*. In addition,

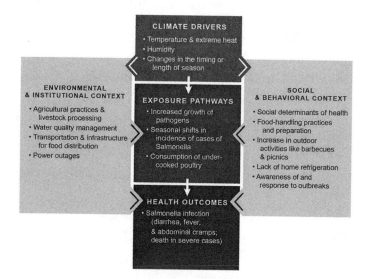

Figure 19.2. *Climate Change and Health*—Salmonella

This conceptual diagram for a Salmonella *example illustrates the key pathways by which humans are exposed to health threats from climate drivers, and potential resulting health outcomes (center boxes). These exposure pathways exist within the context of other factors that positively or negatively influence health outcomes (gray side boxes). Key factors that influence vulnerability for individuals are shown in the right box, and include social determinants of health and behavioral choices. Key factors that influence vulnerability at larger scales, such as natural and built environments, governance and management, and institutions, are shown in the left box. All of these influencing factors can affect an individual's or a community's vulnerability through changes in exposure, sensitivity, and adaptive capacity and may also be affected by climate change.*

climate change impacts on the transport of chemical contaminants or accumulation of pesticides or heavy metals (such as mercury) in food, can also represent significant health threats in the food chain.

How Climate Affects Food Safety

Climate already influences food safety within an agricultural system—prior to, during, and after the harvest, and during transport, storage, preparation, and consumption. Changes in climate factors, such as temperature, precipitation, and extreme weather, are key drivers of pathogen introduction, food contamination, and foodborne disease, as well as changes in the level of exposure to specific contaminants and chemical residues for crops and livestock.

The impact of climate on food safety occurs through multiple pathways. Changes in air and water temperatures, weather-related changes, and extreme events can shift the seasonal and geographic occurrence of bacteria, viruses, pests, parasites, fungi, and other chemical contaminants. For example:

- Higher temperatures can increase the number of pathogens already present on produce and seafood.

- Bacterial populations can increase during food storage, which, depending on time and temperature, can also increase food spoilage rates.

- Sea surface temperature is directly related to seafood exposure to pathogens.

- Precipitation has been identified as a factor in the contamination of irrigation water and produce, which has been linked to foodborne illness outbreaks.

- Extreme weather events, such as dust storms or flooding, can introduce toxins to crops during development.

- Changing environmental conditions and soil properties may result in increases in the incidence of heavy metals in the food supply.

Climate Impacts on Pathogen Prevalence

While climate change affects the prevalence of pathogens harmful to human health, the extent of exposure and resulting illness will depend on individual and institutional sensitivity and adaptive capacity, including human behavior and the effectiveness of food safety regulatory, surveillance, monitoring, and communication systems.

Rising Temperature and Humidity

Climate change will influence the fate, transport, transmission, viability, and multiplication rate of pathogens in the food chain. For example, increases in average global temperatures and humidity will lead to changes in the geographic range, seasonal occurrence, and survivability of certain pathogens.

Ongoing changes in temperature and humidity will not affect all foodborne pathogens equally. The occurrence of some pathogens, such as *Salmonella*, *Escherichia coli* (*E. coli*), and *Campylobacter*, could increase with climate change because these pathogens thrive in warm, humid conditions. For example, *Salmonella* on raw chicken will double in number approximately every hour at 70°F, every 30 minutes at 80°F, and every 22 minutes at 90°F.

Norovirus, the most common cause of stomach flu, can be transmitted by consumption of contaminated food. Although norovirus generally has a winter seasonal peak, changing climate parameters, particularly temperature and rainfall, may influence its incidence and spread. Overall, localized climate impacts could improve health outcomes (fewer cases during warmer winters) or worsen them (elevated transmission during floods), such that projected trends in overall health outcomes for norovirus remain unclear.

Rising ocean temperatures can increase the risk of pathogen exposure from ingestion of contaminated seafood. For example, significantly warmer coastal waters in Alaska from 1997 to 2004 were associated with an outbreak in 2004 of *Vibrio parahaemolyticus*, a bacterium that causes gastrointestinal illnesses when contaminated seafood is ingested. *Vibrio parahaemolyticus* is one of the leading causes of seafood-related gastroenteritis in the United States and is associated with the consumption of raw oysters harvested from warm-water estuaries. Similarly, the emergence of a related bacterium, *Vibrio vulnificus*, may also be associated with high water temperatures. While increasing average water temperatures were implicated in a 2004 outbreak, ambient air temperature also affects pathogen levels of multiple species of Vibrio in shellfish. For example, *Vibrio vulnificus* may increase 10- to 100-fold when oysters are stored at ambient temperatures for 10 hours before refrigeration. Increases in ambient ocean water and air temperatures would accelerate Vibrio growth in shellfish, potentially necessitating changes in postharvest controls to minimize the increased risk of exposure.

Finally, climate change is projected to result in warmer winters, earlier springs, and an increase in the overall growing season in many regions. While there are potential food production benefits from such changes, warmer and longer growing seasons could also alter the timing and occurrence of pathogen transmissions in food and the chance of human exposure.

Extreme Events

In addition to the effects of increasing average temperature and humidity on pathogen survival and growth, increases in temperature and precipitation extremes can contribute to changes in pathogen transmission, multiplication, and survivability. More frequent and severe heavy rainfall events can increase infection risk from most pathogens, particularly when it leads to flooding. Flooding, and other weather extremes, can increase the incidence and levels of pathogens in food production, harvesting, and processing environments. Groundwater and surface water used for irrigation, harvesting, and washing can be contaminated with runoff or flood waters that carry partially or untreated sewage, manure, or other wastes containing foodborne contaminants. The level of *Salmonella* in water is elevated during times of monthly maximum precipitation in the summer and fall months; consequently, the likelihood of *Salmonella* in water may increase in regions experiencing increased total or heavy precipitation events.

Water is also an important factor in food processing. Climate and weather extremes, such as flooding or drought, can reduce water quality and increase the risk of pathogen transfer during the handling and storage of food following harvest.

The direct effect of drought on food safety is less clear. Dry conditions can pose a risk for pathogen transmission due to reduced water quality, increased risk of runoff when rains do occur, and increased pathogen concentration in reduced water supplies if such water is used for irrigation, food processing, or livestock management. Increasing drought generally leads to an elevated risk of exposure to pathogens, such as norovirus and *Cryptosporidium*. However, drought and extreme heat events could also decrease the survivability of certain foodborne pathogens, affecting establishment and transmission, and thus reducing human exposure.

Mycotoxins and Phycotoxins

Mycotoxins are toxic chemicals produced by molds that grow on crops prior to harvest and during storage. Prior to harvest, increasing temperatures and drought can stress plants, making them more susceptible to mold growth. Warm and moist conditions favor mold growth directly and affect the biology of insect vectors that transmit molds to crops. Postharvest contamination is also affected by environmental parameters, including extreme temperatures and moisture. If crops are not dried and stored at low humidity, mold growth and mycotoxin production can increase to very high levels.

Phycotoxins are toxic chemicals produced by certain harmful freshwater and marine algae that may affect the safety of drinking water and shellfish or other seafood. For example, the alga responsible for producing ciguatoxin (the toxin that causes the illness known as "ciguatera fish poisoning") thrives in warm water. Projected increases in sea surface temperatures may expand the endemic range of ciguatoxin-producing algae and increase ciguatera fish poisoning incidence following ingestion. Predicted increases in sea surface temperature of 4.5°F to 6.3°F (2.5°C to 3.5°C) could yield increases in ciguatera fish poisoning cases of 200 to 400 percent.

Once introduced into the food chain, these poisonous toxins can result in adverse health outcomes, with both acute and chronic effects. Current regulatory laws and management strategies safeguard the food supply from mycotoxins and phycotoxins; however, increases in frequency and range of their prevalence may increase the vulnerability of the food safety system.

Climate Impacts on Chemical Contaminants

Climate change will affect human exposure to metals, pesticides, pesticide residues, and other chemical contaminants. However, resulting incidence of illness will depend on the genetic predisposition of the person exposed, type of contaminant, and extent of exposure over time.

Metals and Other Chemical Contaminants

There are a number of environmental contaminants, such as polychlorinated biphenyls, persistent organic pollutants, dioxins, pesticides, and heavy metals, which pose a human health risk when they enter the food chain. Extreme events may facilitate the entry of such contaminants into the food chain, particularly during heavy precipitation and flooding. For example, chemical contaminants in floodwater following Hurricane Katrina included spilled oil, pesticides, heavy metals, and hazardous waste.

Methylmercury is a form of mercury that can be absorbed into the bodies of animals, including humans, where it can have adverse neurological effects. Elevated water temperatures may lead to higher concentrations of methylmercury in fish and mammals. This is related to an increase in metabolic rates and increased mercury uptake at higher water temperatures. Human exposure to dietary mercury is influenced by the amount of mercury ingested, which can vary with the species, age, and size of the fish. If future fish consumption patterns are unaltered, increasing ocean temperature would likely increase mercury exposure in human diets. Methylmercury exposure can affect the development of children, particularly if exposed in utero.

Pesticides

Climate change is likely to exhibit a wide range of effects on the biology of plant and livestock pests (weeds, insects, and microbes). Rising minimum winter temperatures and longer growing seasons are very likely to alter pest distribution and populations. In addition, rising average temperature and CO_2 concentration are also likely to increase the range and distribution of pests, their impact, and the vulnerability of host plants and animals.

Pesticides are chemicals generally regulated for use in agriculture to protect plants and animals from pests; chemical management is the primary means for agricultural pest control in the United States and most developed countries. Because climate and CO_2 will intensify pest distribution and populations, increases in pesticide use are expected. In addition, the efficacy of chemical management may be reduced in the context of climate change. This decline in efficacy can reflect CO_2-induced increases in the herbicide tolerance of certain weeds or climate-induced shifts in invasive weed, insect, and plant pathogen populations, as well as climate-induced changes that enhance pesticide degradation or affect coverage.

Increased pest pressures and reductions in the efficacy of pesticides are likely to lead to increased pesticide use, contamination in the field, and exposure within the food chain. Increased exposure to pesticides could have implications for human health. However, the extent of pesticide use and potential exposure may also reflect climate change induced choices for crop selection and land use.

Pesticide Residues

Climate change, especially increases in temperature, may be important in altering the transmission of vector-borne diseases in livestock by influencing the life cycle, range, and reproductive success of disease vectors. Potential changes in veterinary practices, including an increase in the use of parasiticides and other animal health treatments, are likely to be adopted to maintain livestock health in response to climate-induced changes in pests, parasites, and microbes. This could increase the risk of pesticides entering the food chain or lead to evolution of pesticide resistance, with subsequent implications for the safety, distribution, and consumption of livestock and aquaculture products.

Climate change may affect aquatic animal health through temperature-driven increases in disease. The occurrence of increased infections in aquaculture with rising temperature has been observed for some diseases (such as Ichthyophthirius multifiliis and Flavobacterium columnare) and is likely to result in greater use of aquaculture drugs.

Nutrition

While sufficient quantity of food is an obvious requirement for food security, food quality is essential to fulfill basic nutritional needs. Globally, chronic dietary deficiencies of micronutrients, such as vitamin A, iron, iodine, and zinc, contribute to "hidden hunger," in which the consequences of the micronutrient insufficiency may not be immediately visible or easily observed. This type of micronutrient deficiency constitutes one of the world's leading health risk factors and adversely affects metabolism, the immune system, cognitive development and maturation—particularly in children. In addition, micronutrient deficiency can exacerbate the effects of diseases and can be a factor in prevalence of obesity.

In developed countries with abundant food supplies, such as the United States, the health burden of malnutrition may not be intuitive and is often underappreciated. In the United States, although a number of foods are supplemented with nutrients, it is estimated that the diets of 38 and 45 percent of the population fall below the estimated average requirements for calcium and magnesium, respectively. Approximately 12 percent of the population is at risk for zinc deficiency, including perhaps as much as 40 percent of the elderly. In addition, nutritional deficiencies of magnesium, iron, selenium, and other essential micronutrients can occur in overweight and obese individuals, whose diets might reflect excessive intake of calories and refined carbohydrates but insufficient intake of vitamins and essential minerals.

How Rising CO_2 Affects Nutrition

Though rising CO_2 stimulates plant growth and carbohydrate production, it reduces the nutritional value (protein and minerals) of most food crops. This direct effect of rising CO_2 on the nutritional value of crops represents a potential threat to human health.

Protein

As CO_2 increases, plants need less protein for photosynthesis, resulting in an overall decline in protein concentration in plant tissues. This trend for declining protein levels is evident for wheat flour derived from multiple wheat varieties when grown under laboratory conditions simulating the observed increase in global atmospheric CO_2 concentration since 1900. When grown at the CO_2 levels projected for 2100 (540–958 ppm), major food crops, such as barley, wheat, rice, and potato, exhibit 6 to 15 percent lower protein concentrations relative to ambient levels (315–400 ppm). In contrast, protein content is not anticipated to decline significantly for corn or sorghum.

While protein is an essential aspect of human dietary needs, the projected human health impacts of a diet including plants with reduced protein concentration from increasing CO_2 are not well understood and may not be of considerable threat in the United States, where dietary protein deficiencies are uncommon.

Micronutrients

The ongoing increase in atmospheric CO_2 is also very likely to deplete other elements essential to human health (such as calcium, copper, iron, magnesium, and zinc) by 5 to 10 percent in most plants. The projected decline in mineral concentrations in crops has been attributed to at least 2 distinct effects of elevated CO_2 on plant biology. First, rising CO_2 increases carbohydrate accumulation in plant tissues, which can, in turn, dilute the content of other nutrients, including minerals. Second, high CO_2 concentrations reduce plant demands for water, resulting in fewer nutrients being drawn into plant roots.

The ongoing increase in CO_2 concentrations reduces the amount of essential minerals per calorie in most crops, thus reducing nutrient density. Such a reduction in crop quality may aggravate existing nutritional deficiencies, particularly for populations with preexisting health conditions.

Carbohydrate-to-Protein Ratio

Elevated CO_2 tends to increase the concentrations of carbohydrates (starch and sugars) and reduce the concentrations of protein. The overall effect is a significant increase in the ratio of carbohydrates to protein in plants exposed to increasing CO_2. There is growing evidence that a dietary increase in this ratio can adversely affect human metabolism and body composition.

Distribution and Access

A reliable and resilient food distribution system is essential for access to a safe and nutritious food supply. Access to food is characterized by transportation and availability, which are defined by infrastructure, trade management, storage requirements, government regulation, and other socioeconomic factors.

The shift in recent decades to a more global food market has resulted in a greater dependency on food transport and distribution, particularly for growing urban populations. Consequently, any climate-related disturbance to food distribution and transport may have significant impacts not only on safety and quality but also on food access. The effects of climate change on each of these interfaces will differ based on geographic, social, and economic factors. Ultimately, the outcome of climate-related disruptions and damages to the food transportation system will be strongly influenced by the resilience of the system, as well as the adaptive capacity of individuals, populations, and institutions.

How Extreme Events Affect Food Distribution and Access

Projected increases in the frequency or severity of some extreme events will interrupt food delivery, particularly for vulnerable transport routes. The degree of disruption is related to three factors: a) popularity of the transport pathway, b) availability of alternate routes, and c) timing or seasonality of the extreme event. As an example, the food transportation system in the United States frequently moves large volumes of grain by water. In the case of an extreme weather event affecting a waterway, there are few, if any, alternate pathways for transport. This presents an especially relevant risk to food access if an extreme event, such as flooding or drought, coincides with times of agricultural distribution, such as the fall harvest.

Immediately following an extreme event, food supply and safety can be compromised. Hurricanes or other storms can disrupt food distribution infrastructure, damage food supplies, and limit access to safe and nutritious food, even in areas not directly affected by such events. For example, the Gulf Coast transportation network is vulnerable to storm surges of 23 feet. Following Hurricane Katrina in 2005, where storm surges of 25 to 28 feet were recorded along parts of the Gulf Coast, grain transportation by rail or barge was severely slowed due to physical damage to infrastructure and the displacement of employees. Barriers to food transport may also affect food markets, reaching consumers in the form of increased food costs.

The risk for food spoilage and contamination in storage facilities, supermarkets, and homes is likely to increase due to the impacts of extreme weather events, particularly those that result in power outages, which may expose food to ambient temperatures inadequate for safe storage. Storm-related power grid disruptions have steadily increased since 2000. Between 2002 and 2012, extreme weather caused 58 percent of power outage events, 87 percent of which affected 50,000 or more customers. Power outages are often linked to an increase in illness. For example, in August of 2003, a sudden power outage affected over 60 million people in the northeastern United States and Canada. New York City's Department of Health and Mental Hygiene detected a statistically significant citywide increase in diarrheal illness resulting from consumption of spoiled foods due to lost refrigeration capabilities.

Populations of Concern

Climate change, combined with other social, economic, and political conditions, may increase the vulnerability of many different populations to food insecurity or food-related illness. However, not all populations are equally vulnerable. Infants and young children, pregnant women, the elderly, low-income populations, agricultural workers, and those with weakened immune systems or who have underlying medical conditions are more susceptible to the effects of climate change on food safety, nutrition, and access.

Children may be especially vulnerable because they eat more food by body weight than adults and do so during important stages of physical and mental growth and development. Children are also more susceptible to severe infection or complications from *E. coli* infections, such as hemolytic uremic syndrome. Agricultural field workers, especially pesticide applicators, may experience increased exposure, as pesticide applications increase with rising pest loads, which could also lead to higher pesticide levels in the children of these field workers. People living in low-income urban areas, those with limited access to supermarkets, and the elderly may have difficulty accessing safe and nutritious food after disruptions associated with extreme weather events. Climate change will also affect U.S. Indigenous peoples' access to both wild and cultivated traditional foods associated with their nutrition, cultural practices, local economies, and community health. All of the health impacts described in this chapter can have significant consequences on mental health and well-being.

Emerging Issues

Climate and food allergies. Food allergies in the United States currently affect between 1 and 9 percent of the population, but have increased significantly among children under the age of 18 since 1997. Rising CO_2 levels can reduce protein content and alter protein composition in certain plants, which has the potential to alter allergenic sensitivity. For example, rising CO_2 has been shown to increase the concentration of the Amb a 1 protein—the allergenic protein most associated with ragweed pollen.

Heavy metals. Arsenic and other heavy metals occur naturally in some groundwater sources. Climate change can exacerbate drought and competition for water, resulting in the use of poorer-quality water sources. Because climate and rising CO_2 levels can also influence the extent of water loss through the crop canopy, poorer water quality could lead to changes in the concentrations of arsenic and potentially other heavy metals (such as cadmium and selenium) in plant tissues. Additional information is needed to determine how rising levels of CO_2 and climate change affect heavy metal accumulation in food and the consequences for human exposure.

Foodborne pathogen contamination of fresh produce by insect vectors. Climate change will alter the range and distribution of insects and other microorganisms that can transmit bacterial pathogens, such as *Salmonella*, to fresh produce.

Chapter 20

Temperature-Related Illness

The Earth is warming due to elevated concentrations of greenhouse gases, and will continue to warm in the future. The U.S. average temperatures have increased by 1.3°F to 1.9°F since record keeping began in 1895, heat waves have become more frequent and intense, and cold waves have become less frequent across the nation. Annual average U.S. temperatures are projected to increase by 3°F to 10°F by the end of this century, depending on future emissions of greenhouse gases and other factors. These temperature changes will have direct effects on human health.

Days that are hotter than the average seasonal temperature in the summer or colder than the average seasonal temperature in the winter cause increased levels of illness and death by compromising the body's ability to regulate its temperature or by inducing direct or indirect health complications. Figure 20.1 provides a conceptual model of the various climate drivers, social factors, and environmental and institutional factors that can interact to result in changes in illness and deaths as a result of extreme heat. Increasing concentrations of greenhouse gases lead to an increase of both average and extreme temperatures, leading to an increase in deaths and illness from heat and a potential decrease in deaths from cold. Challenges involved in determining the temperature–death relationship include a lack of consistent diagnoses on death certificates and the fact that the health

This chapter includes text excerpted from "Temperature-Related Death and Illness," GlobalChange.gov, U.S. Global Change Research Program (USGCRP), April 4, 2016.

implications of extreme temperatures are not absolute, differing from location to location and changing over time. Both of these issues can be partially addressed through the use of statistical methods. Climate model projections of future temperatures can be combined with the estimated relationships between temperatures and health in order to assess how deaths and illnesses resulting from temperature could change in the future. The impact of a warming climate on deaths and illnesses will not be realized equally as a number of populations, such as children, the elderly, and economically disadvantaged groups, are especially vulnerable to temperature.

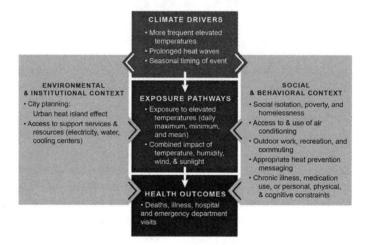

Figure 20.1. *Climate Change and Health—Extreme Heat*

This conceptual diagram illustrates the key pathways by which climate change influences human health during an extreme heat event, and potential resulting health outcomes (center boxes). These exposure pathways exist within the context of other factors that positively or negatively influence health outcomes. Key factors that influence vulnerability at larger scales, such as natural and built environments, governance and management, and institutions, are shown in the left box. All of these influencing factors can affect an individual's or a community's vulnerability through changes in exposure, sensitivity, and adaptive capacity and may also be affected by climate change.

Contribution of Extreme Temperatures to Death and Illness

Temperature extremes most directly affect health by compromising the body's ability to regulate its internal temperature. Loss of internal temperature control can result in a cascade of illnesses, including heat cramps, heat exhaustion, heatstroke, and hyperthermia in the presence of extreme heat, and hypothermia and frostbite in the presence of extreme cold. Temperature extremes can also worsen chronic conditions, such as cardiovascular disease, respiratory disease, cerebrovascular disease, and diabetes-related conditions. Prolonged exposure to high temperatures is associated with increased hospital admissions for cardiovascular, kidney, and respiratory disorders. Exposures to high minimum temperatures may also reduce the ability of the human body to recover from high daily maximum temperatures.

Defining Temperature Exposures

Extreme temperatures are typically defined by some measure, for example, an ambient temperature, heat index (a combination of temperature and humidity), or wind chill (a combination of temperature and wind speed), exceeding predefined thresholds over a number of days. Extremes can be defined by average, minimum, or maximum daily temperatures, by nighttime temperatures, or by daytime temperatures. However, there is no standard method for defining a heat wave or cold wave. There are dramatic differences in the observed relationships between temperature, death, and illness across different regions and seasons; these relationships vary based on average temperatures in those locations and the timing of the heat or cold event. For example, a 95°F day in Vermont will have different implications for health than a 95°F day in Texas, and similarly, a 95°F day in May will have different implications than one in August. Therefore, in some cases, temperature extremes are defined by comparison to some local average (for example, the top 1 percent of warmest days recorded in a particular location) rather than to some absolute temperature (such as 95°F). While temperature extremes are generally determined based on weather station records, the exposure of individuals will depend on their location: urban heat islands, microclimates, and differences between indoor and outdoor temperatures can all lead to differences between weather station data and actual exposure. The indoor environment is particularly important as most people spend the majority of their time inside.

One exception to using relative measures of temperature is that there are some critical physical and weather condition thresholds that are absolute. For example, one combined measure of humidity and temperature is known as the "wet bulb temperature." As the wet bulb temperature reaches or exceeds the threshold of 35°C (95°F), the human body can no longer cool through perspiration, and recent evidence suggests that there is a physical heat tolerance limit in humans to sustained temperatures above 35°C that is similar across diverse climates. The combined effects of temperature and humidity have been incorporated in tools such as heat index tables, which reflect how combinations of heat and relative humidity "feel." The heat index in these tools is often presented with notes about the potential nature and type of health risks different combinations of temperature and humidity may pose, along with confounding conditions, such as exposure to direct sunlight or strong winds.

Variations in heat wave definitions make it challenging to compare results across studies or determine the most appropriate public health warning systems. This is important as the associations between deaths and illnesses and extreme heat conditions vary depending on the methods used for defining the extreme conditions.

Measuring the Health Impact of Temperature

Two broad approaches are used to study the relationship between temperatures and illness and death: direct attribution and statistical methods.

Direct Attribution Studies

With direct attribution, researchers link health outcomes to temperatures based on assigned diagnosis codes in medical records, such as hospital admissions and death certificates. For example, the International Classification of Diseases (ICD-10) contains specific codes for attributing deaths to exposure to excessive natural heat (X30) and excessive natural cold (X31). However, medical records will not include information on the weather conditions at the time of the event or preceding the event. It is generally accepted that direct attribution underestimates the number of people who die from temperature extremes. Reasons for this include difficulties in diagnosing heat-related and cold-related deaths, lack of consistent diagnostic criteria, and difficulty in identifying, or lack of reporting, heat or cold as a factor that worsened a preexisting medical condition. Heat-related deaths are often not reported as such if another cause of death exists, and there is no well-publicized heat wave. An additional challenging factor in deaths classified as X31 (cold) deaths is that a number of these deaths result from situations involving substance use/abuse and/or contact with water, both of which can contribute to hypothermia.

Statistical Studies

Statistical studies measure the impact of temperature on death and illness using methods that relate the number of cases (for example, total daily deaths in a city) to observed weather conditions and other socio-demographic factors. These statistical methods determine whether the temperature conditions were associated with increased deaths or illness above longer-term average levels. These associations establish the relationship between temperature and premature deaths and illness. In some cases, particularly with extreme temperature conditions, the increase in premature deaths and illness can be quite dramatic and the health impact may be referred to in terms of excess deaths or illnesses. Methods for evaluating the impact of temperature in these models vary.

Many studies include all the days in the study period, which makes it possible to capture changes in deaths resulting from small variations of temperatures from their seasonal averages. Other methods restrict the analysis to days that exceed some threshold for extreme heat or cold conditions. Some studies incorporate methods that determine different health relationships for wind, air pressure, and cloud cover, as well as the more common temperature and humidity measures. Another approach is to identify a heat event and compare observed illness and deaths during the event with a carefully chosen comparison period. Many of these methods also incorporate sociodemographic factors (for example, age, race, and poverty) that may affect the temperature–death relationship.

Comparing Results of Direct Attribution and Statistical Studies

Comparing death estimates across studies is therefore complicated by the use of different criteria for temperature extremes, different analytical methods, varying time periods, and different affected populations. Further, it is widely accepted that characteristics of extreme temperature events, such as duration, intensity, and timing in season, directly affect actual death totals. Estimates of the average number of deaths attributable to heat and cold considering all temperatures, rather than just those associated with extreme events, provide an alternative for considering the mortality impact of climate change. Statistical studies can also offer insights into what aspects of a temperature extreme are most important. For example, there are indications that the relationship between high nighttime temperatures and mortality is more pronounced than the relationship for daytime temperatures.

These two methods (direct attribution and statistical approaches) yield very different results for several reasons. First, statistical approaches generally suggest that the actual number of deaths associated with temperature is far greater than those recorded as temperature-related in medical records. Medical records often do not capture the role of heat in exacerbating the cause of death, only recording the ultimate cause, such as a stroke or a heart attack. Statistical methods focus on determining how temperature contributes to premature deaths and illness, and therefore, are not susceptible to this kind of undercount, though they face potential biases due to time-varying factors, such as seasonality. Both methods depend on temperatures measured at weather stations, though the actual temperature exposure of individuals may differ. In short, while the focus on temperature is consistent in both methods, the methods potentially evaluate very different combinations of deaths and weather conditions.

Observed Impact of Temperature on Deaths

A number of extreme temperature events in the United States have led to dramatic increases in deaths, including events in Kansas City and St. Louis in 1980, Philadelphia in 1993, Chicago in 1995, and California in 2006.

Studies in specific communities and for specific extreme temperature events continue to conclude that extreme temperatures, particularly extreme heat, result in premature deaths. This finding is further reinforced by a growing suite of regional- and national-scale studies documenting an increase in deaths following extreme temperature conditions, using both direct attribution and statistical approaches. The connection between heat events and deaths is also evident internationally. The European heat wave of 2003 is an especially notable example, as it is estimated to have been responsible for between 30,000 and 70,000 premature deaths. However, statistical approaches find that elevated death rates are seen even for less extreme temperatures. These approaches find an optimal temperature and show that there are more deaths at any temperatures that are higher or lower than that optimal temperature. Even though the increase in deaths per degree are smaller near the optimum than at more extreme temperatures, because the percentage of days that do not qualify as extreme are large, it can be important to address the changes in deaths that occur for these smaller temperature differences.

An analysis of U.S. deaths from temperature extremes based on death records found an average of approximately 1,300 deaths per year from 2006 to 2010 coded as resulting from extreme cold exposures, and 670 deaths per year coded as resulting from exposure to extreme heat. These results, and those from all similar studies that rely solely on coding within medical records to determine cause of deaths, will underestimate the actual number of deaths due to extreme temperatures. For example, some statistical approaches estimate that more than 1,300 deaths per year in the United States are due to extreme heat. Different approaches to attributing cause of death lead to differences in the relative number of deaths attributed to heat and cold. Studies based on statistical approaches have found that, despite a larger number of deaths being coded as related to extreme cold rather than extreme heat, and a larger mortality rate in winter overall, the relationship between mortality and an additional day of extreme heat is generally much larger than the relationship between mortality and an additional day of extreme cold.

Confounding Factors and Effect Modifiers

While the direct attribution approach underestimates the number of deaths resulting from extreme temperature events, there are a few ways in which the statistical approach may lead to an overestimation. However, any overestimation due to these potential confounding factors and effect modifiers is thought to be much smaller than the direct attribution underestimation.

The first potential overestimation results from the connection between elevated temperatures and other variables that correlate with temperature, such as poor air quality. This connection involves a combination of factors, including stagnant air masses and changes in the atmospheric chemistry that affect the concentrations of air pollutants, such as ozone or particulate matter. If some portion of the deaths during extreme heat events are actually a result of the higher levels of atmospheric pollution that are correlated with these events, then including those deaths in a statistical analysis to determine the relationship of increased heat on human health would result in double counting deaths. However, this issue is often addressed by including air pollution and other correlated variables in statistical modeling.

A second consideration when using statistical approaches to determine the relationship between temperature and deaths is whether some of the individuals who died during the temperature event were already near death, and therefore, the temperature event could be considered to have "displaced" the death by a matter of days rather than having killed a person not otherwise expected to die. This effect is referred to as "mortality displacement." There is still no consensus regarding the influence of mortality displacement on premature death estimates, but this effect generally accounts for a smaller portion of premature deaths as events become more extreme.

Evidence of Adaptation to Temperature Extremes

The impact on human health of a given temperature event (for example, a 95°F day) can depend on where and when it occurs. The evidence also shows larger changes in deaths and hospitalizations in response to elevated temperatures in cities where temperatures are typically cooler as compared with warmer cities. This suggests that people can adapt, at least partially, to the average temperature that they are used to experiencing. Some of this effect can be explained by differences in infrastructure. For example, locations with higher average temperature, such as the Southeast, will generally have greater prevalence and use of air conditioning. However, there is also evidence that there is a physiological acclimatization (the ability to gradually adapt to heat), with changes in sweat volume and timing, blood flow and heat transfer to the skin, and kidney function and water conservation occurring over the course of weeks to months of exposure to a hot climate. For example, as a result of this type of adaptation, heat events later in the summer have less of an impact on deaths than those earlier in the summer, all else being equal, although some of this effect is also due to the deaths of some of the most vulnerable earlier in the season. However, children and older adults remain vulnerable given their reduced ability to regulate their internal temperature and limited acclimatization capacities.

An increased tolerance to extreme temperatures has also been observed over multiyear and multidecadal periods. This improvement is likely due to some combination of physiological acclimatization, increased prevalence and use of air conditioning, and general improvements in public health over time, but the relative importance of each is not yet clear.

Recent changes in urban planning and development programs reflect an adaptive trend implemented partially in response to the anticipated temperature health risks of climate change. For example, because urban areas tend to be warmer than surrounding rural areas (the "urban heat island" effect), there is an increased emphasis on incorporating green space and other technologies, such as cool roofs, in new development or redevelopment projects. Similarly, programs that provide advice and services in preparation for or response to extreme temperatures continue to increase in number and expand the scope of their activity. Continued changes in personal behavior as a result of these efforts, for example, seeking access to air-conditioned areas during extreme heat events or limiting outside activity, may continue to change future exposure to extreme temperatures and other climate-sensitive health stressors, such as outdoor air pollutants and vectors for disease such as ticks or mosquitoes.

Observed Trends in Heat Deaths

The U.S. average temperature has increased by 1.3°F to 1.9°F since 1895, with much of that increase occurring since 1970, though this temperature increase has not been uniform geographically and some regions, such as the Southeast, have seen little increase in temperature and extreme heat over time. This warming is attributable to elevated concentrations of greenhouse gases, and it has been estimated that three-quarters of moderately hot extremes are already a result of this historical warming. As discussed in the previous section, there have also been changes in the tolerance of populations within the United States to extreme temperatures. Changes in mortality due to high temperatures are therefore, a result of the combination of higher temperatures and higher heat tolerance. Use of the direct attribution approach, based on diagnosis codes in medical records, to examine national trends in heat mortality over time is challenging because of changes in classification methods over time. The few studies using statistical methods that have presented total mortality estimates over time suggest that, over the last several decades, reductions in mortality due to increases in tolerance have outweighed increases in mortality due to increased temperatures.

Observed Impact of Temperature on Illness

Temperature extremes are linked to a range of illnesses reported at emergency rooms and hospitals. However, estimates for the national burden of illness associated with extreme temperatures are limited.

Using a direct attribution approach, an analysis of a nationally representative database from the Healthcare Utilization Project (HCUP) produced an annual average estimate of 65,299 emergency visits for acute heat illness during the summer months (May through September)—an average rate of 21.5 visits for every 100,000 people each year. This result was based only on recorded diagnosis codes for hyperthermia and probably underestimates the true number of heat-related healthcare visits, as a wider range of health outcomes is potentially affected by extreme heat. For example, hyperthermia is not the only complication from extreme heat, and not every individual that suffers from a heat illness visits an emergency department. In a national study of Medicare patients from 2004 to 2005, an annual average of 5,004 hyperthermia cases and 4,381 hypothermia cases were reported for inpatient and outpatient visits. None of these studies link health episodes to observed temperature data, thus limiting the opportunity to attribute these adverse outcomes to specific heat events or conditions.

High ambient heat has been associated with adverse impacts for a wide range of illnesses. Examples of illnesses associated with extreme heat include cardiovascular, respiratory, and renal illnesses; diabetes; hyperthermia; mental-health issues; and preterm births. Children spend more time outdoors and have insufficient ability for physiologic adaptation, and thus may be particularly vulnerable during heat waves. Respiratory illness among the elderly population was most commonly reported during extreme heat.

Statistical studies examine the association between extreme heat and illness using data from various healthcare access points (such as hospital admissions, emergency department visits, and ambulance dispatches). The majority of these studies examine the association of extreme heat with cardiovascular and respiratory illnesses. For these particular health outcomes, the evidence is mixed, as many studies observed elevated risks of illness during periods of extreme heat but others found no evidence of elevated levels of illness. The evidence on some of the other health outcomes is more robust. Across emergency department visits and hospital admissions, high temperatures have been associated with renal diseases, electrolyte imbalance, and hyperthermia. These health risks vary not only across types of illness but also for the same illness across different healthcare settings. In general, evidence for associations with morbidity outcomes, other than cardiovascular impacts, is strong.

While there is still uncertainty about how levels of heat-related illnesses are expected to change with projected increases in summer temperature from climate change, advances have been made in surveillance of heat-related illness. For example, monitoring of emergency ambulance calls during heat waves can be used to establish real-time surveillance systems to identify extreme heat events. The increase in emergency visits for a wide range of illnesses during the 2006 heat wave in California points to the potential for using this type of information in real-time health surveillance systems.

Projected Deaths and Illness from Temperature Exposure

Climate change will increase the frequency and severity of future extreme heat events, while also resulting in generally warmer summers and milder winters with implications for human health. Absent further adaptation, these changes are expected to lead to an increase in illness and death from increases in heat, and reductions in illness and death resulting from decreases in cold, due to changes in outcomes, such as heat stroke, cardiovascular disease, respiratory disease, cerebrovascular disease, and kidney disorders.

A warmer future is projected to lead to increases in future mortality on the order of thousands to tens of thousands of additional premature deaths per year across the United States by the end of this century. Studies differ in which regions of the United States are examined and in how they account for factors, such as adaptation, mortality displacement, demographic changes, definitions of heat waves and extreme cold, and air quality factors, and some studies examine only extreme events while others take into account the health effects of smaller deviations from average seasonal temperatures. Despite these differences, there is reasonable agreement on the magnitude of the projected changes. Additionally, studies have projected an increase in premature deaths due to increases in temperature for Chicago, IL; Dallas, TX; the Northeast corridor cities of Boston, MA, New York, NY, and Philadelphia, PA; Washington State; California; or a group of cities including Portland, OR; Minneapolis and St. Paul, MN; Chicago, IL; Detroit, MI; Toledo, Cleveland, Columbus, and Cincinnati, OH; Pittsburgh and Philadelphia, PA; and Washington, DC. However, these regional projections use a variety of modeling strategies, and therefore, show more variability in mortality estimates than studies that are national in scope.

Less is known about how nonfatal illnesses will change in response to projected increases in heat. However, hospital admissions related to respiratory, hormonal, urinary, genital, and renal problems are generally projected to increase. Kidney stone prevalence has been linked to high temperatures, possibly due to dehydration leading to concentration of the salts that form kidney stones. In the United States, an increased rate of kidney stones is observed in southern regions of the country, especially the Southeast. An expansion of the regions where the risk of kidney stones is higher is, therefore, plausible in a warmer future.

The decrease in deaths and illness due to reductions in winter cold have not been studied, as well as the health impacts of increased heat, but the reduction in premature deaths from cold are expected to be smaller than the increase in deaths from heat in the United States. While this is true nationally (with the exception of Barreca 2012), it may not hold for all regions within the country. Similarly, international studies have generally projected a net increase in deaths from a warming climate, though in some regions, decreases in cold mortality may outweigh increases in heat mortality. The projected net increase in deaths is based in part on historical studies that show that an additional extreme hot day leads to more deaths than an additional extreme cold day, and in part on the fact that the decrease in extreme cold deaths is limited as the total number of cold deaths approaches zero in a given location.

It is important to distinguish between generally higher wintertime mortality rates that are not strongly associated with daily temperatures—such as respiratory infections and some cardiovascular disease—from mortality that is more directly related to the magnitude of the cold temperatures. Some recent studies have suggested that factors leading to higher wintertime mortality rates may not be sensitive to climate warming, and that deaths due to these factors are expected to occur with or without climate change. Considering this, some estimates of wintertime mortality may overstate the benefit of climate change in reducing wintertime deaths.

The U.S. population has become less sensitive to heat over time. Factors that have contributed to this change include infrastructure improvements; including increased access and use of air conditioning in homes and businesses; and improved societal responses, including increased access to public health programs and healthcare. Projecting these trends into the future is challenging, but this trend of increasing tolerance is projected to continue, with future changes in adaptive capacity expected to reduce the future increase in mortality.

However, there are limits to adaptation, whether physiological or sociotechnical (for example, air conditioning, awareness programs, or cooling centers). Historically, adaptation has outpaced warming, but most studies project a future increase in mortality even when including assumptions regarding adaptation. Additionally, the occurrence of events such as power outages simultaneous with a heat wave may reduce some of these adaptive benefits. Such simultaneous events can be more common because of the additional demand on the electricity grid due to high air-conditioning usage. Another potential effect is that if current trends of population growth and migration into large urban areas continue, there may be an increasing urban heat island effect which will magnify the rate of warming locally, possibly leading to more heat-related deaths and fewer cold-related deaths.

Projected changes in future health outcomes associated with extreme temperatures can be difficult to quantify. Projections can depend on: 1. the characterization of population sensitivity to temperature event characteristics such as magnitude, duration, and humidity; 2. differences in population sensitivity, depending on the timing and location of an extreme event; 3. future changes in baseline rates of death and illness, as well as human tolerance and adaptive capacity; 4. the changing proportions of vulnerable populations, including the elderly, in the future; and 5. uncertainty in climate projections.

Populations of Concern for Death and Illness from Extreme Temperature

Impacts of temperature extremes are geographically varied and disproportionally affect certain populations of concern. Certain populations are more at risk for experiencing detrimental consequences of exposure to extreme temperatures due to their sensitivity to hot and cold temperatures and limitations to their capacity for adapting to new climate conditions.

Older adults are a rapidly growing population in the United States, and heat impacts are projected to occur in places where older adults are heavily concentrated and therefore most exposed. Older adults are at higher risk for temperature-related mortality and morbidity, particularly those who have preexisting diseases, those who take certain medications that affect thermoregulation or block nerve impulses (for example, beta-blockers, major tranquilizers, and diuretics), those who are living alone, or those with limited mobility. The relationship between increased temperatures and death in older adults is well-understood with strong evidence of heat-related vulnerability for adults over 65 and 75 years of age. An increased risk for respiratory and cardiovascular death is observed in older adults during temperature extremes due to reduced thermoregulation. Morbidity studies have also identified links between increased temperatures and respiratory and cardiovascular hospitalizations in older adults.

Children are particularly vulnerable because they must rely on others to help keep them safe. This is especially true in environments that may lack air conditioning, including homes, schools, or cars. The primary health complications observed in children exposed to extreme heat include dehydration, electrolyte imbalance, fever, renal disease, heat stress, and hyperthermia. Infectious and respiratory diseases in children are affected by both hot and cold temperatures. Inefficient thermoregulation, reduced cardiovascular output, and heightened metabolic rate are physiological factors driving vulnerability in children to extreme heat. Children also spend a considerable amount of time outdoors and participating in vigorous physical activities. High-school football players are especially vulnerable to heat illness. A limited number of studies show evidence of cold-related mortality in children. However, no study has examined the relationship between cold temperature and cause-specific mortality. Pregnant women are also vulnerable to temperature extremes, as preterm birth has been associated with extreme heat. Elevated heat exposure can increase dehydration, leading to the release of labor-inducing hormones. Extreme heat events are also associated with adverse birth outcomes, such as low birth weight and infant mortality.

Where a person lives, works, or goes to school can also make them more vulnerable to health impacts from extreme temperatures. Of particular concern for densely populated cities is the urban heat island effect, where human-made surfaces absorb sunlight during the day and then radiate the stored energy at night as heat. This process will exacerbate any warming from climate change and limit the potential relief of cooler nighttime temperatures in urban areas. In addition to the urban heat island effect, land cover characteristics and poor air quality combine to increase the impacts of high ambient temperatures for city dwellers and further increase the burden on populations of concern within the urban area. The homeless are often more exposed to heat and cold extremes, while also sharing many risk factors with other populations of concern, such as social isolation, psychiatric illness, and other health issues.

Race, ethnicity, and socioeconomic status can affect vulnerability to temperature extremes. Non-Hispanic Black persons have been identified as being more vulnerable than other racial and ethnic groups to detrimental consequences of exposure to temperature extremes. One study found that non-Hispanic Blacks were two and a half times more likely to experience heat-related mortality when compared to non-Hispanic Whites, and non-Hispanic Blacks had a two-fold risk of dying from a heat-related event compared to Hispanics. Evidence of racial differences in heat tolerance due to genetic differences is inconclusive. However, other factors may contribute to increased vulnerability of Black populations, including comorbidities (coexisting

chronic conditions) that increase susceptibility to higher temperatures, disparities in the availability and use of air conditioning and
in heat risk-related land cover characteristics (for example, living in
urban areas prone to heat-island effects), and environmental justice
issues. Overall, the link between temperature extremes, race, ethnicity, and socioeconomic status is multidimensional and dependent
on the outcome being studied. Education level, income, safe housing,
occupational risks, access to healthcare, and baseline health and nutrition status can further distort the association between temperature
extremes, race, and ethnicity.

Outdoor workers spend a great deal of time exposed to temperature
extremes, often while performing vigorous activities. Certain occupational groups, such as agricultural workers, construction workers,
and electricity and pipeline utility workers, are at increased risk for
heat- and cold-related illness, especially where jobs involve heavy
exertion. One study found failure of employers to provide for acclimatization to be the factor most clearly associated with heat-related
death in workers.

Mental, behavioral, and cognitive disorders can be triggered or
exacerbated by heat waves. Specific illnesses impacted by heat include
dementia, mood disorders, neurosis and stress, and substance abuse.
Some medications interfere with thermoregulation, thereby increasing vulnerability to heat. One study in Australia found that hospital
admissions for mental and behavioral disorders increased by 7.3 percent during heat waves above 80°F. Studies have also linked extreme
heat and increased aggressive behavior.

Emerging and Cross-Cutting Issues

Emerging and cross-cutting issues include:

1. Disparate ways that extreme temperature and health are related

2. Urban and rural differences

3. Interactions between impacts and future changes in adaptation

4. Projections of extreme temperature events

The health effects addressed in this chapter are not the only ways
in which heat and health are related. For example, research indicates
that hotter temperatures may lead to an increase in violent crime
and could negatively affect the labor force, especially occupational
health for outdoor sectors. Extreme temperatures also interact with

air quality, which can complicate estimating how extreme temperature events impact human health in the absence of air quality changes. In addition, increased heat may also increase vulnerability to poor air quality and allergens, leading to potential nonlinear health outcome responses. Extreme temperature events, as well as other impacts from climate change, can also be associated with changes in electricity supply and distribution that can have important implications for the availability of heating and air conditioning, which are key adaptive measures.

Though the estimates of the health impact from extreme heat were produced only for urban areas (which provided a large sample size for statistical validity), there is also emerging evidence regarding high rates of heat-related illness in rural areas. Occupational exposure and a lack of access to air conditioning are some of the factors that may make rural populations particularly susceptible to extreme heat. There are quantitative challenges to using statistical methods to estimate mortality impacts of temperatures in rural areas due to lower population density and more dispersed weather stations, but rural residents have also demonstrated vulnerability to heat events.

Other changes in human behavior will also have implications for the linkage between climate and heat-related illness. Changes in building infrastructure as a response to changes in temperature can have impacts on indoor air quality. Similarly, changes in behavior as a result of temperature changes, for example, seeking access to air conditioning, can change exposure to indoor and outdoor pollution and vector-borne diseases.

Finally, projecting climate variability and the most extreme temperature events can be more challenging than projecting average warming. Extreme temperatures may rise faster than average temperatures, with the coldest days warming faster than average for much of the twentieth century, and the warmest days warming faster than average temperatures in the past 30 years. Extremely high temperatures in the future may also reach levels outside of past experience, in which case statistically based relationships may no longer hold for those events. There have been suggestive links between rapid recent Arctic sea ice loss and an increased frequency of cold and warm extremes, but this is an active area of research with conflicting results. In regions where temperature variability increases, mortality will be expected to increase; mortality is expected to decrease in regions where variability decreases.

Chapter 21

Air Quality Impacts

Changes in the climate affect the air we breathe, both indoors and outdoors. Taken together, changes in the climate affect air quality through three pathways—via outdoor air pollution, aeroallergens, and indoor air pollution. The changing climate has modified weather patterns, which in turn have influenced the levels and location of outdoor air pollutants, such as ground-level ozone (O_3) and fine particulate matter. Increasing carbon dioxide (CO_2) levels also promote the growth of plants that release airborne allergens (aeroallergens). Finally, these changes to outdoor air quality and aeroallergens also affect indoor air quality as both pollutants and aeroallergens infiltrate homes, schools, and other buildings.

Climate change influences outdoor air pollutant concentrations in many ways (see Figure 21.1). The climate influences temperatures, cloudiness, humidity, the frequency and intensity of precipitation, and wind patterns, each of which can influence air quality. At the same time, climate-driven changes in meteorology can also lead to changes in naturally occurring emissions that influence air quality (for example, wildfires, wind-blown dust, and emissions from vegetation). Over longer time scales, human responses to climate change may also affect the amount of energy that humans use, as well as how land is used and where people live. These changes would in turn modify emissions (depending on the fuel source) and thus further influence air quality. Some air pollutants, such as ozone, sulfates, and black carbon, also

This chapter includes text excerpted from "Air Quality Impacts," GlobalChange.gov, U.S. Global Change Research Program (USGCRP), April 4, 2016.

cause changes in climate. However, this chapter does not consider the climate effects of air pollutants but instead remains focused on the health effects resulting from climate-related changes in air pollution exposure.

Poor air quality, whether outdoors or indoors, can negatively affect the human respiratory and cardiovascular systems. Outdoor ground-level ozone and particle pollution can have a range of adverse effects on human health. Current levels of ground-level ozone have been estimated to be responsible for tens of thousands of hospital and emergency room visits, millions of cases of acute respiratory symptoms and school absences, and thousands of premature deaths each year in the United States. Fine particle pollution has also been linked to

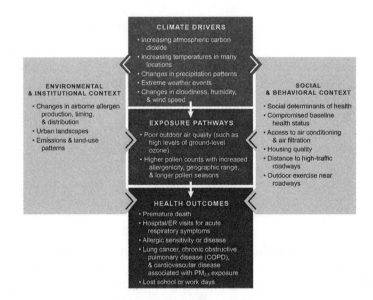

Figure 21.1. *Climate Change and Health—Outdoor Air Quality*

This conceptual diagram for an outdoor air quality example illustrates the key pathways by which humans are exposed to health threats from climate drivers, and potential resulting health outcomes (center boxes). These exposure pathways exist within the context of other factors that positively or negatively influence health outcomes (gray side boxes). Key factors that influence vulnerability for individuals are shown in the right box, and include social determinants of health and behavioral choices. Key factors that influence vulnerability at larger scales, such as natural and built environments, governance and management, and institutions, are shown in the left box. All of these influencing factors can affect an individual's or a community's vulnerability through changes in exposure, sensitivity, and adaptive capacity and may also be affected by climate change.

even greater health consequences through harmful cardiovascular and respiratory effects.

A changing climate can also influence the level of aeroallergens, such as pollen, which in turn adversely affect human health. Rising levels of CO_2 and resulting climate changes alter the production, allergenicity (a measure of how much particular allergens, such as ragweed, affect people), distribution, and seasonal timing of aeroallergens. These changes increase the severity and prevalence of allergic diseases in humans. Higher pollen concentrations and longer pollen seasons can increase allergic sensitization and asthma episodes, thereby limiting productivity at work and school.

Finally, climate change may alter the indoor concentrations of pollutants generated outdoors (such as ground-level ozone), particulate matter, and aeroallergens (such as pollen). Changes in the climate may also increase pollutants generated indoors, such as mold and volatile organic compounds. Most of the air people breathe over their lifetimes will be indoors, since people spend the vast majority of their time in indoor environments. Thus, alterations in indoor air pollutant concentrations from climate change have important health implications.

Climate Impacts on Outdoor Air Pollutants and Health

Changes in the climate affect air pollution levels. Human-caused climate change has the potential to increase ozone levels, may have already increased ozone pollution in some regions of the United States, and has the potential to affect future concentrations of ozone and fine particles (particulate matter smaller than 2.5 microns in diameter, referred to as "PM2.5"). Climate change and air quality are both affected by, and influence, several factors; these include the levels and types of pollutants emitted, how land is used, the chemistry governing how these pollutants form in the atmosphere, and weather conditions.

Ground-Level Ozone

Ozone levels and subsequent ozone-related health impacts depend on:

1. The amount of pollutants emitted that form ozone

2. The meteorological conditions that help determine the amount of ozone produced from those emissions

Both of these factors are expected to change in the future. The emissions of pollutants from anthropogenic (of human origin) sources that form ozone (that is, ozone "precursors") are expected to decrease over the next few decades in the United States. However, irrespective of these changes in emissions, climate change will result in meteorological conditions more favorable to forming ozone. Consequently, attaining national air quality standards for ground-level ozone will also be more difficult, as climate changes offset some of the improvements that would otherwise be expected from emissions reductions. This effect is referred to as the "climate penalty."

Meteorological conditions influencing ozone levels include air temperatures, humidity, cloud cover, precipitation, wind trajectories, and the amount of vertical mixing in the atmosphere. Higher temperatures can increase the chemical rates at which ozone is formed and increase ozone precursor emissions from anthropogenic sources and biogenic (vegetative) sources. Lower relative humidity reduces cloud cover and rainfall, promoting the formation of ozone and extending ozone lifetime in the atmosphere. A changing climate will also modify wind patterns across the United States, which will influence local ozone levels. Over much of the country, the worst ozone episodes tend to occur when the local air mass does not change over a period of several days, allowing ozone and ozone precursor emissions to accumulate over time. Climate change is already increasing the frequency of these types of stagnation events over parts of the United States, and further increases are projected. Ozone concentrations near the ground are strongly influenced by upward and downward movement of air ("vertical mixing"). For example, high concentrations of ozone near the ground often occur in urban areas when there is downward movement of air associated with high pressure ("subsidence"), reducing the extent to which locally emitted pollutants are diluted in the atmosphere. In addition, high concentrations of ozone can occur in some rural areas resulting from downward transport of ozone from the stratosphere or upper troposphere to the ground.

Aside from the direct meteorological influences, there are also indirect impacts on U.S. ozone levels from other climate-influenced factors. For instance, higher water vapor concentrations due to increased temperatures will increase the natural rate of ozone depletion, particularly in remote areas, thus decreasing the baseline level of ozone. Additionally, potential climate-driven increases in nitrogen oxides (NOx) created by lightning or increased exchange of naturally produced ozone in the stratosphere to the troposphere could also affect ozone in those areas of the country most influenced by background ozone concentrations. Increased occurrences of wildfires due to climate change can also lead to increased ozone concentrations near the ground.

There is natural year-to-year variability in temperature and other meteorological factors that influence ozone levels. While global average temperature over 30-year climatic timescales is expected to increase, natural interannual variability will continue to play a significant role in year-to-year changes in temperature. Over the next several decades, the influence of climate change on meteorological parameters affecting average levels of ozone is expected to be smaller than the natural interannual variability.

To address these issues, most assessments of climate impacts on meteorology and associated ozone formation concurrently simulate global and regional chemical transport over multiple years using coupled models. This approach can isolate the influence of meteorology in forming ozone from the effect of changes in emissions. The consensus of these model-based assessments is that accelerated rates of photochemical reaction, increased occurrence of stagnation events, and other direct meteorological influences are likely to lead to higher levels of ozone over large portions of the United States. At the same time, ozone levels in certain regions are projected to decrease as a result of climate change, likely due to localized increases in cloud cover, precipitation, and/or increased dilution resulting from deeper mixed layers. These climate-driven changes in projected ozone vary by season and location, with climate and air quality models showing the most consistency in ozone increases due to climate change in the northeastern United States.

Generally, ozone levels will likely increase across the United States if ozone precursors are unchanged. This climate penalty for ozone will offset some of the expected health benefits, that would otherwise result from the expected ongoing reductions of ozone precursor emissions, and could prompt the need for adaptive measures (for example, additional ozone precursor emissions reductions) to meet national air quality goals.

Air pollution epidemiology studies describe the relationship between a population's historical exposure to air pollutants and the risk of adverse health outcomes. Populations exposed to ozone air pollution are at greater risk of dying prematurely, being admitted to the hospital for respiratory hospital admissions, being admitted to the emergency department, and suffering from aggravated asthma, among other impacts.

Air pollution health impact assessments combine risk estimates from these epidemiology studies with modeled changes in future or historical air quality changes to estimate the number of air-pollution-related premature deaths and illness. Future ozone-related human health impacts attributable to climate change are projected to lead to hundreds to thousands of premature deaths, hospital admissions, and cases of acute respiratory illnesses per year in the United States in 2030.

Health outcomes that can be attributed to climate change impacts on air pollution are sensitive to a number of factors noted above—including the climate models used to describe meteorological changes (including precipitation and cloud cover), the models simulating air quality levels (including wildfire incidence), the size and distribution of the population exposed, and the health status of that population. Moreover, there is emerging evidence that air pollution can interact with climate-related stressors, such as temperature, to affect the human physiological response to air pollution. For example, the risk of dying from exposure to a given level of ozone may increase on warmer days.

Particulate Matter

Particulate matter (PM) is a complex mixture of solid- or liquid-phase substances in the atmosphere that arise from both natural and human sources. Principal constituents of PM include sulfate, nitrate, ammonium, organic carbon, elemental carbon, sea salt, and dust. These particles (also known as "aerosols") can either be directly emitted or can be formed in the atmosphere from gas-phase precursors. PM smaller than 2.5 microns in diameter (PM2.5) is associated with serious chronic and acute health effects, including lung cancer, chronic obstructive pulmonary disease (COPD), cardiovascular disease, and asthma development and exacerbation. The elderly are particularly sensitive to short-term particle exposure, with a higher risk of hospitalization and death.

As is the case for ozone, atmospheric PM2.5 concentrations depend on emissions and on meteorology. Emissions of sulfur dioxide (SO_2), NOx, and black carbon are projected to decline substantially in the United States over the next few decades due to regulatory controls, which will lead to reductions in sulfate and nitrate aerosols.

Climate change is expected to alter several meteorological factors that affect PM2.5, including precipitation patterns and humidity; although, there is greater consensus regarding the effects of meteorological changes on ozone than on PM2.5. Several factors, such as increased humidity, increased stagnation events, and increased biogenic emissions are likely to increase PM2.5 levels, while increases in precipitation, enhanced atmospheric mixing, and other factors could decrease PM2.5 levels. Because of the strong influence of changes in precipitation and atmospheric mixing on PM2.5 levels, and because there is more variability in projected changes to those variables, there is no consensus yet on whether meteorological changes will lead to a net increase or decrease in PM2.5 levels in the United States.

As a result, while it is clear that PM2.5 accounts for most of the health burden of outdoor air pollution in the United States, the health effects of climate-induced changes in PM2.5 are poorly quantified. Some studies have found that changes in PM2.5 will be the dominant driver of air quality-related health effects due to climate change, while others have suggested a potentially more significant health burden from changes in ozone.

Particulate matter resulting from natural sources (such as plants, wildfires, and dust) is sensitive to daily weather patterns, and those fluctuations can affect the intensity of extreme PM episodes. Wildfires are a major source of PM, especially in the western United States during summer. Because winds carry PM2.5 and ozone precursor gases, air pollution from wildfires can affect people even far downwind from the fire location. PM2.5 from wildfires affects human health by increasing the risk of premature death and hospital and emergency department visits.

Climate change has already led to an increased frequency of large wildfires, as well as longer durations of individual wildfires and longer wildfire seasons in the western United States. Future climate change is projected to increase wildfire risks and associated emissions, with harmful impacts on health. The area burned by wildfires in North America is expected to increase dramatically over the 21st century due to climate change. By 2050, changes in wildfires in the western United States are projected to result in 40 percent increases of organic carbon and 20 percent increases in elemental carbon aerosol concentrations. Wildfires may dominate summertime PM2.5 concentrations, offsetting even large reductions in anthropogenic PM2.5 emissions.

Likewise, dust can be an important constituent of PM, especially in the southwest United States. The severity and spatial extent of drought has been projected to increase as a result of climate change, though the impact of increased aridity on airborne dust PM has not been quantified.

Climate Impacts on Aeroallergens and Respiratory Diseases

Climate change may alter the production, allergenicity, distribution, and timing of airborne allergens (aeroallergens). These changes contribute to the severity and prevalence of allergic disease in humans.

The very young, those with compromised immune systems, and the medically uninsured bear the brunt of asthma and other allergic illnesses. While aeroallergen exposure is not the sole, or even necessarily the most significant factor associated with allergic illnesses, that relationship is part of a complex pathway that links aeroallergen exposure to the prevalence of allergic illnesses, including asthma episodes. On the other hand, climate change may reduce adverse allergic and asthmatic responses in some areas. For example, as some areas become drier, there is the potential for a shortening of the pollen season due to plant stress.

Aeroallergens and Rates of Allergic Diseases in the United States

Aeroallergens are substances present in the air that, once inhaled, stimulate an allergic response in sensitized individuals. Aeroallergens include tree, grass, and weed pollen; indoor and outdoor molds; and other allergenic proteins associated with animal dander, dust mites, and cockroaches. Ragweed is the aeroallergen that most commonly affects persons in the United States.

Allergic diseases develop in response to complex and multiple interactions among both genetic and nongenetic factors, including a developing immune system, environmental exposures (such as ambient air pollution or weather conditions), and socioeconomic and demographic factors. Aeroallergen exposure contributes to the occurrence of asthma episodes, allergic rhinitis or hay fever, sinusitis, conjunctivitis, urticaria (hives), atopic dermatitis or eczema, and anaphylaxis (a severe, whole-body allergic reaction that can be life-threatening). Allergic illnesses, including hay fever, affect about one-third of the U.S. population, and more than 34 million Americans have been diagnosed with asthma. These diseases have increased in the United States over the past 30 years. The prevalence of hay fever has increased from 10 percent of the population in 1970 to 30 percent in 2000. Asthma rates have increased from approximately 8 to 55 cases per 1,000 persons to approximately 55 to 90 cases per 1,000 persons over that same time period; however, there is variation in reports of active cases of asthma as a function of geography and demographics.

Climate Impacts on Aeroallergen Characteristics

Climate change contributes to changes in allergic illnesses as greater concentrations of CO_2, together with higher temperatures and changes in precipitation, extend the start or duration of the growing season, increase the quantity and allergenicity of pollen, and expand the spatial distribution of pollens.

Historical trends show that climate change has led to changes in the length of the growing season for certain allergenic pollens. For instance, the duration of pollen release for common ragweed (Ambrosia artemisiifolia) has been increasing as a function of latitude in recent decades in the midwestern region of North America. Latitudinal effects on increasing season length were associated primarily with a delay in first frost during the fall season and lengthening of the frost-free period. Studies in controlled indoor environments find that increases in temperature and CO_2 result in earlier flowering, greater floral numbers, greater pollen production, and increased allergenicity in common ragweed. In addition, studies using urban areas as proxies for both higher CO_2 and higher temperatures demonstrate earlier flowering of pollen species, which may lead to a longer total pollen season.

Climate Variability and Effects on Allergic Diseases

Climate-change related alterations in local weather patterns, including changes in minimum and maximum temperatures and rainfall, affect the burden of allergic diseases. The role of weather on the initiation or exacerbation of allergic symptoms in sensitive persons is not well understood. So-called "thunderstorm asthma" results as allergenic particles are dispersed through osmotic rupture, a phenomenon where cell membranes burst. Pollen grains may, after contact with rain, release part of their cellular contents, including allergen-laced fine particles. Increases in the intensity and frequency of heavy rainfall and storminess over the coming decades is likely to be associated with spikes in aeroallergen concentrations and the potential for related increases in the number and severity of allergic illnesses.

Potential nonlinear interactions between aeroallergens and ambient air pollutants (including ozone, nitrogen dioxide, sulfur dioxide, and fine particulate matter) may increase health risks for people who are simultaneously exposed. In particular, preexposure to air pollution (especially ozone or fine particulate matter) may magnify the effects of aeroallergens, as prior damage to airways may increase the permeability of mucous membranes to the penetration of allergens; although, existing evidence suggests greater sensitivity but not necessarily a direct link with ozone exposure. A report noted remaining uncertainties across the epidemiologic, controlled human exposure, and toxicology studies on this emerging topic.

Climate Impacts on Indoor Air Quality and Health an Emerging Issue

Climate change may worsen existing indoor air problems and create new problems by altering outdoor conditions that affect indoor conditions and by creating more favorable conditions for the growth and spread of pests, infectious agents, and disease vectors that can migrate indoors. Climate change can also lead to changes in the mixing of outdoor and indoor air. Reduced mixing of outdoor and indoor air limits penetration of outdoor pollutants into the indoor, but also leads to higher concentrations of pollutants generated indoors since their dilution by outdoor air is decreased.

Indoor air contains a complex mixture of chemical and biological pollutants or contaminants. Contaminants that can be found indoors include carbon monoxide (CO), fine particles (PM2.5), nitrogen dioxide, formaldehyde, radon, mold, and pollen. Indoor air quality varies from building to building and over the course of a day in an individual building.

Public and environmental health professionals have known for decades that poor indoor air quality is associated with adverse respiratory and other health effects. Since most people spend about 90 percent of their time indoors, much of their exposures to airborne pollutants (both those influenced by climate change and those driven by other factors) happen indoors.

Outdoor Air Changes Reflected in Indoor Air

Indoor air pollutants may come from indoor sources or may be transported into the building with outdoor air. Indoor pollutants of outdoor origin may include ozone, dust, pollen, and fine particulate matter. Even if a building has an outdoor air intake, some air will enter the building through other openings, such as open windows or under doors, or through cracks in the buildings, bypassing any filters and bringing outdoor air pollutants inside. If there are changes in airborne pollutants of outdoor origin, such as pollen and mold and fine PM from wildfires, there will be changes in indoor exposures to these contaminants. Although indoor fine PM levels from wildfires are typically lower than outdoors (about 50%), because people spend most of their time indoors, most of their exposure to and health effects from wildfire particles (about 80%) will come from particles inhaled indoors. Climate-induced changes in indoor-outdoor temperature differences may somewhat reduce the overall intake of outdoor pollutants into buildings for certain regions and seasons.

Most exposures to high levels of ozone occur outdoors; however, indoor exposures, while lower, occur for much longer time periods. Indoors, ozone concentrations are usually about 10 to 50 percent of outdoor concentrations; however, since people spend most of their time indoors, most of their exposure to ozone is from indoor air. Thus, about 45 to 75 percent of a person's overall exposure to ozone will occur indoors. About half of the health effects resulting from any outdoor increases in ozone will be due to indoor ozone exposures. The elderly and children are particularly sensitive to short-term ozone exposure; however, they may spend even more time indoors than the general population, and, consequently, their exposure to ozone is at lower levels for longer periods than the general public. In addition, ozone entering a building reacts with some organic compounds to produce secondary indoor air pollutants. These reactions lower indoor ozone concentrations but introduce new indoor air contaminants, including other respiratory irritants.

Climate-related increases in droughts and dust storms may result in increases in indoor transmission of dust-borne pathogens, as the dust penetrates the indoor environment. Dust contains particles of biologic origin, including pollen and bacterial and fungal spores. Some of the particles are allergenic. Pathogenic fungi and bacteria can be found in dust both indoors and outdoors. For example, in the southwestern United States, spores from the fungi Coccidiodes, which can cause valley fever, are found indoors. The geographic range where Coccidiodes is commonly found is increasing. Climate changes, including increases in droughts and temperatures, may be contributing to this spread and to a rise in valley fever.

Legionnaires' disease is primarily contracted from aerosolized water contaminated with Legionella bacteria. Legionella bacteria are naturally found outdoors in water and soil; they are also known to contaminate treated water systems in buildings, as well as building cooling systems, such as swamp coolers or cooling towers. Legionella can also be found indoors inside plumbing fixtures, such as showerheads, faucets, and humidifiers. Legionella can cause outbreaks of a pneumonia known as "Legionnaires' disease," which is a potentially fatal infection. Exposure can occur indoors when a spray or mist of contaminated water is inhaled, including mist or spray from showers and swamp coolers. The spread of Legionella bacteria can be affected by regional environmental factors. Legionnaires' disease is known to follow a seasonal pattern, with more cases in late summer and autumn, potentially due to warmer and damper conditions. Cases of Legionnaires' disease are rising in the United States, with an increase

317

of 192 percent from 2000 to 2009. If climate change results in sustained higher temperatures and damper conditions in some areas, there could be increases in the spread and transmission of Legionella.

Contaminants Generated Indoors

Although research directly linking indoor dampness and climate change is not available, information on building science, climate change, and outdoor environmental factors that affect indoor air quality can be used to project how climate change may influence indoor environments. Climate change could result in increased indoor dampness in at least two ways:

1. If there are more frequent heavy precipitation events and other severe weather events (including high winds, flooding, and winter storms) that result in damage to buildings, allowing water or moisture entry

2. If outdoor humidity rises with climate change, indoor humidity and the potential for condensation and dampness will likely rise.

Outdoor humidity is usually the largest contributor to indoor dampness on a yearly basis. Increased indoor dampness and humidity will in turn increase indoor mold, dust mites, bacteria, and other bio-contamination indoors, as well as increase levels of volatile organic compounds (VOCs) and other chemicals resulting from the off-gassing of damp or wet building materials. Dampness and mold in U.S. homes are linked to approximately 4.6 million cases of worsened asthma and between 8 and 20 percent of several common respiratory infections, such as acute bronchitis. If there are climate-induced rises in indoor dampness, there could be increases in adverse health effects related to dampness and mold, such as asthma exacerbation.

Additionally, power outages due to more frequent extreme weather events, such as flooding, could lead to a number of health effects. Heating, ventilation, and air conditioning (HVAC) systems will not function without power; therefore, many buildings could have difficulty maintaining indoor temperatures or humidity. Loss of ventilation, filtration, air circulation, and humidity control can lead to indoor mold growth and increased levels of indoor contaminants, including VOCs, such as formaldehyde. Power outages are also associated with increases in hospital visits from carbon monoxide (CO) poisoning, primarily due to the incorrect use of backup and portable generators that contaminate indoor air with carbon monoxide. Following floods, CO poisoning is also associated with the improper indoor use of wood-burning appliances, and other combustion appliances designed for use outdoors. There were at least nine deaths from carbon monoxide poisoning related to power outages from 2000 to 2009.

Climate factors can influence populations of rodents that produce allergens and can harbor pathogens, such as *hantaviruses*, which can cause *Hantavirus* pulmonary syndrome (HPS). *Hantaviruses* can be spread to people by rodents that infest buildings, and limiting indoor exposure is a key strategy to prevent the spread of *hantavirus*. Climate change may increase rodent populations in some areas, including indoors, particularly when droughts are followed by periods of heavy rain and with increases in temperature and rainfall. Also, extreme weather events, such as heavy rains and flooding, may drive some rodents to relocate indoors. Increases in rodent populations may result in increased indoor exposures to rodent allergens and related health effects. In addition, climate factors may also influence the prevalence of *hantaviruses* in rodents. This is a complex dynamic because climate change may influence rodent populations, ranges, and infection rates.

Populations of Concern

Certain groups of people may be more susceptible to harm from air pollution due to factors including age, access to healthcare, baseline health status, or other characteristics. In the contiguous United States, Blacks or African Americans, women, and the elderly experience the greatest baseline risk from air pollution. The young, older adults, asthmatics, and people whose immune systems are compromised are more vulnerable to indoor air pollutants than the general population. Lower socioeconomic status and housing disrepair have been associated with higher indoor allergen exposures, though higher-income populations may be more exposed to certain allergens, such as dust mites.

Nearly 6.8 million children in the United States are affected by asthma, making it a major chronic disease of childhood. It is also the main cause of school absenteeism and hospital admissions among children. In 2008, 9.3 percent of American children between the ages of 2 to 17 were reported to have asthma. The onset of asthma in children has been linked to early allergen exposure and viral infections, which act in concert with genetic susceptibility. Children can be particularly susceptible to allergens due to their immature respiratory and immune systems, as well as indoor or outdoor activities that contribute to aeroallergen exposure.

A study of children in California found that racial and ethnic minorities are more affected by asthma. Among minority children, the prevalence of asthma varies with the highest rates among Blacks and American Indians/Alaska Natives (17%), followed by non-Hispanic or non-Latino Whites (10%), Hispanics (7%), and Asian Americans (7%).

Minority adults and children also bear a disproportionate burden associated with asthma as measured by emergency department visits, lost work and school days, and overall poorer health status. Twice as many Black children had asthma-related emergency department visits and hospitalizations when compared with White children. Fewer Black and Hispanic children reported using preventative medication, such as inhaled corticosteroids (ICS), as compared to White children. Black and Hispanic children also had more poorly controlled asthma symptoms, leading to increased emergency department visits and greater use of rescue medications rather than routine daily use of ICS, regardless of symptom control.

Children living in poverty were 1.75 times more likely to be hospitalized for asthma than their nonpoor counterparts. When income is accounted for, no significant difference was observed in the rate of hospital admissions by race or ethnicity. This income effect may be related to access and use of healthcare and appropriate use of preventive medications, such as ICS.

People with preexisting medical conditions—including hypertension, diabetes, and chronic obstructive pulmonary disorder—are at greater risk for outdoor air pollution-related health effects than the general population. Populations with irregular heartbeats (atrial fibrillation) who were exposed to air pollution and high temperatures experience increased risk. People who live or work in buildings without air conditioning and other ventilation controls or in buildings that are unable to withstand extreme precipitation or flooding events are at greater risk of adverse health effects. Other health risks are related to exposures to poor indoor air quality from mold and other biological contaminants and chemical pollutants emitted from wet building materials. While the presence of air conditioning has been found to greatly reduce the risk of ozone-related deaths, communities with a higher percentage of unemployment and a greater population of Blacks are at greater risk.

Part Four

International Travel and Infectious Diseases

Chapter 22

International Adoption: Health Guidance and the Immigration Process

For Parents: Overseas Medical Exam and Vaccinations for Your Adopted Child
Medical Exam

The medical examination process for your adopted child begins overseas with a visit to a panel physician. A panel physician is a Department of State-designated medical doctor who performs medical exams overseas for immigrants (including international adoptees), refugees, and migrants coming into the United States. Panel physicians, who are located in many countries in the world, must refer to the Centers for Disease Control and Prevention (CDC) guidelines on medical exams. Panel physicians are trained in the technical instructions that the CDC provides.

The purpose of the overseas medical exam is to identify applicants, including adoptees, with Class A conditions (illnesses that prevent

This chapter includes text excerpted from "International Adoption: Health Guidance and the Immigration Process," Centers for Disease Control and Prevention (CDC), March 29, 2012. Reviewed May 2019.

immigration to the United States). Children with these conditions must be treated or get a waiver before they can get a visa to come to the United States.

The visa medical exam differs from a normal physical that you may be used to. The visa medical exam includes:

- A physical exam

- A series of vaccines*

- A screening for tuberculosis (TB) (skin test/chest X-ray examination)

- A blood test for syphilis (not routinely done for children under the age of 15 unless there is reason to suspect infection)

Some adopted children can receive an affidavit to have their vaccinations delayed until after they arrive in the United States. Children who receive an affidavit must receive the required vaccines once they arrive in the United States.

Once the medical exam is completed, the panel physician will give you a sealed packet containing the medical exam forms. When you arrive in the United States, give the sealed packet to the Customs and Border Protection (CBP) officer. The CBP officer is an immigration official who will process your paperwork when you first enter the United States. During the medical exam, you should ask for an extra copy of the medical exam forms and give them to your child's medical provider in the United States.

Children should also receive a medical exam once they enter the United States.

Vaccinations

Vaccinations are an important part of the overseas medical examination. The Immigration and Nationality Act requires that all immigrant visa applicants, including adopted children, show proof of having received certain vaccinations named in the law, as well as others recommended by the Advisory Committee on Immunization Practices, before they may be granted an immigrant visa. Vaccination requirements depend on the age of your child.

For Parents: Finding a Medical Provider in the United States

Once you have brought your child into the United States, you need to find a medical provider with whom you feel comfortable taking your child for medical care. CDC encourages parents to schedule their child's medical visit within a few weeks of arrival. Your child's first medical visit in the United States will be more detailed than his or her visa medical exam. Since the visa medical exam only screens for certain diseases, it may not give you a complete picture of your child's health. The first U.S. medical exam will help you find out about any other health issues your child may have and allow for timely treatment, if needed.

Your child's first medical visit in the United States should:

- Check growth and development

- Test hearing and vision

- Screen for these diseases, if needed:

  - Human immunodeficiency viruses (HIV)/acquired immunodeficiency syndrome (AIDS)

  - Syphilis

  - Hepatitis B

  - Illnesses caused by parasites

  - TB tuberculin skin test (TST)

Your child must also get vaccines if she or he did not receive them overseas. Parents are required to get their children vaccinated within 30 days of arrival.

Your child's medical provider may also want to learn about your child's medical history. If you have any forms or papers with details about your child's medical background, bring them to the first visit.

If you are looking for a medical provider, you may want to consider pediatricians who focus on treating international adoptees. They tend to have more experience with medical conditions seen in children adopted overseas.

Chapter 23

Refugee Health Guidelines

Infectious diseases know no borders. People come and go between the United States and Mexico to visit, work, and live. The movement of people and products between the two countries creates a unique binational environment for preventing and controlling diseases spread through food and water, from insects or animals, and between people.

Border Crossings

In 2016, 185 million northbound crossings took place at 25 land ports of entry along the 2,000-mile border between the United States and Mexico.

Tourism

Mexico is the top foreign tourist destination for U.S. travelers.

In 2016, 31 million people traveled from the United States to Mexico, and 18.7 million Mexicans traveled to the United States.

This chapter contains text excerpted from the following sources: Text in this chapter begins with excerpts from "About Binational Health," Centers for Disease Control and Prevention (CDC), February 1, 2013. Reviewed May 2019; Text beginning with the heading "Guidelines for Predeparture and Postarrival Medical Screening and Treatment of U.S.-Bound Refugees" is excerpted from "Refugee Health Guidelines," Centers for Disease Control and Prevention (CDC), March 29, 2012. Reviewed May 2019.

Residence

- Mexico is the number one country of residence for U.S. expatriates. In 2016, one million U.S. citizens lived in Mexico.

- In 2016, 36.3 million people of Mexican origin lived in the United States,

- In 2015, within 100 kilometers (62 miles) of the United States-Mexico border, 7.7 million people lived in 44 U.S. counties across the 4 border states, and 6.7 million lived in 80 Mexican border "municipios" (counties or cities).

Guidelines for Predeparture and Postarrival Medical Screening and Treatment of U.S.-Bound Refugees

Many health conditions may affect the health of refugees; therefore, the Centers for Disease Control and Prevention (CDC) provides guidelines for healthcare providers who may see refugees at any point during the resettlement process. These guidelines aim to:

- Promote and improve the health of the refugee

- Prevent disease

- Familiarize refugees with the U.S. healthcare system

There are two major categories of refugee health guidelines—overseas and domestic.

- The overseas medical screening guidelines are intended to provide panel physicians guidance on the overseas predeparture presumptive treatments for malaria and intestinal parasites. These screenings are usually conducted days to weeks before the refugee departs from her or his country of asylum.

- The domestic medical screening guidelines are provided for state public health departments and medical providers in the United States who conduct the initial medical screening for refugees. These screenings are usually conducted 30 to 90 days postarrival in the United States.

All the guidelines are based on current medical knowledge and the advice of experts in refugee health. Both domestic and overseas medical screening guidelines are to provide healthcare providers with currently accepted best practices, but should not be considered mandates. The guidelines, and revisions to current guidelines.

The CDC Technical Instructions should not be confused with the domestic or overseas guidelines. The Technical Instructions focus on the required medical screening of refugees and immigrants for diseases of public health significance, such as tuberculosis, in accordance with U.S. immigration law. The Technical Instructions are meant to be used by panel physicians who perform the overseas screening and civil surgeons in the United States who conduct the medical exams for adjustment of visa status.

Medical Screening of Asylees

Asylees are persons who meet the definition of a refugee but are already in the United States or are seeking admission at a U.S. port of entry. From 2000 to 2010, the top 10 countries of origin for people granted asylum in the United States were China, Colombia, Haiti, India, Ethiopia, Iraq, Armenia, Albania, Iran, and Somalia. Those who are living in the United States or are seeking admission at a U.S. port of entry when they apply for asylum are recommended to have a domestic medical exam once they have been granted asylum status. When an asylee applies for adjustment of status, an I-693 medical examination (including vaccinations) by a civil surgeon is required. Once an asylee has been granted asylum status, their family members may follow to join them in the United States, and therefore, these family members would undergo the required medical examination overseas prior to immigration.

Currently, there are very little data available about the health problems of asylees after they migrate to the United States. Many asylum seekers originate in, or transfer through, countries with public health issues similar to those facing refugees arriving through the U.S. Refugee Admissions Program. Therefore, the CDC recommends that medical providers screening asylees should apply the same screening and treatment recommendations as according to the CDC Refugee Domestic Guidelines when performing a medical evaluation of an asylee. For individuals who have been in the United States for more than one year, special attention should be paid to diseases with long latency and associated severe morbidities, such as tuberculosis, hepatitis B, and *Strongyloides* infection.

Chapter 24

Screening Internationally Adopted Children, Migrants, and Travelers for Infectious Diseases

Each year, parents in the United States adopt more than 5,000 children from all over the world. Adopting a child is a wonderful and exciting event for families. The health of the adopted child is one of many issues that parents need to address during the adoption process. Parents should be prepared for possible challenges during the adoption process and be aware that sometimes the process can be lengthy.

Children born in other areas of the world may have different health problems from those of children raised in the United States. Children may have been exposed to vaccine-preventable diseases that are rare in the United States. Some children are adopted from countries with high rates of diseases, such as tuberculosis, hepatitis, and human

This chapter contains text excerpted from the following sources: Text in this chapter begins with excerpts from "International Adoption: Health Guidance and the Immigration Process," Centers for Disease Control and Prevention (CDC), March 29, 2012. Reviewed May 2019; Text beginning with the heading "Travel Preparation for Adoptive Parents and Their Families" is excerpted from "International Adoption," Centers for Disease Control and Prevention (CDC), June 12, 2017.

immunodeficiency virus (HIV)/acquired immunodeficiency syndrome (AIDS). For all these reasons, knowing as much as possible about a child's health will help parents get the right treatment and care for their child. Ensuring that adopted children are healthy will also help prevent the spread of disease in families and communities in the United States.

Travel Preparation for Adoptive Parents and Their Families

A pretravel clinic visit is strongly recommended for prospective adoptive parents. In preparation, the travel health provider must know the disease risks in the adopted child's country of origin and the medical and social histories of the adoptee (if available), as well as which family members will be traveling, their immunization and medical histories, the season of travel, the length of stay in the country, and the itinerary while in country. Family members who remain at home, including extended family, should be current on their routine immunizations. Protection against measles, varicella, tetanus, diphtheria, pertussis, hepatitis A, hepatitis B, and polio must be ensured for everyone who will be in the household or in close contact by providing care for the adopted child. Measles immunity or two doses of measles-mumps-rubella (MMR) vaccine separated by ≥28 days should be documented for all people born in or after 1957. Varicella vaccine should be given to those without a history of varicella disease or documentation of two doses of varicella vaccine ≥3 months apart. Adults who have not received tetanus-diphtheria-acellular pertussis (Tdap) vaccine, including adults >65 years old, should receive a single dose of Tdap to protect against Bordetella pertussis in addition to tetanus and diphtheria. Unprotected family members and close contacts of the adopted child should be immunized against hepatitis A virus (HAV) before the child's arrival. Most adult family members and caretakers will need to be immunized with hepatitis B vaccine, since it has only been routinely given since 1990.

Overseas Medical Examination of the Adopted Child

All immigrants, including children adopted internationally by United States citizens, must undergo a medical examination in their country of origin, performed by a physician designated by the Department of State. The medical examination is used primarily to detect diseases or risk behaviors that may make the immigrant ineligible for a visa. Prospective adoptive parents should not rely on this medical examination to detect all possible disabilities and illnesses. Laboratory results from the country of origin may be unreliable. This examination should not replace the evaluation that is recommended once the child comes to the United States.

If the adopted child is from a polio-endemic area, family members and caretakers should ensure they have completed the recommended age-appropriate polio vaccine series. A one-time inactivated polio booster for adults who have completed the primary series in the past is recommended if they are traveling to these areas and can be considered for adults who remain at home but who will be in close contact caring for the child. Additional polio vaccination requirements for long-term travelers (staying >4 weeks) and residents departing from countries with polio transmission may affect travel.

Prospective adoptive parents and any children traveling with them should receive advice on travel safety, food safety, immunization, malaria chemoprophylaxis, diarrhea prevention and treatment, and other travel-related health issues, as outlined elsewhere in this book. Instructions on car seats, injury prevention, food safety, and air travel apply equally to the adoptive child, so the travel health provider should also be familiar with and provide information on these child-specific issues.

Follow-Up Medical Examination after Arrival in the United States

The adopted child should have a medical examination within two weeks of arrival in the United States or earlier if the child has fever, anorexia, diarrhea, vomiting, or other medical concerns. Items to consider during medical examination of an adopted child include the following:

- **Temperature** (fever requires further investigation)

- **General appearance:** alert, interactive

- **Anthropometric measurements:** weight/age, height/age, weight/height, head circumference/age, body mass index

- **Facial features:** length of palpebral fissures, philtrum, upper lip (fetal alcohol syndrome: short palpebral fissures, thin upper lip, indistinct philtrum), other facial features suggestive of a genetic syndrome

- **Hair:** texture, color, areas of alopecia with dry patches (tinea capitis)

- **Eyes:** jaundice, pallor, strabismus, visual acuity screen

- **Ears:** hearing screen, otitis media

- **Mouth:** palate, thrush, presence of a uvula, teeth (number and condition)

- **Neck:** thyroid (enlargement secondary to hypothyroidism, iodine deficiency), lymph nodes

- **Heart:** murmurs

- **Chest:** symmetry, Tanner stage breasts

- **Abdomen:** liver or spleen enlargement

- **Skin:** Mongolian spots, scars, bacillus Calmette-Guérin (BCG) scar, birthmarks, molluscum contagiosum, tinea capitis, tinea corporis

- **Lymph nodes:** enlargement suggestive of TB or other infections

- **Back:** scoliosis, sacral dimple

- **Genitalia:** Tanner stage, presence of both testicles, findings of sexual abuse

- **Extremities:** presence of bowing (rickets) or deformities

- **Neurologic:** presence and quality of reflexes

In addition, all children should receive a developmental screening by a clinician with experience in child development to determine if immediate referrals should be made for a more detailed neurodevelopmental examination and therapies. Further evaluation will depend on the country of origin, the age of the child, previous living conditions, nutritional status, developmental status, and the adoptive family's specific questions. Concerns raised during the preadoption medical review may dictate further investigation.

Screening for Infectious Diseases

The current panel of tests for infectious diseases recommended by the American Academy of Pediatrics (AAP) for screening internationally adopted children is as follows:

- HAV serologic testing (IgG and IgM)

- Hepatitis B virus (HBV) serologic testing (repeat at six months if initial testing is negative)

- Hepatitis C antibody (repeat at six months if initial testing is negative)

- Syphilis serologic testing (treponemal and nontreponemal testing)

- HIV 1 and 2 serologic testing (antigen/ antibody)

- Complete blood cell count with differential and red blood cell indices

- Stool examination for ova and parasites (three specimens)

- Stool examination for Giardia intestinalis and *Cryptosporidium* antigen (one specimen)

- Tuberculin skin test (TST) (all ages) or interferon-γ release assay (IGRA) (for children >5 years of age) (repeat at six months if initial test is negative)

Additional screening tests may be useful, depending on the child's country of origin or specific risk factors. These screens may include Chagas disease serologic tests, malaria smears, or serologic testing for schistosomiasis, strongyloidiasis, and filariasis.

Gastrointestinal Parasites

Gastrointestinal parasites are commonly seen in international adoptees, but the prevalence varies by birth country and age. The highest rates of infection have been reported from Ukraine and Ethiopia and increase with older age. Giardia intestinalis is the most common parasite identified. Three stool samples collected in the early morning, two to three days apart and placed in a container with preservative are recommended for ova and parasite analysis. Only one of these samples needs to be analyzed for Giardia antigen and *Cryptosporidium* antigen. Although theoretically possible, transmission of intestinal parasites from internationally adopted children to family and school contacts has not been reported; however, good hand hygiene is recommended to prevent infection. Stool samples should be cultured for enteric bacterial pathogens for any child with fever and bloody diarrhea. Unlike refugees, internationally adopted children are not treated for parasites before departure.

Hepatitis A

HAV serology (IgG and IgM) should be considered for all internationally adopted children to identify children who may be acutely infected and shedding virus and to make decisions regarding HAV immunization. In 2007 and early 2008, multiple cases of hepatitis A secondary to exposure to newly arrived internationally adopted children were reported in the United States. Some of these cases involved extended family members who were not living in the household. Identification of acutely infected toddlers new to the United States is necessary to prevent further transmission. If a child is found to have acute infection, HAV vaccine or immunoglobulin can be given to close contacts to prevent infection. In addition, it is cost-effective to identify children with past infection with serologic testing since they would not need to receive the HAV vaccine.

Hepatitis B

All internationally adopted children should be screened for HBV infection with serology for hepatitis B surface antigen (HBsAg) and hepatitis B surface antibody to determine past infection, current infection, or protection due to vaccination. HBV infection has been reported in one to five percent of newly arrived adoptees. Because of widespread use of the HBV vaccine, the prevalence of HBV infection has decreased over the years. Children found to be positive for HBsAg should be retested six months later to determine if the child has a chronic infection. Results of a positive HBsAg test should be reported to the state health department. HBV is highly transmissible within the household. All members of households adopting children with chronic HBV infection must be immunized and should have follow-up antibody titers to determine whether levels consistent with immunity have been achieved. Children with chronic HBV infection should receive additional tests for HBV e antigen, HBV e antibody, hepatitis D virus antibody, viral load, and liver function. They should be vaccinated for hepatitis A if they are not immune. They should also have a consultation with a pediatric gastroenterologist. Repeat screening at six months after arrival should be done on all children who initially test negative for HBV surface antibody.

Hepatitis C

Routine screening for hepatitis C virus (HCV) should be done, since most children with HCV infection are asymptomatic, screening for risk factors is not possible, effective treatments are available, and close follow-up of infected patients is needed to identify long-term complications. Antibody testing with an EIA should be done for screening. Since maternal antibody may be present in children <18 months of age, Polymerase chain reaction (PCR) testing should be done if the EIA is positive. Children with HCV infection should be referred to a gastroenterologist for further evaluation, management, and treatment.

Syphilis

Screening for *Treponema pallidum* is recommended for all internationally adopted children. Initial screening is done with both non-treponemal and treponemal tests. Treponemal tests remain positive for life in most cases even after successful treatment and are specific for treponemal diseases, which include syphilis and other diseases (such as yaws, pinta, and bejel) that can be seen in some countries. In children with a history of syphilis, the child's initial evaluation, treatment (antibiotic type and treatment duration), and follow-up testing are rarely available; therefore, a full evaluation for disease must be undertaken and anti treponemal treatment given dependent upon the results.

Human Immunodeficiency Virus

Human immunodeficiency virus (HIV) screening is recommended for all internationally adopted children. Positive HIV antibodies in children younger than 18 months of age may reflect maternal antibody and not an infection. Assaying for HIV DNA with PCR will confirm the diagnosis of HIV in the infant or child. Standard screening for HIV is with enzyme-linked immunosorbent assay (ELISA) antibody testing, but some experts recommend PCR for any infant aged <6 months on arrival. If PCR testing is done, two negative results from assays administered one month apart, at least one of which is done after the age of four months, are necessary to exclude infection. Children with HIV infection should be referred to a specialist. Some experts recommend repeating the screen for HIV antibodies 6 months after arrival if the initial testing is negative.

Chagas Disease

Screening for Chagas disease should be considered for children arriving from a country endemic for Chagas disease. Chagas disease is endemic throughout much of Mexico, Central America, and South America. The risk of Chagas disease varies by region within endemic countries. Although the risk of Chagas disease is likely low in adopted children from endemic countries, treatment of infected children is effective. Serologic testing when the child is aged 9 to 12 months will avoid possible false-positive results from maternal antibody. Testing by PCR can be done in children younger than 9 months of age. If a child tests positive for Chagas disease, the child should be referred to a specialist for further evaluation and management.

Malaria

Routine screening for malaria is not recommended for internationally adopted children. However, thick and thin malaria smears should be obtained immediately for any febrile child newly arrived from a malaria-endemic area.

Tuberculosis

All internationally adopted children should be screened for tuberculosis (TB) after arriving in the United States. Internationally adopted children are at four to six times the risk for TB than their United States-born peers. The TST is indicated for all children, regardless of their BCG status. TST results must be interpreted carefully for internationally adopted children; guidelines may be found in the bibliography. For children aged ≥5 years, IGRA (such as QuantiFERON-TB Gold) is an acceptable screening alternative to the TST. IGRA has the advantage of not requiring a follow-up visit for testing or requiring individual interpretation of results (although results may be termed "indeterminate" by the laboratory). In addition, they appear to be more specific than the TST for Mycobacterium tuberculosis infection in children who have had BCG vaccination. The TST remains the most widely used screening test for TB in children. A chest radiograph and complete physical examination to assess for pulmonary and extrapulmonary TB are indicated for all children with positive TB screening results. Hilar lymphadenopathy is a more sensitive finding for TB in young children than are pulmonary infiltrates or cavitation. A repeat TST three to six months after arrival is recommended for children who initially test negative. Children who have a positive TST or IGRA result but have no evidence of active disease have latent tuberculosis infection (LTBI) and should generally be treated with isoniazid for nine months. In consultation with TB experts, a shorter-course LTBI treatment regimen may be considered. If active disease is found, every effort should be made to isolate the organism and determine sensitivities, particularly if the child is from a region of the world with a high rate of multidrug-resistant TB.

Eosinophilia

A complete blood count with a differential should be done on all internationally adopted children. An eosinophil count >450 cells/mm3 in an internationally adopted child may warrant further evaluation. Intestinal parasite screening will identify some helminths that may cause eosinophilia. Further investigation of the eosinophilia might include serologic evaluation for *Strongyloides stercoralis*, Toxocara canis, Ancylostoma spp., and *Trichinella spiralis*. For children arriving from countries endemic for Schistosoma spp. and filariasis, serologic testing should be done for these diseases as well.

Screening for Noninfectious Diseases

Several screening tests for noninfectious diseases should be performed in all or in select internationally adopted children. All children should have a complete blood count with a differential, hemoglobin electrophoresis, and glucose-6-phosphate dehydrogenase (G6PD) deficiency screening. Serum levels of thyroid-stimulating hormone and lead should be measured in all internationally adopted children. Testing for serum levels of iron, iron-binding capacity, transferrin, ferritin, and total vitamin D 25 hydroxy should be considered. All children should have vision and hearing screening and a dental evaluation. In certain circumstances, neurologic and psychological testing may also be considered.

Chapter 25

Preventing Spread of Disease on Commercial Aircraft

This chapter provides cabin crew with practical methods to protect themselves, passengers, and other crew members when someone onboard is sick with a possible contagious disease. Included are instructions to protect yourself and others, manage a sick traveler, clean contaminated areas, and take actions after flight.

When interacting with a sick and potentially infectious traveler (passenger or crew), follow the steps in this chapter to reduce the risk of onboard disease transmission. Be sure to follow your company's policy for managing in-flight medical emergencies.

This general guidance is NOT designed for:

Noncontagious illnesses or emergencies, such as chest pain, possible stroke, asthma, or diabetic complications.

Identifying a Sick and Potentially Infectious Traveler

Since illness is not yet known to be contagious when symptoms first appear, treat any bodily fluids (such as diarrhea, vomit, or blood) as

This chapter includes text excerpted from "Preventing Spread of Disease on Commercial Aircraft: Guidance for Cabin Crew," Centers for Disease Control and Prevention (CDC), January 21, 2016.

potentially infectious. Once you identify a sick and potentially infectious passenger, use appropriate infection control measures.

Suspect a contagious disease when a traveler (passenger or crew) has:

- A fever (when an individual has a measured temperature of 100.4°F [38°C] or greater, feels warm to the touch, or gives a history of feeling feverish) and one or more of these signs or symptoms:

  - Skin rash

  - Difficulty breathing

  - Persistent cough

  - Decreased consciousness or confusion of recent onset

  - New unexplained bruising or bleeding (without previous injury)

  - Persistent diarrhea

  - Persistent vomiting (other than air sickness)

  - Headache with a stiff neck

  - Appears obviously unwell

- Has a fever that has persisted for more than 48 hours

- Has symptoms or other indications of communicable disease, as the Centers for Disease Control and Prevention (CDC) may announce through posting of a notice in the Federal Register.

The U.S. Code of Federal Regulations [42 CFR 70.11 and 71.21] contain requirements for reporting death and illness to the CDC that occur on domestic flights between U.S. states and territories, and on international flights arriving at the United States.

General Infection Control Measures
Protecting Yourself and Others

- Treat all bodily fluids (such as diarrhea, vomit, or blood) like they are infectious.

- Handwashing is the single most important infection control measure.

- Wash hands often with soap and water for at least 20 seconds after assisting sick travelers or touching potentially contaminated bodily fluids or surfaces. Also, wash hands when visibly soiled.

- Use alcohol-based hand sanitizer (containing at least 60% alcohol) if soap and water are not available.

- Avoid touching your mouth, eyes, and nose with unwashed or gloved hands.

Personal Protective Equipment

- Protect yourself by using personal protective equipment (PPE) when tending to a sick traveler. After use, PPE must be carefully removed to avoid contaminating your skin or clothing. Soiled items must be placed in a biohazard bag (or plastic bag labeled "biohazard" if a biohazard bag is not available).

- Always wash hands or use an alcohol-based hand sanitizer after removing any PPE.

Disposable Gloves (Gloves Do Not Replace Proper Handwashing)

- Wear disposable gloves when:
  - Tending to a sick traveler
  - Touching bodily fluids (such as blood, vomit, or diarrhea)
  - Touching potentially contaminated surfaces, such as in bathrooms

- Remove gloves carefully to avoid contaminating yourself or your clothing.

- Properly dispose soiled gloves in a biohazard bag (or plastic bag labeled "biohazard" if a biohazard bag is not available); do not reuse gloves.

- After removing gloves, wash your hands with soap and water or use an alcohol-based hand sanitizer.

Facemasks

- Face masks should be considered:

- For crew when you are helping sick travelers with respiratory symptoms, such as coughing or sneezing

- For sick travelers to help reduce the spread of respiratory germs

- For people sitting near sick travelers (with respiratory symptoms) when the sick traveler cannot tolerate wearing a mask

- Face masks are not needed:

  - For a sick traveler complaining of nausea or vomiting. This could result in choking or a blocked airway.

  - For sick travelers who cannot tolerate a face mask or refuse one. In this case, ask sick travelers to cover their coughs or sneezes.

Infection Control Guidance

- Minimize the number of people directly exposed to sick travelers. If possible, designate one crew member to interact with the sick traveler.

- Keep interactions with sick travelers as brief as possible. Provide a plastic bag for disposal of used tissues, air sickness bag(s), or other contaminated items.

- Encourage sick travelers to wash their hands or use an alcohol-based hand sanitizer (if available).

- If possible, separate the sick traveler from others by six feet or move adjacent passengers without compromising flight safety or exposing additional passengers.

- Use infection control measures based on symptoms.

Reporting Illness or Death

Reporting illness or death is required as per federal regulations. Crew need to report all sick travelers with certain symptoms on flights to or within the United States to the pilot as soon as possible. Refer to the CDC Death and Disease Reporting Tool for information on reportable illnesses. For assistance, contact the CDC quarantine station closest to your arrival city.

Table 25.1. Infection Control

Possible Symptoms	Illness Category (Examples of Possible Diseases Transmitted)	How Infection Spreads	Infection Control Measures (Use in Addition to General Infection Control Measures)
Coughing, sneezing, fever, rash, or difficulty breathing	Respiratory (e.g., measles, tuberculosis, influenza, whooping cough [pertussis], meningococcal disease, and Middle East respiratory syndrome [MERS])	Via droplets in the air or from contact with contaminated surfaces	Ask sick travelers to cover their mouth with a tissue if coughing or sneezing. Offer a facemask for persistent cough, if available, but do not give masks to travelers who say they are nauseated or vomiting due to risk of choking.
Nausea, stomach pain, vomiting, fever, or diarrhea	Gastrointestinal (e.g., norovirus and cholera)	Contact with contaminated surfaces, stool or vomit, or from contaminated food or water	Seat sick travelers with diarrhea or vomiting close to a bathroom, if possible. Restrict the use of that bathroom to only sick traveler(s), if possible. Disinfect, per company policy, if restriction is not possible. Provide air-sickness bags if travelers say they are nauseated or vomiting.
Visible bleeding, whether due to injury or not	Bloodborne (e.g., HIV, hepatitis B and C, and viral hemorrhagic fevers, including Ebola)	Contact with open cuts, scrapes, or mucous membranes (lining of mouth, eyes, or nose).	If sick travelers are actively bleeding, such as from an injury or nosebleed, provide first aid according to your airline's guidelines. Provide towels, tissues, or other items to absorb blood, if possible.

Targeting Clean-Up In-Flight

- Employees should put on PPE in the universal precaution kit (UPK) before cleaning or disinfecting any area.
- Take the following actions in areas contaminated with diarrhea, vomit, blood, or other bodily fluids.
  - For hard (nonporous) surfaces, such as tray tables, TV monitors, seat arms, windows, and walls, remove any visible contamination and clean and disinfect the area with products approved by your company.
  - For soft (porous) surfaces, such as carpeted floor or seat cushions, remove as much of the contaminant as possible, cover the area with an absorbent substance, and contain the area as much as possible. Remove the absorbent substance and any remaining material, and then clean and disinfect the area with products approved by your company.

Bagging and Disposal

- Carefully place all contaminated items inside a biohazard bag (or plastic bag labeled "biohazard" if a biohazard bag is not available). Tie or tape the bag shut securely to avoid any leaking. Keep the bag in a secure place until it can be safely collected for disposal.
- Dispose all waste according to your company policy.
- For areas not contaminated with diarrhea, vomit, blood, or other bodily fluids, routine cleaning and disinfection should be performed.

Postflight Measures

- Properly dispose contaminated items. Notify cleaning crew of areas contaminated with diarrhea, vomit, blood, or other bodily fluids, needing more than routine cleaning or possible removal. For example:
  - Soft materials (e.g., seat cushion)
  - Hard surfaces, such as armrests and tray tables
  - Bathroom(s) used by a sick traveler
- Remind cleaning crew this situation may require additional PPE, and they should follow company policy for such situations.

- If the sick traveler changed seats, ensure both areas are adequately cleaned.

- Consult a healthcare provider, as needed.

  - Risk of infection depends on many factors, including the type of disease, flight duration, level of exposure, and your level of immunity.

  - Follow company policy for reporting contact with a sick passenger or potentially infectious materials, such as items contaminated with diarrhea, vomit, blood, or other bodily fluids.

  - After the flight, you could choose to consult with your private healthcare provider if you develop symptoms (such as fever, rash, persistent cough, vomiting, or diarrhea) or have other concerns that have not been addressed.

  - The CDC will collaborate with your airline's occupational medicine consultant to provide guidance for certain confirmed infectious diseases, such as measles.

  - The state health department where your flight arrived or where you live may also contact you to ensure your well-being and prevent further spread of the identified contagious disease.

Sick Crew Members

If you have a possible contagious illness, please follow your company policy and do not report to work until you have recovered in order to avoid exposing others. If you develop symptoms of a contagious illness during a flight, discontinue your work duties as soon as it is safe to do so and follow the procedures outlined for sick passengers. Do not prepare or serve food or beverages if you have symptoms of an illness that could be contagious.

Immunizations and Healthy Travel Tips

- Be prepared. Many contagious diseases can be prevented by vaccines. To protect yourself, be up-to-date on all routine immunizations, as well as recommended immunizations and other preventive measures, such as preventive treatment for malaria, specific to your destination(s).

- Get vaccinated.
- Postpone travel when you are sick.
- Follow healthy travel tips.
- Read travel health notices.

Chapter 26

Guidance for Cruise Ships

Chapter Contents

Section 26.1

Varicella (Chickenpox) Management

This section includes text excerpted from "Guidance for Cruise Ships on Varicella (Chickenpox) Management," Centers for Disease Control and Prevention (CDC), July 14, 2016.

Varicella, commonly known as "chickenpox," is a frequent cause of outbreaks onboard cruise ships. Varicella is highly communicable, and secondary attack rates can be as high as 90 percent. Complications occur more frequently in people older than 15 years of age, and since crew members and most cruise ship passengers are adults, outbreaks have the potential to involve serious illness. Travelers at highest risk for severe disease are immunocompromised persons or pregnant women without a history of varicella disease or vaccination. A substantial proportion of crew members are from tropical countries that do not have routine varicella vaccination programs, where infection generally occurs at a later age than in temperate climates. Because of this differing epidemiology of varicella disease and low rates of immunization, crew members are more likely to be susceptible to varicella than the general adult population in the United States.

This section provides guidance to cruise ships for the reporting, investigation, management, and control of varicella-related illness and deaths in passengers and crew members of cruise ships traveling on voyages destined for U.S. ports.

Varicella Vaccination Practices in the United States

The Centers for Disease Control and Prevention (CDC) recommends two doses of varicella vaccine given at 12 to 15 months and 4 to 6 years for people aged <13 years of age. The single-antigen varicella vaccine (VARIVAX) or the combination measles, mumps, rubella, and varicella (ProQuad) vaccine can be used. Recommendations from the Advisory Committee on Immunization Practices (ACIP) on the prevention of varicella can be found here (www.cdc.gov/mmwr/preview/mmwrhtml/rr5604a1.htm). Additionally, ACIP recommendations for the use of ProQuad have been published.

For people aged over 13 years of age who have no contraindication, two doses of varicella vaccine should be given 4 to 8 weeks apart. Only single-antigen varicella vaccine can be used.

Managing Passengers and Crew with Varicella
Varicella Disease

Varicella-zoster virus (VZV) causes two distinct diseases: varicella (chickenpox) as the primary infection and, later, when VZV reactivates, herpes zoster (shingles). Clinical signs and symptoms of varicella in unvaccinated people include fever and rash. The rash is generalized and pruritic (itchy), generally occurring 14 to 16 days after exposure (range 10–21 days). It rapidly progresses within 24 hours from macules (flat lesions) and papules (bumps) to vesicular lesions (blisters) and crusts. Skin lesions are present simultaneously in several stages of development and are superficial; the vesicles contain a clear fluid. The rash spreads from head to trunk and extremities, with the highest concentration of vesicles usually on the trunk. In healthy children, the clinical course is generally mild. Adults may have more severe disease and a higher incidence of complications such as pneumonia and encephalitis. Varicella in previously vaccinated persons ("breakthrough" infection) is usually mild, without fever, and characterized by an atypical rash, with fewer than 50 lesions that are mostly maculopapular, with few or no vesicular lesions.

Varicella is highly contagious. In households, secondary attack rates among susceptible household contacts may reach 85 to 90 percent. Person-to-person transmission is by direct contact with vesicular fluid, inhalation of aerosolized fluid from skin lesions of acute cases, or inhalation of infected respiratory tract secretions. The incubation period is 10 to 21 days (commonly 14–16 days). The contagious period is from 1 to 2 days before the rash appears until all lesions have crusted, or, in vaccinated people, until no new lesions appear within a 24-hour period.

Isolation of Infectious People Onboard

Passengers who develop varicella en route should be medically evaluated (see next section) and remain isolated in their cabins until all lesions have crusted over or no new lesions appear within a 24-hour period (usually 5 to 7 days after rash onset).

Crew members with suspected varicella should take the following actions:

- Self-isolate in their cabins or quarters.

- Notify their supervisors and report their illness to the ship's infirmary in accordance with shipboard protocols.

351

- If varicella is diagnosed following medical evaluation, remain isolated in their cabins or quarters until all lesions have crusted over or no new lesions appear within a 24-hour period (usually 5 to 7 days after rash onset).

Only crew members with evidence of immunity to varicella should care for passengers or other crew members under isolation.

Medical Evaluation and Management

Updated resources for clinicians, and guidance on the medical evaluation and management of persons with varicella are available on the CDC's webpage about Chickenpox (Varicella) for Healthcare Providers (www.cdc.gov/chickenpox/hcp/index.html) and page about the Control and Investigation of Varicella Outbreaks.

Diagnostic Tests

Laboratory confirmation is not routinely required, since the typical varicella rash has a highly characteristic appearance. However, as vaccination rates increase, a higher proportion of cases may occur in vaccinated people, who usually have atypical disease. Clinical diagnosis in atypical disease may be more difficult, and laboratory confirmation may be useful.

Skin lesions are the preferred specimen for laboratory confirmation of varicella. The following are guidelines for cruise ships regarding collecting and shipping specimens to be sent to state or local health departments or the CDC once the ship arrives at a U.S. port:

- **Vesicular lesions:** Remove the top of the vesicle, swab the base vigorously enough to ensure cell collection, put the dry swab into a snap-cap tube or other closable container, and ship at room temperature.

- **Scabs:** Collect several dry scabs from crusted-over lesions and place each in a separate, small Ziploc© bag or other container for shipping. No transport medium is needed, and specimens may be stored indefinitely at room temperature.

Additional resources on laboratory testing for varicella are available on the CDC's page about Collecting Specimens for Varicella Zoster Virus (VZV) Testing.

Management of Passengers and Crew Members with Varicella upon Disembarkment

A disembarking cruise ship passenger with varicella whose lesions have not crusted over should be advised to wear clothes that cover the lesions (e.g., long sleeves, long pants) and a facemask, if tolerated. People with varicella should stay at home or in hotel isolation in the city of disembarkment and should not travel commercially until all lesions have crusted over or no new lesions appear within a 24-hour period.

The CDC quarantine station with jurisdiction over the port of entry will notify local public-health authorities if varicella is a reportable disease in that state.

Crew members should remain in isolation (shipboard or in a hotel) until their rash has crusted over or no new lesions appear within a 24-hour period.

Managing Passengers and Crew Members Following Exposure to an Ill Person

Identify all passengers and crew members who may have been exposed to a person suspected of having varicella.

A varicella case contact is a person who has had greater than five minutes of face-to-face contact with a varicella case during the infectious period, from one to two days before rash onset until lesions are crusted (generally five to seven days after rash onset) or direct contact with the fluid from skin lesions of patients with varicella or herpes zoster.

Assess crew members and passenger contacts for evidence of immunity to varicella. Evidence of immunity includes:

- Written documentation of receipt of two doses of varicella-containing vaccine

- Serologic evidence of immunity or confirmed disease

- Birth in the United States before 1980

- A diagnosis or history of varicella or herpes zoster verified by a healthcare provider or the cruise ship clinician based on the patient's description of the illness.

Identify high-risk susceptible passenger and crew-member contacts with contraindications to vaccination (i.e., pregnant, immunocompromised (i.e., with HIV infection or diabetes, etc.), those with a malignant condition affecting the bone marrow or lymphatic systems, or people taking oral steroids or other immunosuppressant medications).

Provide postexposure prophylaxis (as indicated below) to all susceptible contacts.

Postexposure Prophylaxis
Varicella Vaccine

To prevent illness, a first dose of varicella vaccine should be administered within three days of exposure (possibly up to five days) to all susceptible contacts who lack evidence of immunity except those who are pregnant or immunocompromised.

A second dose should be given at the ACIP-recommended intervals:

- At least 3 months for people less than 13 years of age

- At least 4 weeks for people over 13 years of age. Only single-antigen varicella vaccine may be used for vaccination of people in this age group.

Vaccination is still recommended beyond five days to prevent infection from future exposures and further spread of disease. Contacts with written documentation of receipt of one dose of varicella vaccine may be vaccinated with a second dose—except for those who are pregnant or immunocompromised—if the time interval between doses is appropriate, per ACIP-recommended intervals.

Varicella Zoster Immune Globulin

High-risk susceptible contacts for whom varicella vaccine is contraindicated (i.e., pregnant women or immunocompromised persons) should be evaluated for administration of varicella zoster immune globulin (VZIG). VZIG should be administered as soon as possible, but may still be effective if administered as late as 10 days after exposure.

The VZIG product licensed in the United States is Varicella Zoster Immune Globulin (Human) (VariZIG) and is available on an as-needed basis.

If administration of VZIG is needed, contact the CDC for further assistance with management of people receiving VZIG.

Surveillance and Management of Contacts

Recommend contacts among passengers and crew members monitor their health for up to 21 days (or 28 days if VZIG is received) after the last exposure to an active case and report fever or rash to the shipboard infirmary immediately.

Susceptible crew members who receive the first dose of varicella vaccine within 3 to 5 days of exposure may return to work immediately after vaccination; these people do not need to be separated from others, but should be monitored daily for signs and symptoms of varicella for up to 21 days after their last exposure to an active varicella case. Active surveillance of crew members requires that supervisors question all susceptible crew member contacts daily about the presence of a fever or rash. If the exposure date is unknown, active surveillance should be conducted through 27 days after rash onset of the last case (i.e., one incubation period after the end of the infectious period of the last case).

From the eighth day after the first exposure through the 21st day (or 28 days if VZIG is received as administration of VZIG can extend the incubation period) after last exposure to the case, susceptible crew members who do not receive varicella vaccine or received it more than 5 days after exposure and persons who do receive VZIG should have no passenger contact, minimize contact with other crew members, and be placed under active surveillance for signs and symptoms of varicella. Contact with other crew members during this period should be limited to those who have evidence of immunity to varicella.

Isolate any crew member who develops a fever within 21 days (or 28 days if VZIG is received) after contact with a varicella case and observe for rash onset. If a rash develops, then continue isolation until all lesions are crusted or no new lesions appear within a 24-hour period. If a rash does not develop within 2 days of fever onset, the crew member may be released from isolation but should minimize contact with others and continue active surveillance until a total of 21 days (or 28 days if VZIG is received) has passed since exposure.

Conduct passive surveillance for rash illness aboard the ship until 27 days after the rash onset date of the last case. Passive surveillance is defined as monitoring clinic visits for rash illnesses suggestive of varicella.

Preventing Varicella in Crew Members

Crew members whose work activities involve contact with ill passengers or crew members with varicella should have evidence of immunity to varicella. The following precautions are recommended for all people who come in contact with varicella cases, regardless of immune status.

355

Standard precautions (that apply to all patients, regardless of suspected or confirmed diagnosis or presumed infection status):

- Practice good hand hygiene. Wash hands often for at least 20 seconds with soap and warm water. If soap and water are not available and hands are not visibly soiled, an alcohol-based hand cleaner can be used as an interim measure.

- Avoid direct contact with the ill person while interviewing, escorting, or providing other assistance.

- Keep interactions with ill people as brief as possible.

- Limit the number of people who interact with ill people. To the extent possible, the ill person should receive care and meals from a single person.

- Ask the ill person to follow good cough and sneeze etiquette and hand hygiene and to wear a face mask while in contact with others, if it can be tolerated.

- If a face mask cannot be tolerated, provide tissues and ask the ill person to cover his or her mouth and nose when coughing or sneezing. Used tissues should be disposed of immediately in a disposable container (plastic bag) or a washable trash can.

Contact precautions (intended to prevent transmission of infectious agents, including epidemiologically important microorganisms, which are spread by direct or indirect contact with the patient or the patient's environment):

- Standard precautions:

  - Gloves: crew members should wear impermeable, disposable gloves if they need to have direct contact with ill people or potentially contaminated surfaces, rooms, or lavatories used by ill passengers and crew members. Crew members should wash their hands with soap and water after removing gloves. Gloves should be discarded in the trash and should not be washed or saved for reuse. Crew members should avoid touching their faces with gloved or unwashed hands.

Airborne precautions:

- Standard precautions:

  - In physician offices and similar settings, masking the patient, placing the patient in a private room with the door closed, and providing N95 or higher-level respirators or masks for healthcare personnel will reduce the likelihood of airborne transmission.

- Use of N95 respirators or face masks is not generally recommended for cruise ship crew members for general work activities.

- Whenever possible, nonimmune healthcare workers should not care for patients with airborne vaccine-preventable diseases (e.g., measles, mumps, and varicella).

Additional Recommendations
Medication and Supplies

Dispensers of alcohol-based hand sanitizers should be conveniently located; where sinks are available to ensure that supplies for hand washing (i.e., soap, disposable towels) are consistently available.

Ships should carry a sufficient quantity of medical supplies to meet day-to-day needs. Contingency plans are recommended for rapid resupply in outbreak situations.

Cleaning and Disinfection

Environmental management of varicella should include routine cleaning and disinfection strategies, as well as more frequent cleaning of commonly touched surfaces, such as handrails, countertops, and doorknobs.

- Ship-wide cleaning or disinfection is not recommended.

- Clean equipment, appliances, and surfaces soiled by discharges from the patient's nose and throat with soap and water and disinfect by using an alcohol- or chlorine-based disinfectant or ordinary cleaning or disinfecting solutions.

For additional recommendations on infection-control practices by the CDC and the Healthcare Infection Control Practices Advisory Committee (HICPAC), please refer to the CDC webpage Guidelines for Environmental Infection Control in Health-Care Facilities.

Reporting

Quarantine regulations found in the U.S. Code of Federal Regulations (CFR) Title 42, Part 71 require ships destined for a U.S. port of entry from a foreign country or possession to report to the CDC quarantine station at or nearest the next intended U.S. port of arrival any shipboard death or reportable illness among passengers or crew, including passengers or crew who have disembarked or who have been removed.

The Maritime Conveyance Illness or Death Investigation Form is the preferred method of reporting varicella cases. Ships may submit this form by email, fax, or phone; find instructions on the CDC's webpage Guidance for Cruise Ships: How to Report Onboard Death or Illness to the CDC.

The CDC quarantine station of jurisdiction will continue to review and evaluate varicella reports; however, for routine cases, this guidance should be sufficient for the ship to conduct case and contact management. Under certain conditions, additional quarantine-station involvement may be indicated. Criteria for an enhanced response include but are not limited to:

- Varicella cases requiring hospitalization

- Any death attributed to varicella disease

- A varicella outbreak (defined as three cases in adults or five cases in children on the same vessel in the past 42 days)

- A request from the cruise line for CDC assistance

Section 26.2

Influenza-Like Illness Management

This section includes text excerpted from "Guidance for Cruise Ships on Influenza-Like Illness (ILI) Management," Centers for Disease Control and Prevention (CDC), August 22, 2016.

Reducing the Spread of Influenza

Commercial maritime travel is characterized by the movement of large numbers of people in closed and semi-closed settings. Like other close-contact environments, these settings can facilitate the transmission of influenza viruses and other respiratory viruses from person to person through droplet spread or potentially through contact with contaminated surfaces.

The Centers for Disease Control and Prevention (CDC) recommends that efforts to reduce the spread of influenza and other respiratory diseases on cruise ships focus on encouraging crew members and passengers to:

- Get vaccinated annually for influenza

- Postpone travel when sick

- Take everyday steps to protect themselves and others while traveling

Specific management should include early identification and isolation of crew members and passengers with influenza-like illness (ILI), encouraging good respiratory hygiene and cough etiquette, use of influenza antiviral medications for treatment of people with suspected or confirmed influenza, and use of antiviral chemoprophylaxis during influenza outbreaks, if indicated, for high-risk people exposed to influenza.

Influenza Vaccination of Crew and Passengers

The CDC recommends that all people six months of age and older be vaccinated each year with the influenza vaccine.

Crew members should be vaccinated yearly. Vaccination of passengers, especially those at high risk for influenza complications, is recommended at least two weeks before cruise ship travel, if influenza vaccine is available and the person has not already been vaccinated with the current year's vaccine.

Managing Passengers and Crew with Influenza-Like Illness

Signs and symptoms of influenza include acute onset of some or all of these signs and symptoms: fever or feeling feverish, chills, cough, sore throat, runny or stuffy nose, muscle or body aches, headache, fatigue (tiredness), and sometimes diarrhea or vomiting. Fever (a temperature of 100°F [37.8°C] or higher) will not always be present in people with influenza, especially not in elderly or immunosuppressed people. Cruise ship medical personnel should consider someone to have a fever if the sick person feels warm to the touch, gives a history of feeling feverish, or has an actual measured temperature of 100°F (37.8°C) or higher. Because the signs and symptoms of influenza are not specific and most people who have a respiratory illness are not tested for influenza, ILI has been defined for surveillance purposes as an illness with fever or feverishness plus either a cough or sore throat in the absence of another diagnosis.

Sick people should be advised to seek healthcare if they are at high risk of developing severe illness from influenza or if they are concerned about their illness. People with underlying chronic medical conditions can experience exacerbation of those conditions with influenza.

Respiratory Hygiene and Cough Etiquette

People with ILI should be advised of the importance of covering coughs and sneezes with a tissue. Used tissues should be disposed of immediately in a disposable container (e.g., plastic bag) or a washable trash can. Passengers and crew members should be reminded to wash their hands often with soap and water, especially after coughing or sneezing. If soap and water are not available, they can use an alcohol-based hand sanitizer.

Managing Passengers or Crew with Influenza-Like Illness upon Boarding and While Onboard

Any passenger who has ILI at the time of embarkation should be advised not to travel until at least 24 hours after resolution of fever without the use of fever-reducing medications (e.g., acetaminophen, ibuprofen, paracetamol). Aspirin should not be used to treat influenza signs or symptoms in children or adolescents younger than 19 years of age because of the risk of Reye syndrome.

Passengers with ILI who nonetheless decide to board, as well as passengers who become sick with ILI en route, should remain isolated in their cabins or quarters (with the exception of clinic visits, if needed), until at least 24 hours after resolution of fever without the use of fever-reducing medications.

Crew members with ILI should take the following actions:

- Notify their supervisors

- Report to the infirmary for medical evaluation, according to shipboard protocols

- Remain isolated in their cabins or quarters until at least 24 hours after resolution of fever without the use of fever-reducing medications

- Continue to practice respiratory hygiene, cough etiquette, and hand hygiene after returning to work, because respiratory viruses can continue to be shared for several days after fever resolves

Passengers and crew members who are in a high-risk group for complications from influenza or who are experiencing severe illness should seek medical care as soon as possible and be evaluated for possible influenza testing and antiviral treatment.

While temporarily in common areas, passengers and crew members with ILI should be encouraged to remain as far away from others as possible (at least six feet), and either wear face masks or cover their mouths and noses with a tissue.

Managing Passengers or Crew with Influenza-Like Illness upon Disembarkment

A disembarking cruise ship passenger or crew member who has ILI or who has had fever within the 24 hours before disembarking should be advised to take the same precautions: to stay inside home or hotel in the city of disembarkment and to refrain from further travel until at least 24 hours after she or he is free of fever without the use of fever-reducing medications.

If a passenger or crew member with ILI is taken to a healthcare facility off the ship, the facility should be informed before arrival.

Managing Passengers and Crew Following Exposure to a Person with Influenza-Like Illness

Passengers and crew members who may have been exposed to a person suspected of having influenza should monitor their health for 4 to 5 days after the exposure. Passengers and crew members who develop ILI while still onboard should notify the ship infirmary immediately and remain isolated in their cabins or quarters until at least 24 hours after resolution of fever without the use of fever-reducing medications. Sick travelers should be advised to seek healthcare if they are at high risk of developing severe illness from influenza or if they are concerned about their illness.

361

Influenza Diagnostic Tests

The CDC's influenza website also includes recommendations for the clinical use of influenza diagnostic tests, information on available tests, specimen collection, and guidance on interpretation of influenza testing results. Respiratory specimens should ideally be collected within three to four days of illness onset. The Infectious Diseases Society of America (IDSA) recommends use of rapid influenza molecular assays in outpatients with suspected influenza and provides recommendations for respiratory specimen collection and influenza testing.

Healthcare providers should understand the advantages and limitations of influenza tests, and proper interpretation of negative results of rapid influenza diagnostic tests (antigen-detection tests). Rapid influenza diagnostic tests without an analyzer device have low to moderate sensitivity compared with real-time polymerase chain reaction (RT-PCR), and false negative results can occur frequently. Rapid influenza diagnostic tests that use a digital analyzer reader device have moderately high sensitivity compared with RT-PCR, but false negative results can still occur. Negative rapid influenza diagnostic test results do not exclude a diagnosis of influenza; clinical diagnosis of influenza should be considered; however, positive test results are useful to establish a diagnosis of influenza and to provide evidence of influenza in passengers and crew members aboard ships.

Use of Antiviral Treatment and Chemoprophylaxis for People at High Risk for Complications

Early antiviral treatment with neuraminidase inhibitors (oral oseltamivir, inhaled zanamivir or IV peramivir) is recommended for people with suspected or confirmed influenza who have severe illness or are at high risk for influenza complications, including people with asthma, diabetes, and heart disease.

Baloxavir marboxil is a new antiviral medication with a different mechanism of action from the neuraminidase inhibitors, and is approved for early treatment of uncomplicated influenza in people aged 12 years and older. A single oral dose of baloxavir is equivalent to 5 days of twice daily oral oseltamivir; however, baloxavir is not recommended for pregnant women, lactating mothers, or people with severe influenza, including hospitalized patients, because of the lack of data in these groups. Antiviral treatment recommendations are available.

Antiviral treatment also can be considered, on the basis of clinical judgment, for outpatients with uncomplicated, suspected, or confirmed influenza who are not known to be at increased risk for developing severe or complicated illness if antiviral treatment can be initiated within 48 hours of illness onset; treatment of these cases may be particularly advisable in an outbreak setting on a cruise ship.

Antiviral chemoprophylaxis can be considered for prevention of influenza in exposed people who are at high risk for complications or could be given to all contacts on a cruise ship when the outbreak threshold is met or exceeded. Additional information about antiviral chemoprophylaxis is available in the IDSA guidelines.

Outbreak Control

A combination of measures can be implemented to control influenza outbreaks, including isolation and early antiviral treatment of sick people, infection-control efforts, antiviral chemoprophylaxis of exposed people, crew member and passenger notifications, and active surveillance for new cases. Recommendations for controlling institutional influenza outbreaks are available in the IDSA guidelines.

Preventing Influenza in Crew Members

In addition to annual influenza vaccination, the following recommendations should be followed, when possible, by crew members whose work activities involve contact with passengers and other crew members who have ILI.

- Maintain a distance of six feet from the sick person while interviewing, escorting, or providing other assistance.
- Keep interactions with sick people as brief as possible.
- Limit the number of people who interact with sick people. To the extent possible, the sick person should receive care and meals from a single person.
- Avoid touching your eyes, nose, and mouth.
- Wash your hands often with soap and water. If soap and water are not available, use an alcohol-based hand sanitizer.
- Ask the sick person to consider wearing a face mask, and provide one if wearing it can be tolerated.
- Provide tissues and access to soap and water and ask the sick person to:

- Cover his or her mouth and nose with a tissue (or face mask) when coughing or sneezing.

- Throw away used tissues immediately in a disposable container (plastic bag) or a washable trash can.

- Wash his or her hands often with soap and water for 20 seconds.

    - If soap and water are not available, the sick person should use an alcohol-based hand sanitizer.

Reporting

The CDC requests that cruise ships submit a cumulative ILI report (even if no deaths or ILI cases have occurred), preferably during the final 24 hours of the voyage or as soon as an outbreak is suspected, as described below. These reports should be made once per voyage by completing the one-page Maritime Conveyance Cumulative Influenza/ Influenza-like Illness (ILI) Form and clicking on the gray "Send Via Email" box in the top left corner.

The CDC requests that cruise lines immediately report any of the following events to the CDC quarantine station having jurisdiction over the next U.S. port of entry:

- Outbreaks of influenza or ILI (exceeding 1.380 cases per 1,000 traveler days) among passengers or crew members (instructions for calculating ILI threshold are available on the CDC Quarantine and Isolation website)

- Hospitalization (ashore or at sea) caused by, or suspected to be associated with, influenza or ILI onboard the vessel

In addition, the CDC emphasizes that any death, including those caused by or suspected to be associated with influenza or ILI, that occurs aboard a cruise ship destined for a U.S. port must be reported to the CDC immediately. Report ILI hospitalizations or deaths by submitting an individual Maritime Conveyance Illness or Death Investigation Form for each hospitalization or death, or report by telephone.

Vessel captains may request assistance from the CDC to evaluate or control influenza outbreaks as needed. If the ship will not be arriving imminently at a U.S. seaport, CDC quarantine officials will provide guidance to cruise ship officials regarding management and isolation of the sick person or people and recommendations for other passengers and crew members. Before the ship arrives, inform the respective CDC quarantine station if any support is needed, including hospitalization of sick people and laboratory testing of clinical specimens.

For influenza cases requiring hospitalization, CDC quarantine officials will work with the cruise line and local and state health departments to facilitate medical transportation of the patient upon arrival. In outbreak situations, CDC staff may also help with disease control and containment measures, passenger and crew notification, surveillance activities, communicating with local public-health authorities, obtaining and testing laboratory specimens, and provide additional guidance as needed.

For ships on international voyages, if an illness occurred on board, the Maritime Declaration of Health should be completed and sent to the competent authority, according to the 2005 International Health Regulations and the national legislation of the country of disembarkation. Before entering a seaport, cruise ships may also be required to report the ship's previous itinerary.

Additional Recommendations
Personal Protective Equipment

Crew members and other staff who may have contact with people with ILI should be instructed in the proper use, storage, and disposal of personal protective equipment (PPE). Improper use or handling of PPE can increase disease transmission risk.

Crew members should wear impermeable, disposable gloves if they need to have direct contact with sick people or potentially contaminated surfaces, rooms, or lavatories used by sick passengers and crew members. Crew members should wash their hands with soap and water or use an alcohol-based hand sanitizer after removing gloves. Used gloves should be discarded in the trash and should not be washed or saved for reuse. Crew members should avoid touching their faces with gloved or unwashed hands.

Use of N95 respirators or face masks is not generally recommended for cruise ship crew members for general work activities. Use of face masks can be considered for cruise ship workers who cannot avoid close contact with people with ILI. Crew members who use N95 respirators should receive annual fit testing. Crew members who provide healthcare to passengers or other crew members (e.g., onboard nurses and physicians) should follow the CDC's prevention strategies for seasonal influenza in healthcare settings.

Supplies

Ships should ensure the availability of conveniently located dispensers of alcohol-based hand sanitizer. Where sinks are available, ships should ensure that supplies for handwashing (i.e., soap, disposable towels) are consistently available.

Ships should carry a sufficient quantity of PPE, such as face masks, N95 respirators, and disposable gloves, for use in controlling the spread of influenza or other diseases.

Ships should carry a sufficient quantity of medical supplies to meet day-to-day needs. Contingency plans are recommended for rapid resupply during outbreaks. Stocking oral oseltamivir and inhaled zanamivir for antiviral treatment or chemoprophylaxis of influenza virus infection is recommended.

Ships are encouraged to carry sterile viral transport media and sterile swabs to collect nasopharyngeal and nasal specimens. These optimal recommendations can be modified to reflect individual ship capabilities and characteristics.

Cleaning and Disinfection

During influenza outbreaks, in addition to routine cleaning and disinfection strategies, cruise ships may consider more frequent cleaning of commonly touched surfaces such as handrails, countertops, and doorknobs. Surfaces contaminated by the respiratory secretions of a sick person (e.g., in the sick person's living quarters or work area, and in isolation rooms) should also be cleaned. The primary mode of influenza virus transmission is believed to be through respiratory droplets that are spread from an infected person through coughing or sneezing to a susceptible close contact within about six feet; therefore, widespread disinfection to control influenza outbreaks is unlikely to be effective.

Chapter 27

Animal Importing

The Centers for Disease Control and Prevention (CDC) regulations govern the importation of animals and animal products capable of causing human disease. Pets taken out of the United States are subject upon return to the same regulations as those entering for the first time.

The CDC does not require general certificates of health for pets for entry into the United States. However, health certificates may be required for entry into some states or may be required by airlines for pets. You should check with officials in your state of destination and with your airline prior to your travel date.

Animals Regulated by Centers for Disease Control and Prevention
Bringing a Dog into the United States

All dogs must appear healthy to enter the United States. Depending upon what country the dogs are coming from, they may need a valid rabies vaccination certificate. The rules for bringing your dog into the United States are covered under U.S. regulations.

These rules apply to all dogs, including puppies, service animals, and emotional support dogs. These rules also apply whether you are just visiting the United States with your dog; importing dogs into the United States; or traveling out of the United States and returning with your dog after a temporary visit, such as a vacation or holiday; or

This chapter includes text excerpted from "Bringing an Animal into the United States," Centers for Disease Control and Prevention (CDC), September 1, 2016.

for shopping or visiting friends and relatives. If you do not follow the CDC's rules, your dog may not be allowed to enter the United States.

Bringing a Cat into the United States

A general certificate of health is not required by the CDC for entry of pet cats into the United States; although, some airlines or states may require them. However, pet cats are subject to inspection at ports of entry and may be denied entry into the United States if they have evidence of an infectious disease that can be transmitted to humans. If a cat appears to be ill, further examination by a licensed veterinarian at the owner's expense might be required at the port of entry.

Cats are not required to have proof of rabies vaccination for importation into the United States. However, some states require vaccination of cats for rabies, so it is a good idea to check with state and local health authorities at your final destination.

All pet cats arriving in the state of Hawaii and the territory of Guam, even from the U.S. mainland, are subject to locally imposed quarantine requirements.

Bringing a Turtle, Snake, or Lizard into the United States

The Centers for Disease Control and Prevention does not regulate snakes or lizards, but they do limit imports of small turtles, tortoises, and terrapins and their viable eggs. Turtles with a carapace (shell) length of less than four inches and turtle eggs may not be imported for any commercial purpose. An individual may import as many as six small turtles or six eggs or any combination totaling six or fewer turtles and turtle eggs for noncommercial purposes. This rule was implemented in 1975 after it was discovered that small turtles frequently transmitted *Salmonella* to humans, particularly to young children.

Turtles with a shell length that is less than four inches and viable turtle eggs may not be imported for commercial purposes. The U.S. Fish and Wildlife Service (USFWS) regulates the importation of reptiles.

Bringing a Monkey into the United States

Monkeys and other nonhuman primates (NHP) may not be imported as pets under any circumstances. Importation for permitted purposes is strictly controlled through a registration process. The CDC's

Division of Global Migration and Quarantine (DGMQ) administers these regulations.

These regulations are in place to protect U.S. residents from severe infections that can spread from monkeys to humans. These diseases include:

- Ebola Reston

- B virus (Cercopithecine herpesvirus 1)

- Monkeypox

- Yellow fever

- Simian immunodeficiency virus

- Tuberculosis

- Other diseases not yet known or identified

Since 1975, the Federal Quarantine Regulations (42 CFR 71.53) have restricted the importation of NHP. Importers must register with the CDC, implement disease control measures, and may import and distribute NHP for only bona fide scientific, educational, or exhibition purposes, as defined in the regulations. These restrictions also apply to the reimportation of NHP originating in the United States.

Other federal, state, and local authorities may have regulations that apply to NHP.

Bringing a Civet into the United States

Civets may not be imported into the United States. They are prohibited because they may carry the severe acute respiratory syndrome (SARS) virus.

About civets: A civet is a meat-eating mammal. In general, a civet has a somewhat cat-like appearance with a small head, long body, and long tail; although, a civet is not in fact a cat. Its muzzle is long and often pointed, rather like that of an otter or a mongoose. Excluding its tail, a civet ranges from about 17 inches to 28 inches long and weighs between 3 to 10 pounds. There are several species of civets; they are native to most of Africa, the Spanish peninsula, southern China, and Southeast Asia.

Civet oil is often requested for import into the United States for use in the perfume industry.

Bringing an African Rodent into the United States

A person may not import into the United States any live or dead rodent of African origin, including any rodents that were caught in Africa and then shipped directly to the United States or shipped to other countries before being imported to the United States. The ban also applies to rodents whose native habitat is in Africa, even if those rodents were born elsewhere. These animals may still be imported for scientific, exhibition, or educational purposes with a valid permit issued by the CDC.

Bringing Bats into the United States

Certain animals, such as bats, insects, and snails, are known to carry zoonotic diseases. Bats are known to carry rabies and histoplasmosis. Importing such animals for any reason requires permits from the CDC and the U.S. Fish and Wildlife Service. The CDC permits are issued by the CDC's etiologic agent import program. Because bats can be infected with and transmit rabies, permits are not granted for importing bats as pets.

Etiological agents, hosts, or vectors of human disease, including microorganisms, insects, biological materials, tissue, certain live animals (e.g., live bats), and animal products may require a CDC permit for importation or transfer within the United States. The CDC's Office of Health and Safety administers these regulations:

- Import instructions and permits for live bats
- Etiologic agent and vector species

Animals Not Regulated by Centers for Disease Control and Prevention

Bringing Fish into the United States

There are no CDC regulations regarding the importation of live fish. However, importers should visit the United States Fish and Wildlife Service for specific requirements on fish that are considered endangered or injurious. Visit the United States Department of Agriculture (USDA) for import restrictions on live fish; fertilized eggs; and gametes susceptible to spring viremia of carp (SVC), an extremely contagious viral disease of carp. The National Marine Fisheries Service (NMFS) may also have regulations.

Bringing Small Mammals and Non-African Rodents into the United States

Unless they are included in a specific embargo, such as civets and African rodents, or known to carry disease transmissible to humans, these animals are not covered under the CDC's regulations.

However, state or local regulations may apply. Pet ferrets, for example, are prohibited in California. Any animal known to carry a disease that can be transmitted to people (zoonotic disease) is subject to regulation 42 CFR 71.

Additionally, animals carrying diseases of risk to domestic or wild animals are subject to regulations from the U.S. Fish and Wildlife Service, as they may be considered injurious species.

Bringing Horses into the United States

If the horse is not known to carry any diseases transmissible to humans, no CDC regulations would apply. However, the United States Department of Agriculture requires various periods of quarantine depending on the country of origin of the horse. In countries with prevalent screwworm, the quarantine period is 7 days. Horses coming from countries with African horse sickness are quarantined for 60 days.

Chapter 28

Traveling with Pets

Taking your dog or cat on a flight abroad? Make sure you have your pet's documents when traveling internationally and returning home to the United States. Leave yourself plenty of time before the trip to take care of your pet's required medical care and paperwork. Remember to start the process early.

First Stop—Your Vets Office

If you are traveling internationally, tell your veterinarian about your plans as soon as possible. Together, you can make sure your pet meets the requirements for your destination country and is healthy enough to travel. Requirements may include:

- Blood tests
- Vaccinations
- Microchips for identification

Airlines and countries often have different requirements, so make sure you know what the specific ones are.

Research How to Fly with Your Pet

Give yourself plenty of time to do your homework before your trip. A great place to start is the Pet Travel website of the U.S.

This chapter includes text excerpted from "Traveling with Pets," Centers for Disease Control and Prevention (CDC), September 1, 2016.

Department of Agriculture's Animal and Plant Health Inspection Service (APHIS).

Airlines

Different airlines have different rules about whether and how a pet can travel. Depending on the airline, your pet may be able to travel on your flight either in the cabin or in the cargo hold. Confirm this ahead of time with your airline.

On airlines that permit pets to travel, only small dogs and cats that can fit in special carriers under the seat are allowed in the cabin. Their owners must care for them during any layovers. Some airlines may not allow them in the cabin and will transport them as cargo in a heated and ventilated hold. Cats and dogs may travel and rest better this way, since it is quieter and darker, according to the International Air Transport Association (IATA).

Another way for your pet to travel is on a separate flight as an air cargo shipment. If this is your preference or a requirement based on your dog's size or the destination country's rules, then get your pet used to the shipping kennel ahead of time. Make sure the door latches securely to avoid any mishaps in transit. Ask your veterinarian for advice about when to give food and water. If a pet is traveling as an air cargo shipment, you must make arrangements for pickup at the final destination.

Some U.S. carriers do not allow pets to be shipped between May and September, the hottest months for animals to travel in the Northern Hemisphere. No matter what time of year, safety is always a concern when pets travel by airplane. If it is absolutely necessary for a dog or cat to travel in cargo, the animal must be in a sturdy container with enough room to stand and sit, to turn around normally while standing, and to lie down in a natural position.

When waiting for a connecting flight, you may have to care for a pet traveling with you in the cabin, while the airline staff or ground handlers care for a pet traveling in cargo.

Consider Your Pets Comfort

Loading and unloading can be the most stressful part of travel for animals. Consider these tips:

- Get your pet used to its carrier before the flight.

- Purchase flights with fewer connections or layovers.

- Pick departure and arrival times to avoid extreme heat or cold. For example, planning a nighttime arrival to a hot destination may be better for your pet.

- Consult with your veterinarian. The International Air Transport Association discourages the use of sedatives or tranquilizers because they could harm animals while in flight.

- Walk your pet before leaving home and again before checking in.

- If your pet is allowed in the cabin, check in as late as possible to reduce stress.

- If your pet will be transported as cargo, check in early so it can go to the quiet and dimly lit hold of the plane.

Requirements for Dogs Arriving in the United States

Whether returning or coming to the United States, all dogs must appear healthy. If your dog is coming from a high-risk country for rabies, they must have valid rabies vaccination certificates to enter the United States.

- Dogs must be at least 12 weeks old to get the rabies vaccination.

- If this is your dog's first rabies vaccination, you will have to wait 28 days before traveling to allow the vaccine to take effect.

- If you are not sure or do not have proof your dog was vaccinated before, have your dog vaccinated and wait 28 days before traveling.

- If your adult dog's rabies booster is current, you can travel without waiting 28 days.

- Your dog's rabies vaccination certificate must be valid for the duration of your trip.

Some states may require other vaccinations and health certificates. Check with your destination state's health department before you leave on your trip.

Some airlines, cities, or states restrict certain breeds, so be sure to check before you travel. The U.S. Department of Agriculture has additional restrictions for some dogs arriving in the United States, such as working dogs.

Requirements for Cats Arriving in the United States

Cats do not need rabies vaccinations to enter the United States. However, most states and many other countries require them for cats. Be sure to check your destination's requirements, and ask your veterinarian before traveling.

Other Kinds of Pets

If your pet is not a cat or dog, there may be different requirements. Some animals, such as primates (monkeys and apes) or African rodents, would not be allowed back into the United States. Even if they originally came from the United States, they cannot be brought back here as pets.

Illness or Death of a Pet during Travel

Despite all precautions, pets sometimes get sick or even die on an airplane. Public health officials are required to make sure an animal did not die of a disease that can spread to people. They may have to do an animal autopsy or conduct other tests, at your cost, to figure out the cause of death. The animal's remains often cannot be returned to you after this testing.

Think of Different Options

Make sure your pet is healthy enough to travel by air. If you have any doubts, consider leaving your pet with a trusted friend, family member, or boarding kennel during your trip, or consider taking another mode of transportation.

With careful planning, your pet will arrive both at its destination and return home healthy and safe.

Chapter 29

Importing Animal Products

Persons who plan to bring wild animal products, such as hunting trophies, bushmeat, or other products into the United States, must meet the following regulations and rules.

Hunting Trophies

Trophies of Nonhuman Primates

Nonhuman primate trophy materials require a Centers for Disease Control and Prevention (CDC) permit unless the bearer presents proof that the items have been rendered noninfectious. Acceptable proof that items have been rendered noninfectious include veterinary or taxidermy certificates. Persons who plan to import unprocessed trophy materials from nonhuman primates should review the permit requirements and complete an application form, and both can be found on the CDC's website.

Trophies of Animals under Import Restriction

Some trophy animals are under CDC import restriction because they pose a risk for infecting humans. The animals restricted by the

---

This chapter includes text excerpted from "Bringing Animal Products into the United States," Centers for Disease Control and Prevention (CDC), September 1, 2016.

CDC include African rodents, bats, civets, and small turtles. For details on restricted animals, please visit the CDC's website. These animal trophies may be imported if the body has been sufficiently processed to render it noninfectious.

Trophy materials from animals other than those listed above are not restricted by the CDC unless they are known or suspected to be capable of transmitting human disease. Additional information about animals restricted by the CDC can be found in the Code of Federal Regulations 42 CFR 71.54.

Both the U.S. Fish and Wildlife Service and international treaty (the Convention on International Trade in Endangered Species of Wild Fauna and Flora, or CITES) ban the importation of trophies from endangered species. The National Marine Fisheries Service (NMFS) website provides additional information on endangered marine species.

As with animal trophy materials, animal tissue used for other means must be properly processed to render it noninfectious. Some products that are more difficult to render noninfectious, such as goat-skin drums from Haiti, which have been associated with anthrax, may not be imported.

Bushmeat

Bushmeat is raw or processed meat derived from wild animals, such as cane rats, duiker antelope, nonhuman primates, and bats. Many U.S. federal agencies have restrictions on the importation of bushmeat. Most bushmeat is illegal to ship, mail, or carry into the United States. Upon reaching the U.S. borders, bushmeat will be confiscated and destroyed. Persons who carry or import bushmeat may be fined.

Although some countries and ethnic groups consider snails to be bushmeat, smoked snails are allowed if they are declared.

Animal species restricted by the CDC include certain turtles, non-human primates, bats, civets, and African rodents.

Other Products from Restricted Animals

As with animal trophy materials, animal products from restricted animals used for other means must be properly processed to render it noninfectious. Civet oil imported for use in the perfume industry is among these products.

Rendering Animal Products Noninfectious

A veterinary or taxidermy certificate should be included with the trophy, stating that the animal has been rendered noninfectious by:

- Heat (heated to an internal temperature of 70°C (158°F) or placed in boiling water for a minimum of 30 minutes)

- Preservation in formalin

- Chemically treated in acidic or alkaline solutions (soaking in a solution below pH 3.0 or above pH 11.5 for 24 hours)

- The use of hypertonic salts

  - Soaking, with agitation, in a 4 percent (w/v) solution of washing soda (sodium carbonate, Na_2CO_3) maintained at pH 11.5 or above for at least 48 hours

  - Soaking, with agitation, in a formic acid solution (100kg salt [NaCl] and 12 kg formic acid per 1,000 liters water) maintained at below pH 3.0 for at least 48 hours; wetting and dressing agents may be added.

- Gamma irradiation at a dose of at least 20 kilos Gray at room temperature (20°C or higher)

- Ethylene oxide

- In the case of raw hides, salting for at least 28 days with sea salt containing 2 percent washing soda (sodium carbonate, Na_2CO_3)

- For bones only, the following methods are acceptable:

  - Dry heat at 82.2°C (180°F) for 30 minutes

  - Soaking in boiling water for 20 minutes

  - Soaking in a 0.1 percent chlorine bleach solution for 2 hours

  - Soaking in a 5 percent acetic acid solution for 2 hours OR

  - Soaking in a 5 percent hydrogen peroxide solution for 2 hours

- Or, any other method approved by the CDC

Chapter 30

Importation of Human Remains

Blood and other bodily fluids that leak from containers can cause a risk to human health. Under the authority 42 Council on Foreign Relations (CFR) § 71.32(b), persons, carriers, and things, Centers for Disease Control and Prevention (CDC) has issued guidance for importing human remains into the United States that are intended for interment (e.g., burial or placement in a tomb) or subsequent cremation after entry into the United States. Under 42 CFR § 71.55, additional regulations governing the importation of the remains of a person who died from a quarantinable communicable disease already exist.

This chapter outlines all of the CDC's requirements about importing human remains intended for interment or subsequent cremation, regardless of the cause of death. This chapter includes the basic requirement that all human remains be shipped in a leakproof container. All human remains imported to the United States must also be accompanied by a death certificate (in English or accompanied by an English translation) stating the cause of death.

Germs that can cause disease could be present in the blood or other bodily fluids of a deceased person even if the stated cause of death is not a contagious disease. Such germs include human immunodeficiency

This chapter includes text excerpted from "Guidance for Importation of Human Remains into the United States for Interment or Subsequent Cremation," Centers for Disease Control and Prevention (CDC), April 9, 2019.

virus (HIV), hepatitis B virus, hepatitis C virus, and other germs that can be present in bodily fluids. This chapter is based on medical standard precautions to prevent exposure to infectious diseases carried in the blood and other bodily fluids.

This requirement is intended to protect the public, as well as federal, airline, and airport employees from potential exposure to blood and other bodily fluids during transportation, inspection, or storage of human remains.

This guidance applies to human remains (i.e., the whole body or portion of the body of a deceased human being) intended for interment (e.g., burial or placement in a tomb) or subsequent cremation after entry into the United States.

There are no importation requirements into the United States if human remains consist entirely of the following:

- Cremated human remains

- Clean (free of any tissues or blood) dry bones or bone fragments

- Human hair

- Clean (free of any tissues or blood) human teeth, fingernails, or toenails

This does not apply to the following items that are addressed under other U.S. federal regulations:

- Patient specimens or diagnostic specimens

- Any agent, substance, or vector already regulated by the CDC under 42 CFR § 71.54 Import regulations for infectious biological agents, infectious substances, and vectors

- Tissues or organs that are legally imported into the United States for the purpose of transplantation, as these items are regulated by the U.S. Food and Drug Administration (FDA)

Requirements for Importing Human Remains through a United States Port That Are Intended for Interment or Subsequent Cremation

Human remains intended for interment or cremation after entry into the United States must be accompanied by a death certificate stating the cause of death. If the death certificate is in a language other than English, then it should be accompanied by an English language translation. If a death certificate is not available in time for returning the remains, the U.S. embassy or consulate should provide a consular mortuary certificate stating whether the person died from a quarantinable communicable disease.

If the cause of death was a quarantinable communicable disease, the remains must meet the standards for importation found in 42 CFR Part 71.55 and may be cleared, released, and authorized for entry into the United States only under the following conditions:

- The remains are cremated.

- The remains are properly embalmed and placed in a hermetically sealed casket.

- The remains are accompanied by a permit issued by the CDC Director. The CDC permit (if applicable) must accompany the human remains at all times during shipment.

- Permits for the importation of the remains of a person known or suspected to have died from a quarantinable communicable disease may be obtained through the CDC Division of Global Migration and Quarantine by calling the CDC Emergency Operations Center at 770-488-7100. If a CDC permit is obtained to allow importation of human remains, the CDC may impose additional conditions for importation beyond those listed above.

If the cause of death was anything other than a quarantinable communicable disease, then the remains may be cleared, released, and authorized for entry into the United States under the following conditions:

- The remains meet the standards for importation found in 42 CFR Part 71.55, (i.e., the remains are cremated, or properly embalmed and placed in a hermetically sealed casket, or are accompanied by a permit issued by the CDC Director).

- The remains are shipped in a leakproof container.

Under 42 CFR § 71.32(b), the CDC may also require additional measures, including detention, disinfection, disinfestation, fumigation, or other related measures, if it has reason to believe that the human remains are or may be infected or contaminated with a communicable disease and that such measures are necessary to prevent the introduction, transmission, or spread of communicable diseases into the United States.

Part Five

Medical Diagnosis and Treatment of Infectious Diseases

Chapter 31

Diagnostic Tests

Chapter Contents

Section 31.1

Infectious Disease Diagnostic Techniques

This section includes text excerpted from "Diagnostic Techniques,"
Centers for Disease Control and Prevention (CDC),
December 7, 2012. Reviewed May 2019.

The Infectious Diseases Pathology Branch (IDPB) of the Centers for Disease Control and Prevention (CDC) uses a variety of diagnostic techniques in the evaluation of tissue specimens, including morphologic, antigenic, and nucleic acid methodologies. These tests are employed as needed based upon review of the case data and histopathology.

Immunohistochemistry

Immunohistochemistry (IHC) offers several distinct advantages over traditional identification methods. This technique is rapidly expanding the diagnostic capability of the pathologist.

IHC permits rapid agent identification. The technique employs specific antibodies, which localize to the antigens of the etiologic agent of interest. Since this technique uses formalin-fixed tissues, specimen transport is simplified, allowing retrospective studies and minimizing laboratory worker exposure to infectious agents.

IHC is a sensitive and specific test methodology for many microorganisms, and unlike some traditional staining methods, this method results in direct, highly interpretable visual evidence of the presence of an infectious agent within tissues. In addition, IHC detects organisms that are difficult to culture and those that cannot be cultured.

IHC provides invaluable information for clinical diagnosis and the study of pathogenesis. The IDPB has developed many specific IHC assays for emerging or reemerging infectious diseases. Currently, IDPB has diagnostic IHC assays for more than 100 etiologic agents, including viral, bacterial, parasitic, and fungal organisms. For a number of agents, IHC tests may provide the only reliable methods of detection.

Special Stains

Special stains are useful for detecting bacteria, fungi, and parasites in tissues and culture materials. However, they may not confer a specific diagnosis of an organism, and each stain differs in its level of sensitivity.

Molecular

The Infectious Diseases Pathology Branch currently possesses a battery of polymerase chain reaction (PCR)-based tests for the detection of many bacteria, viruses, fungi, and parasites. IDPB molecular tests have been optimized for formalin-fixed paraffin-embedded tissues.

Microbiology

For some cases of unexplained illness, the IDPB possesses limited capability for viral culture of etiologic agents. This technique is dependent on freshly frozen tissues or body fluids and permits additional studies such as immunofluorescence methods or electron microscopy.

Electron Microscopy

Electron microscopy (EM) studies are conducted on cell cultures, tissues, and body fluids. Both thin section and negative stain EM are available to assist in the diagnosis and characterization of pathogens. Electron microscopy examination is conducted on glutaraldehyde-fixed tissues or bodily fluids, formalin-fixed paraffin-embedded tissue blocks, prepared EM sections, images, and grids.

Section 31.2

Bacteria Culture Test

This section includes text excerpted from "Bacteria Culture Test," MedlinePlus, National Institutes of Health (NIH), April 22, 2019.

What Is a Bacteria Culture Test?

Bacteria are a large group of one-celled organisms. They can live on different places in the body. Some types of bacteria are harmless or even beneficial. Others can cause infections and disease. A bacteria culture test can help find harmful bacteria in your body.

During a bacteria culture test, a sample will be taken from your blood, urine, skin, or other parts of your body. The type of sample depends on the location of the suspected infection. The cells in your sample will be taken to a lab and put in a special environment in a lab to encourage cell growth. Results are often available within a few days. But some types of bacteria grow slowly, and it may take several days or longer.

What Is It Used For?

Bacteria culture tests are used to help diagnose certain types of infections. The most common types of bacteria tests and their uses are listed below.

Throat Culture

- Used to diagnose or rule out strep throat
- Test procedure:
  - Your healthcare provider will insert a special swab into your mouth to take a sample from the back of the throat and tonsils.

Urine Culture

- Used to diagnose a urinary tract infection and identify the bacteria causing the infection
- Test procedure:
  - You will provide a sterile sample of urine in a cup, as instructed by your healthcare provider.

Sputum Culture

Sputum is a thick mucus that is coughed up from the lungs. It is different from spit or saliva.

- Used to help diagnose bacterial infections in the respiratory tract. These include bacterial pneumonia and bronchitis.
- Test procedure:
  - You may be asked to cough up sputum into a special cup as instructed by your provider, or a special swab may be used to take a sample from your nose.

Blood Culture

- Used to detect the presence of bacteria or fungi in the blood
- Test procedure:
  - A healthcare professional will take a blood sample. The sample is most often taken from a vein in your arm.

Stool Culture

Another name for stool is "feces."

- Used to detect infections caused by bacteria or parasites in the digestive system. These include food poisoning and other digestive illnesses.
- Test procedure:
  - You will provide a sample of your feces in a clean container as instructed by your healthcare provider.

Wound Culture

- Used to detect infections on open wounds or burn injuries
- Test procedure:
  - Your healthcare provider will use a special swab to collect a sample from the site of your wound.

Why Do I Need a Bacteria Culture Test?

Your healthcare provider may order a bacteria culture test if you have symptoms of a bacterial infection. The symptoms vary depending on the type of infection.

Why Do I Have to Wait So Long for My Results?

Your test sample does not contain enough cells for your healthcare provider to detect an infection. So your sample will be sent to a lab to allow the cells to grow. If there is an infection, the infected cells will multiply. Most disease-causing bacteria will grow enough to be seen within one to two days, but it can take some organisms five days or longer.

Will I Need to Do Anything to Prepare for the Test?

There are many different types of bacteria culture tests. Ask your healthcare provider if you need to do anything to prepare for your test.

Are There Any Risks to the Test?

There are no known risks to having a swab or blood test or to providing a urine or stool sample.

What Do the Results Mean?

If enough bacteria is found in your sample, it likely means you have a bacterial infection. Your healthcare provider may order additional tests to confirm a diagnosis or determine the severity of the infection. Your provider may also order a "susceptibility test" on your sample. A susceptibility test is used to help determine which antibiotic will be most effective in treating your infection. If you have questions about your results, talk to your healthcare provider.

Section 31.3

Rapid Influenza Diagnostic Test

This section includes text excerpted from "Guidance for Clinicians on the Use of Rapid Influenza Diagnostic Tests," Centers for Disease Control and Prevention (CDC), December 21, 2010. Reviewed May 2019.

Rapid influenza diagnostic tests (RIDTs) are immunoassays that can identify the presence of influenza A and B viral nucleoprotein antigens in respiratory specimens and display the result in a qualitative way (positive versus negative). In the United States, a number of RIDTs are commercially available. The reference standards for laboratory confirmation of influenza virus infection are reverse transcription-polymerase chain reaction (RT-PCR), or viral culture. RIDTs can yield results in a clinically relevant time frame, i.e., approximately 15 minutes or less. However, RIDTs have limited sensitivity to detect influenza virus infection and negative test results should be interpreted with caution given the potential for false negative results.

Use of Rapid Influenza Diagnostic Tests in Clinical Decision-Making

RIDTs may be used to help with diagnostic and treatment decisions for patients in clinical settings, such as whether to prescribe antiviral medications. However, due to the limited sensitivities and predictive values of RIDTs, negative results of RIDTs do not exclude influenza virus infection in patients with signs and symptoms suggestive of influenza. Therefore, antiviral treatment should not be withheld from patients with suspected influenza, even if they test negative. Testing is not needed for all patients with signs and symptoms of influenza to make antiviral treatment decisions. Once influenza activity has been documented in the community or geographic area, a clinical diagnosis of influenza can be made for outpatients with signs and symptoms consistent with suspected influenza, especially during periods of peak influenza activity in the community.

Use of Rapid Influenza Diagnostic Tests for Public-Health Purposes to Detect Influenza Outbreaks

RIDTs can be useful to identify influenza virus infection as a cause of respiratory outbreaks in any setting, but especially in institutions (i.e., nursing homes, chronic care facilities, and hospitals), cruise ships, summer camps, schools, and so on. Positive RIDT results from one or more ill persons with suspected influenza can support decisions to promptly implement prevention and control measures for influenza outbreaks. However, negative RIDT results do not exclude influenza virus infection as a cause of a respiratory outbreak because of the limited sensitivity of these tests. Testing respiratory specimens from several persons with suspected influenza will increase the likelihood of detecting influenza virus infection if influenza virus is the cause of the outbreak. Public-health authorities should be notified of any suspected institutional outbreak and respiratory specimens should be collected from ill persons (whether positive or negative by RIDT) and sent to a public health laboratory for more accurate influenza testing.

Interpretation of Rapid Influenza Diagnostic Test Results

The reliability of RIDTs depends largely on the conditions under which they are used. Understanding some basic considerations can minimize being misled by false-positive or false-negative results.

- Sensitivities of RIDTs are generally 40 to 70 percent, but a range of 10 to 80 percent has been reported compared to viral culture or RT-PCR. Specificities of RIDTs are approximately 90 to 95 percent (range 85 to 100%). Thus false-negative results occur more commonly than false-positive results.

  - Negative results of RIDTs do not exclude influenza virus infection and influenza should still be considered in a patient if clinical suspicion is high based upon history, signs, symptoms, and clinical examination.

- False-positive (and true-negative) results are more likely to occur when disease prevalence in the community is low, which is generally at the beginning and end of the influenza season and during the summer.

  - The negative predictive value of an RIDT (the proportion of patients with negative results who do not have influenza) is highest when influenza activity is low.

  - The positive predictive value of an RIDT (the proportion of patients with positive results who have influenza) is lowest when influenza activity is low.

- False-negative (and true-positive) results are more likely to occur when disease prevalence is high in the community.

  - The positive predictive value of an RIDT (the proportion of patients with positive results who have influenza) is highest when influenza activity is high.

  - The negative predictive value of an RIDT (the proportion of patients with negative results who do not have influenza) is lowest when influenza activity is high.

Minimize False Results

- Collect specimens as early in the illness as possible (ideally less than four days from illness onset).

- Follow the manufacturer's instructions, including acceptable specimens and handling.

- Follow-up negative results with confirmatory tests (RT-PCR or viral culture) if a laboratory-confirmed influenza diagnosis is desired.

Clinicians should contact their local or state health department for information about current influenza activity.

Advantages and Disadvantages of Rapid Influenza Diagnostic Tests
Advantages

- Produce quick result in 15 minutes or less, simple to perform

- Some RIDTs are approved for office/bedside use

Disadvantages

- Suboptimal test sensitivity and false negative results are common, especially when influenza activity is high

- Although specificity is high, false positive results can also occur, especially during times when influenza activity is low

- Some RIDTs distinguish between influenza A or B virus infection while others do not. RIDTs that provide results on type of influenza virus (e.g., influenza A or B virus), do not provide information on influenza A virus subtype (e.g., A/H1N1 versus A/H3N2) or specific strain information (e.g., degree of similarity to vaccine strains)

Section 31.4

Test for Drug-Resistant Diseases

This section includes text excerpted from "Laboratory Testing
and Resources," Centers for Disease Control and
Prevention (CDC), September 10, 2018.

Laboratory tests can help guide patient treatment, detect emerging
threats, and prevent the spread of antibiotic resistance. The Centers
for Disease Control and Prevention's (CDC) Antibiotic Resistance Laboratory Network (AR Lab Network) supports nationwide lab capacity
to:

- Rapidly detect antibiotic resistance in healthcare, food, and the
  community

- Inform local responses to prevent spread and protect people

The AR Lab Network includes labs in 50 states, five cities, and
Puerto Rico, including seven regional labs and the National Tuberculosis Molecular Surveillance Center (National TB Center).

Types of Resistance Tests
Colonization Screening

Colonization screening is a process set up to detect and reduce the
risk of germs spreading in a healthcare facility (in this case, germs
with unusual resistance). Some people can carry germs without becoming sick or showing symptoms, known as "colonization."
People who are colonized can spread germs to others without knowing it. When unusual resistance is identified in a patient, healthcare
workers screen other patients to see if they are colonized with the same
resistant germ. This can prompt additional infection-control actions
reducing the risk of spread and protect patients.

Identification of Pathogens

Laboratories work to identify and confirm the genus and species of
pathogens (disease-causing germs) with resistance. These are often
the first tests performed by the AR Lab Network. This is done through
one of two methods:

- **Biochemical tests:** Classifying a particular species by the way
  it uses different biological chemicals, such as proteins or sugars

- **Mass spectrometry:** A specialized technique that looks for a pathogen's protein "fingerprint"

Molecular Testing

Molecular testing is a collection of techniques used to detect specific genes within a germ, including those that have and can share resistance. These tests can be used to diagnose infections and guide treatment for patients.

Phenotypic Carbapenemase Test

A phenotypic carbapenemase test uses culture (a medium to grow bacteria) instead of the molecular test method to determine if the pathogen produces an enzyme called "carbapenemase." If carbapenemase is produced, then a carbapenem antibiotic is ineffective and will not kill the pathogen.

Susceptibility Testing

Susceptibility testing is a type of lab test that cultures (grows) the pathogen in order to show how sensitive the germ is to different antibiotics. These tests can be used to help select the best drug choice for a drug-resistant infection, and also provide data to monitor how a pathogen's resistance profile might change over time.

Whole Genome Sequencing

Whole genome sequencing (WGS) is a laboratory procedure that provides a very precise DNA fingerprint that can help link cases to one another, allowing an outbreak to be detected and solved sooner.

Chapter 32

Pharmacological Treatment for Infectious Disease

Chapter Contents

Section 32.1

Antibiotic Class Definitions

This section includes text excerpted from "Antibiotic Resistance Patient Safety Atlas," Centers for Disease Control and Prevention (CDC), November 15, 2016.

The Outpatient Antibiotic Prescription data section of the Patient Safety Atlas provides data on oral antibiotic prescriptions dispensed to outpatients in U.S. community pharmacies.

Antibiotics are usually classified or grouped by their chemical structure. Some antibiotic classes work by killing bacteria and others work by preventing the ability of bacteria to multiply.

All of these antibiotics are currently included in the AR Patient Safety Atlas national data, but not all are available in the map format of state data.

Table 32.1. Antibiotics and Their Functions

Class	Examples	How They Work
Penicillins	penicillin, amoxicillin	Penicillins kill bacteria by preventing formation of the bacterial cell wall.
Macrolides	azithromycin, erythromycin	Macrolides prevent bacteria from multiplying by keeping bacteria from making proteins.
Cephalosporins	cephalexin, cefdinir	Cephalosporins kill bacteria by preventing formation of the bacterial cell wall.
Fluoroquinolones	ciprofloxacin, levofloxacin	Fluoroquinolones kill bacteria by keeping bacteria from making DNA
Beta-lactams with increased activity	amoxicillin/ clavulanate, ceftazidime/ avibactam	Beta-lactams with increased activity are combinations that consist of two different drugs: a penicillin or cephalosporin and a beta-lactamase inhibitor. The penicillin or cephalosporin kills bacteria by preventing formation of the bacterial cell wall. The beta-lactamase inhibitor has little antibiotic activity on its own. Its job is to protect the penicillin or cephalosporin from being destroyed by an enzyme some bacteria produce. This protection increases the activity of the penicillin or cephalosporin.

Table 32.1. Continued

Class	Examples	How They Work
Tetracyclines	tetracycline, doxycycline	Tetracyclines prevent bacteria from multiplying by keeping bacteria from making proteins.
Trimethoprim sulfamethoxazole	Trimethoprim sulfamethoxazole	Trimethoprim and sulfamethoxazole work together to inhibit the ability of bacteria to make folic acid, which is necessary to make DNA and proteins. This prevents bacteria from multiplying.
Urinary antiinfectives	nitrofurantoin	Depends of the specific drug. For nitrofurantoin, depending on the concentration, it either kills bacteria or prevents them from multiplying by keeping bacteria from making DNA, proteins, and the bacterial cell wall.
Lincosamides	clindamycin	Lincosamides prevent bacteria from multiplying by keeping bacteria from making proteins.

Section 32.2

How to Use Antibiotics Safely

This section includes text excerpted from "Be Antibiotics Aware: Smart Use, Best Care," Centers for Disease Control and Prevention (CDC), November 9, 2018.

Antibiotic resistance is one of the most urgent threats to the public's health. Antibiotic resistance occurs when bacteria develop the ability to defeat the drugs designed to kill them. Each year in the United States, at least two million people get infected with antibiotic-resistant bacteria, and at least 23,000 people die as a result.

Antibiotics save lives, but any time antibiotics are used, they can cause side effects and lead to antibiotic resistance. About 30 percent of antibiotics, or 47 million prescriptions, are prescribed unnecessarily in doctors' offices and emergency departments in the United States, which makes improving antibiotic prescribing and use a national priority.

Helping healthcare professionals improve the way they prescribe antibiotics, and improving the way we take antibiotics, helps keep us healthy now, helps fight antibiotic resistance, and ensures that these life-saving drugs will be available for future generations.

When Antibiotics Are Needed

Antibiotics are only needed for treating certain infections caused by bacteria. We rely on antibiotics to treat serious infections, such as pneumonia, and life-threatening conditions including sepsis, the body's extreme response to an infection. Effective antibiotics are also needed for people who are at high risk for developing infections. Some of those at high risk for infections include patients undergoing surgery, patients with end-stage kidney disease, or patients receiving cancer therapy (chemotherapy).

When Antibiotics Are Not Needed

Antibiotics do not work on viruses, such as those that cause colds, flu, bronchitis, or runny noses, even if the mucus is thick, yellow, or green.

Antibiotics are only needed for treating infections caused by bacteria, but even some bacterial infections get better without antibiotics. Antibiotics aren't needed for many sinus infections and some ear infections. Antibiotics save lives, and when a patient needs antibiotics, the benefits usually outweigh the risk of side effects and antibiotic resistance. When antibiotics aren't needed, they won't help you, and the side effects could still cause harm. Common side effects of antibiotics can include:

- Rash
- Dizziness
- Nausea
- Diarrhea
- Yeast infections

More serious side effects include *Clostridioides difficile* infection (also called *C. difficile* or *C. diff*), which causes severe diarrhea that can lead to severe colon damage and death. People can also have severe and life-threatening allergic reactions.

What You Can Do to Feel Better

Talk with your healthcare professional about the best treatment for your or your loved one's illness. If you need antibiotics, take them exactly as prescribed. Talk with your healthcare professional if you have any questions about your antibiotics, or if you develop any side effects especially severe diarrhea, since that could be a *C. difficile* infection, which needs to be treated immediately.

Respiratory viruses usually go away in a week or two without treatment. Ask your healthcare professional about the best way to feel better and get relief from symptoms while your body fights off the virus. To stay healthy and keep others healthy:

- Clean your hands.

- Cover coughs.

- Stay home when sick.

- Get recommended vaccines, such as the flu vaccine.

Section 32.3

Antiviral Agents

This section includes text excerpted from "Antiviral Agents," LiverTox®, National Institutes of Health (NIH), May 3, 2019.

The antivirals are a large and diverse group of agents that are typically classified by the virus infections for which they are used, their chemical structure, and their mode of action. Most antiviral agents have been developed in the last 20 to 25 years, many as a result of major research efforts to develop therapies and means of prevention of human immunodeficiency virus (HIV) infection and acquired immunodeficiency syndrome (AIDS). Some of the agents developed to treat HIV infection, AIDS, and its complications were found to also inhibit other viruses, and the novel approaches taken in the development of antiretroviral therapy (ART) have been applied to develop therapies of other viral infections.

Antiretroviral Agents for Human Immunodeficiency Virus Infection

The antiretroviral agents include nucleoside analogues with reverse transcriptase activity (such as tenofovir, emtricitabine, lamivudine, abacavir, stavudine, didanosine, and zidovudine); nonnucleoside reverse transcriptase inhibitors (such as delavirdine, efavirenz, etravirine, nevirapine, and rilpivirine); protease inhibitors (atazanavir, darunavir, indinavir, ritonavir, tipranavir, and many others); and miscellaneous agents such as maraviroc, that inhibit binding of the HIV virus to its T-cell receptor (CCR5 coreceptor antagonist); enfuvirtide, that blocks the uptake of HIV into cells (fusion inhibitor); and integrase inhibitors (raltegravir, elvitegravir, and dolutegravir) that block the integrase enzyme of HIV.

Hepatitis B Agents

The agents active against the hepatitis B virus (HBV) include several nucleoside analogs that are also active against and used to treat HIV infection (tenofovir, emtricitabine, and lamivudine) as well as agents that are poorly if at all active against HIV (adefovir, entecavir, and telbivudine). Alpha interferon and peginterferon (its long-acting pegylated form) are also active against hepatitis B, but are no longer commonly used for this indication.

Hepatitis C Agents

The agents active against hepatitis C virus (HCV) include interferon alfa (1992) and peginterferon (2000), which are used in combination with ribavirin, a nucleoside analog that potentiates the effects of interferon against hepatitis C by unclearly defined mechanisms. Progress in the treatment of hepatitis C began to accelerate in 2010 with the introduction of the first direct-acting anti-HCV agents, two HCV-specific protease inhibitors: boceprevir and telaprevir. While combinations of these protease inhibitors with peginterferon and ribavirin yielded high response rates (60 to 75%), the regimens were poorly tolerated, expensive, and prolonged (courses were typically for 48 weeks).

Beginning in 2013, new direct-acting anti-HCV agents with potent activity against different regions of the virus were introduced, which in combination obviated the need for interferon and yielded sustained response rates of greater than 90 percent with 12 to 24 weeks of treatment. The direct-acting agents were directed against 3 components of HCV: HCV protease (NS3) inhibitors included simeprevir (2013), paritaprevir (2015), grazoprevir (2016) and glecaprevir (2017); HCV RNA polymerase (NS5B) inhibitors included sofosbuvir (2013), a nucleoside analog, and dasabuvir (2015), a nonnucleoside inhibitor; and HCV NS5A inhibitors included daclatasvir (2015), elbasvir (2016), ledipasvir (2014), ombitasvir (2015), velpatsvir (2016) and pibrentasvir (2017). Combinations of 2 or 3 of these achieve sustained response rates of greater than 90 percent, with relatively short courses of therapy (8, 12, to 16 weeks) and without the need of interferon and its difficult and dose-limiting side effects. These combinations are available under brand names such as Harvoni, Technive, Viekira Pak, Zepatier, Epclusa, and Mavyret. Newer agents and different combination products are likely to be developed in the near future. Many of the earlier combinations are likely to be discontinued as newer regimens are more effective, better tolerated, and active against all genotypes and in patients with renal disease, HIV infection, or cirrhosis.

Herpes Virus Agents

The agents active against various herpes viruses (herpes simplex, varicella zoster, and cytomegalovirus) include acyclovir and related acyclic nucleoside analogues, such as valacyclovir, cidofovir, famciclovir, ganciclovir, and valganciclovir, and other miscellaneous agents such as foscarnet.

Influenza Agents

The agents active against influenza A virus include amantadine and rimantadine, which act on viral uncapping, and three neuraminidase inhibitors osteomavir (oral), zanamivir (by inhalation), and peramivir (intravenous). These agents are used during influenza outbreaks, generally for a brief period only, but are effective in prevention as well as amelioration of influenza infection.

The following drug records are discussed individually:

Drugs for Human Immunodeficiency Virus Infection, in the Subclass Antiretroviral Agents

- Fusion inhibitors (HIV)
  - Enfuvirtide, Maraviroc
- Integrase inhibitors (HIV)

- Bictegravir, Dolutegravir, Elvitegravir, Raltegravir
- Monoclonal Antibodies
- Ibalizumab
- Nonnucleoside reverse transcriptase inhibitors (HIV)
  - Delavirdine, Doravirine, Efavirenz, Etravirine, Nevirapine, Rilpivirine
- Nucleoside analogues (HIV)
  - Abacavir, Didanosine, Emtricitabine, Lamivudine, Stavudine, Tenofovir, Zidovudine
- Protease inhibitors (HIV)
  - Amprenavir, Atazanavir, Darunavir, Fosamprenavir, Indinavir, Lopinavir, Nelfinavir, Ritonavir, Saquinavir, Tipranavir

Drugs for Hepatitis B

Alpha interferon, Adefovir, Emtricitabine, Entecavir, Lamivudine, Telbivudine, Tenofovir

Drugs for Hepatitis C

- Interferon-based therapies
  - Alpha Interferon and Peginterferon, Ribavirin
- HCV NS5A inhibitors
  - Daclatasvir, Elbasvir, Ledipasvir, Ombitasvir, Pibrentasvir, Velpatasvir
- HCV NS5B (polymerase) inhibitors
  - Dasabuvir, Sofosbuvir
- HCV Protease inhibitors
  - Asunaprevir, Boceprevir, Glecaprevir, Grazoprevir, Paritaprevir, Simeprevir, Telaprevir, Voxilaprevir
- Combination therapies
  - Epclusa, Harvoni, Mavyret, Technive, Viekira Pak, Vosevi, Zepatier

Drugs for Herpes Virus Infections (Herpes Simplex Virus, Cytomegalovirus, Others)

- Acyclovir, Cidofovir, Famciclovir, Foscarnet, Ganciclovir, Letermovir, Valacyclovir, Valganciclovir

Drugs for Influenza

- Amantadine, Baloxavir, Oseltamivir, Peramivir, Rimantadine, Zanamivir

Section 32.4

Fighting Flu with Antiviral Drugs

This section includes text excerpted from "Fighting Flu with Antiviral Drugs," Centers for Disease Control and Prevention (CDC), January 30, 2019.

Most of the United States is reporting widespread flu activity according to the Centers for Disease Control and Prevention (CDC). Flu activity is expected to continue nationally for a number of weeks.

What can you do to protect yourself and your loved ones? If you have not received a flu vaccine, it is not too late! Flu vaccines reduce the risk of flu illness and potentially serious flu complications that can result in hospitalization and death. Flu activity usually peaks between December and February, although activity can last as late as May.

If You Get Sick with Flu, Antiviral Drugs Can Be Used to Treat Your Illness

Antiviral drugs are prescription medicines that fight against flu viruses in your body. They are different from antibiotics, which fight against bacterial infections. Antiviral drugs can lessen fever and flu symptoms, and shorten the time you are sick by about one day. They also may reduce the risk of complications, such as ear infections in children, respiratory complications requiring antibiotics in adults, and hospitalization.

For people at high risk of serious flu complications, early treatment with an antiviral drug can mean having milder illness instead of more severe illness that might require a hospital stay. For adults hospitalized with flu illness, some studies have reported that early antiviral treatment can reduce their risk of death.

Patients at high risk of developing serious flu complications include pregnant women, people 65 years and older, and children younger than 5 years but especially younger than 2 years. High-risk flu patients also include people with certain underlying medical conditions, including heart disease and diabetes, people with neurological or neurodevelopmental conditions, and people with weakened immune systems.

Studies show that flu antiviral drugs work best for treatment when you take them within two days of getting sick. Starting them later can still be helpful, especially if the sick person has a high-risk health condition or is very sick from flu. Doctors can choose to prescribe antivirals to treat people with mild flu illness who are not at high risk of flu complications if the patient has experienced flu symptoms for two days or less.

There Is a New Antiviral Drug Available This Flu Season

Baloxavir marboxil (trade name Xofluza®) is a new flu antiviral drug approved by the U.S. Food and Drug Administration (FDA) on October 24, 2018. Baloxavir joins oseltamivir (available as a generic or under the trade name Tamiflu®), zanamivir (trade name Relenza®), and peramivir (trade name Rapivab®) as antiviral medications for treating flu. Baloxavir is a pill, given as a single dose by mouth.

Antiviral Drugs Are Not a Substitute for Getting a Flu Vaccine

Getting a flu vaccine is the first and best step you can take to prevent influenza. There are many benefits to flu vaccination. Flu vaccination can keep you from getting sick with the flu, and reduce your risk of flu-associated complications, including hospitalization. Flu vaccination can be lifesaving in children. It can also help prevent serious medical events associated with some chronic conditions such as diabetes and heart and lung disease. Early treatment with antiviral drugs is important for people who are very sick with flu and people who get sick with flu who are at high risk of serious complications.

Bolster Your Flu-Fighting Arsenal

Good health habits can help stop the spread of flu. Everyday preventive actions include handwashing with soap and water. If soap and water are not available, use an alcohol-based hand rub. Avoid touching your eyes, nose, and mouth. Germs spread this way. Cover your nose and mouth with a tissue when you cough and sneeze. Use a disinfectant to clean surfaces and objects that may be contaminated with flu viruses. If you get sick, limit contact with others as much as possible to keep from infecting them.

Chapter 33

Antimicrobial Drug Resistance

Chapter Contents

Section 33.1

What Is Antibiotic Resistance?

This section contains text excerpted from the following sources:
Text in this section begins with excerpts from "About Antimicrobial
Resistance," Centers for Disease Control and Prevention (CDC),
September 10, 2018; Text beginning with the heading "Why Should
I Care about Antibiotic Resistance?" is excerpted from "Antibiotic
Resistance Questions and Answers," Centers for Disease Control and
Prevention (CDC), September 25, 2017.

Antibiotic resistance happens when germs like bacteria and fungi
develop the ability to defeat the drugs designed to kill them. That
means the germs are not killed and continue to grow.

Infections caused by antibiotic-resistant germs are difficult, and
sometimes impossible, to treat. In most cases, antibiotic-resistant
infections require extended hospital stays, additional follow-up doctor
visits, and costly and toxic alternatives.

Antibiotic resistance does not mean the body is becoming resistant
to antibiotics; it is that bacteria have become resistant to the antibiotics designed to kill them.

Antibiotic Resistance Threatens Everyone

Antibiotic resistance has the potential to affect people at any stage
of life, as well as the healthcare, veterinary, and agriculture industries,
making it one of the world's most urgent public health problems.

Each year in the United States, at least two million people are
infected with antibiotic-resistant bacteria, and at least 23,000 people
die as a result.

No one can completely avoid the risk of resistant infections, but
some people are at greater risk than others (for example, people with
chronic illnesses). If antibiotics lose their effectiveness, then we lose
the ability to treat infections and control public health threats.

Many medical advances are dependent on the ability to fight infections using antibiotics, including joint replacements, organ transplants, cancer therapy, and treatment of chronic diseases like diabetes,
asthma, and rheumatoid arthritis.

Why Should I Care about Antibiotic Resistance?

Antibiotic resistance is one of the most urgent threats to the public's
health. Antibiotic resistant bacteria can cause illnesses that were once

easily treatable with antibiotics to become untreatable, leading to dangerous infections. Antibiotic-resistant bacteria are often more difficult to kill and more expensive to treat. In some cases, the antibiotic-resistant infections can lead to serious disability or even death.

Why Are Bacteria Becoming Resistant to Antibiotics?

Overuse and misuse of antibiotics allows the development of antibiotic-resistant bacteria. Every time a person takes antibiotics, sensitive bacteria (bacteria that antibiotics can still attack) are killed, but resistant bacteria are left to grow and multiply. This is how repeated use of antibiotics can increase the number of drug-resistant bacteria.

Antibiotics are not effective against viral infections like the common cold, flu, most sore throats, bronchitis, and many sinus and ear infections. Widespread use of antibiotics for these illnesses is an example of how overuse of antibiotics can promote the spread of antibiotic resistance. Smart use of antibiotics is key to controlling the spread of resistance.

How Do Bacteria Become Resistant to Antibiotics?

Bacteria can become resistant to antibiotics through several ways. Some bacteria can "neutralize" an antibiotic by changing it in a way that makes it harmless. Others have learned how to pump an antibiotic back outside of the bacteria before it can do any harm. Some bacteria can change their outer structure so the antibiotic has no way to attach to the bacteria it is designed to kill.

After being exposed to antibiotics, sometimes one of the bacteria can survive because it found a way to resist the antibiotic. If even one bacterium becomes resistant to antibiotics, it can then multiply and replace all the bacteria that were killed off. That means that exposure to antibiotics provides selective pressure making the surviving bacteria more likely to be resistant. Bacteria can also become resistant through mutation of their genetic material.

How Should I Use Antibiotics to Protect Myself and My Community from Antibiotic Resistance?

Here is what you can do to help prevent antibiotic resistance:

- Tell your healthcare professional you are concerned about antibiotic resistance

413

- Ask your healthcare professional if there are steps you can take to feel better and get symptomatic relief without using antibiotics

- Take the prescribed antibiotic exactly as your healthcare professional tells you

- Safely throw away leftover medication

- Ask your healthcare professional about vaccines recommended for you and your family to prevent infections that may require an antibiotic

- Never skip doses

- Never take an antibiotic for a viral infection like a cold or the flu

- Never pressure your healthcare professional to prescribe an antibiotic

- Never save antibiotics for the next time you get sick

- Never take antibiotics prescribed for someone else

How Can Healthcare Professionals Help Prevent the Spread of Antibiotic Resistance?

Healthcare professionals can prevent the spread of antibiotic resistance by:

- Prescribing an antibiotic only when it is likely to benefit the patient

- Prescribing an antibiotic that targets the bacteria that is most likely causing their patient's illness when an antibiotic is likely to provide benefit

- Encouraging patients to use the antibiotic as instructed

- Collaborating with each other, office staff, and patients to promote appropriate antibiotic use

Section 33.2

Emergence of Antifungal Resistance

This section includes text excerpted from "Antifungal
Resistance," Centers for Disease Control and
Prevention (CDC), September 27, 2018.

Antifungal drugs save lives by treating dangerous fungal infections,
just as antibacterial drugs (antibiotics) are used to treat bacterial infections. Unfortunately, germs such as bacteria and fungi can develop
the ability to defeat the drugs designed to kill them. This is known as
"antimicrobial resistance." That means the germs are not killed and
continue to grow. When this occurs with fungi that no longer respond
to antifungal drugs, it is called "antifungal resistance." Antifungal
resistance is especially a concern for patients with invasive infections
such as those caused by the fungus Candida, a yeast, which can cause
serious health problems, including disability and death.

More information is needed about the risk antifungal resistance poses on human health and how many people are sickened by
drug-resistant fungal infections each year. The Centers for Disease
Control and Prevention (CDC) and its partners are working to:

- Better understand why and how antifungal resistance emerges

- Increase awareness among medical and public-health
  communities about these infections

- Develop better methods to prevent and control drug-resistant
  fungal infections

Fungal Infections Are a Serious Problem in Healthcare Settings

Invasive fungal infections can cause disability and death. Patients
can get fungal infections while receiving care for something else in
a healthcare facility. For example, the fungus Candida is a leading
cause of healthcare-associated bloodstream infections in U.S. hospitals. These infections are also costly for patients and healthcare
facilities. Each case of Candida bloodstream infection (also known
as "candidemia") is estimated to result in an additional 3 to 13 days
of hospitalization and $6,000 to $29,000 in healthcare costs. What is
also concerning is when we find antifungal resistance in some types
of Candida, which makes them harder to treat.

Antifungal Resistance Makes Infections Harder to Treat

Antifungal resistance is a particular problem with Candida infections. Some types of Candida are increasingly resistant to first-line and second-line antifungal medications such as fluconazole and the echinocandins (anidulafungin, caspofungin, and micafungin). About 7 percent of all Candida bloodstream isolates (pure samples of a germ) tested at the CDC are resistant to fluconazole. More than 70 percent of these resistant isolates are the species Candida glabrata or Candida krusei.

The CDC's surveillance data indicate that the proportion of Candida isolates that are resistant to fluconazole has remained fairly constant over the past 20 years. Echinocandin resistance, however, appears to be emerging, especially among Candida glabrata isolates. The CDC's surveillance data indicate that approximately 3 percent of Candida glabrata isolates are resistant to echinocandins. This is especially concerning as echinocandins are the first-line treatment for Candida glabrata, which already has high levels of resistance to fluconazole.

Multidrug-resistant Candida infections (those that are resistant to both fluconazole and an echinocandin) have very few remaining treatment options. The primary treatment option is Amphotericin B, a drug that can be toxic for patients who are already very sick. Not surprisingly, there is growing evidence to suggest that patients who have drug-resistant candidemia are less likely to survive than patients who have candidemia that can be treated by antifungal medications. We must act to prevent further resistance from developing and to prevent the spread of these infections. Emerging antifungal resistance has been identified in species such as Candida auris. Isolates of C. auris sent to the CDC are almost all resistant to fluconazole, and up to one-third are resistant to amphotericin B, usually reserved as a last-resort treatment. Most C. auris isolates are susceptible to echinocandins. However, echinocandin resistance can develop while the patient is being treated. C. auris is also a concerning public-health issue because it is difficult to identify with standard laboratory methods and because it spreads easily in healthcare settings, such as hospitals and long-term care facilities.

Antifungal Resistance in Aspergillus

Although the most common antifungal resistance occurs in Candida species, resistance in other types of less common fungi is also a problem. In Aspergillus (a mold) infections, emerging resistance to the first-line treatment threatens the effectiveness of lifesaving medications.

In general, Aspergillus infections are associated with high rates of death, especially in patients with weakened immune systems or underlying disease. Aspergillus is the leading cause of invasive mold infections, with an estimated 300,000 cases worldwide every year. Depending on location, up to 12 percent of Aspergillus infections are estimated to be resistant to antifungal medications. In a large U.S. study, antifungal resistance was identified in up to 7 percent of Aspergillus specimens from patients with stem cell and organ transplants.

Resistant Aspergillus infections can develop in people who have taken certain antifungal medications. However, resistant infections are also found in people who have not taken antifungal medications. This demonstrates that antifungal resistance in Aspergillus is likely acquired before entering the healthcare setting and is partially driven by environmental sources. For example, research shows that agricultural use of azole fungicides to treat crop diseases, which are similar to azole medications such as fluconazole, can lead to the growth of resistant strains of Aspergillus in soil and other places in the environment. If people with weakened immune systems breathe in antifungal-resistant Aspergillus spores, then they could develop infections that are difficult to treat. There is a potential for resistant infections if people with weak immune systems breathe in spores. More research is needed about how Aspergillus becomes resistant and how to prevent people from getting resistant Aspergillus infections.

What Causes Antifungal Resistance

Some species of fungi are naturally resistant to treatment with certain types of antifungal medications. Other species can develop resistance over time due to improper antifungal use—for example, dosages too low or treatment courses that are not long enough.

Some studies have indicated that antibacterial medications may also contribute to antifungal resistance. This resistance could occur for a variety of reasons. For example, antibacterial drugs can reduce good and bad bacteria in the gut, which creates favorable conditions for Candida growth. It is not yet known if decreasing the use of all or certain antibiotics can reduce Candida infections, but appropriate use of antibacterial and antifungal medications is one of the most important factors in fighting drug resistance.

What You Can Do

Antifungal resistance is a growing threat. Everyone has a role to play in preventing fungal infections and reducing antifungal resistance.

- The CDC is:

    - Tracking trends in antifungal resistance through the Emerging Infections Program by conducting multicenter candidemia surveillance and performing species confirmation and antifungal susceptibility testing on Candida bloodstream isolates

    - Using genetic sequencing and developing new laboratory tests to identify and understand specific mutations associated with antifungal resistance in Candida

    - Summarizing antifungal prescribing patterns across different healthcare facilities to understand opportunities to promote appropriate use of antifungals

- Healthcare facility executives and infection control staff can:

    - Assess antifungal use as part of their antibiotic stewardship programs

    - Ensure adherence to guidelines for hand hygiene, prevention of catheter-associated infections, and environmental infection control

- Doctors and other hospital staff can:

    - Prescribe antifungal medications appropriately

    - Test for antifungal resistance for patients with invasive disease who are not improving with first-line antifungal medications

    - Stay aware of resistance patterns, including antifungal resistance, in your facility and community

    - Document the dose, duration, and indication for every antifungal prescription

    - Participate in and lead efforts within your hospital to improve antifungal prescribing practices

    - Follow hand hygiene and other infection prevention and control guidelines with every patient

- Hospital patients can:

  - Clean their hands

  - Be sure everyone cleans their hands before entering your room

  - If you have a catheter, ask each day if it is necessary

  - Talk to your healthcare provider about your risk for certain infections, especially if you have a weakened immune system

  - Learn more about using antibiotics, including when they are needed and when they are not

Section 33.3

Surveillance of Antimicrobial Resistance Patterns and Rates

This section contains text excerpted from the following sources: Text beginning with the heading "The Threat of Antibiotic Resistance" is excerpted from "Antibiotic Resistance Threats in the United States," Centers for Disease Control and Prevention (CDC), April 23, 2013. Reviewed May 2019; Text under the heading "Biggest Threats and Data" is excerpted from "Biggest Threats and Data," Centers for Disease Control and Prevention (CDC), September 10, 2018.

The Threat of Antibiotic Resistance

Antibiotic resistance is a worldwide problem. New forms of antibiotic resistance can cross international boundaries and spread between continents with ease. Many forms of resistance spread with remarkable speed. World health leaders have described antibiotic-resistant microorganisms as "nightmare bacteria" that "pose a catastrophic threat" to people in every country in the world.

Statistics

Each year in the United States, at least 2 million people acquire serious infections with bacteria that are resistant to one or more of the antibiotics designed to treat those infections. At least 23,000 people die each year as a direct result of these antibiotic-resistant infections. Many more die from other conditions that were complicated by an antibiotic-resistant infection.

In addition, almost 250,000 people each year require hospital care for *Clostridium difficile (C. difficile)* infections. In most of these infections, the use of antibiotics was a major contributing factor leading to the illness. At least 14,000 people die each year in the United States from *C. difficile* infections. Many of these infections could have been prevented.

Antibiotic-resistant infections add considerable and avoidable costs to the already overburdened U.S. healthcare system. In most cases, antibiotic-resistant infections require prolonged and/or costlier treatments, extend hospital stays, necessitate additional doctor visits and healthcare use, and result in greater disability and death compared with infections that are easily treatable with antibiotics. The total economic cost of antibiotic resistance to the U.S. economy has been difficult to calculate. Estimates vary but have ranged as high as $20 billion in excess direct healthcare costs, with additional costs to society for lost productivity as high as $35 billion a year (2008 dollars).

Use of Antibiotics

The use of antibiotics is the single most important factor leading to antibiotic resistance around the world. Antibiotics are among the most commonly prescribed drugs used in human medicine. However, up to 50 percent of all the antibiotics prescribed for people are not needed or are not optimally effective as prescribed. Antibiotics are also commonly used in food animals to prevent, control, and treat disease and to promote the growth of food-producing animals. The use of antibiotics for promoting growth is not necessary and the practice should be phased out. Recent guidance from the U.S. Food and Drug Administration (FDA) describes a pathway toward this goal.

It is difficult to directly compare the amount of drugs used in food animals with the amount used in humans, but there is evidence that more antibiotics are used in food production.

The other major factor in the growth of antibiotic resistance is spread of the resistant strains of bacteria from person to person, or from the nonhuman sources in the environment, including food.

420

Prevent Infections

There are four core actions that will help fight these deadly infections:

- Preventing infections and preventing the spread of resistance
- Tracking resistant bacteria
- Improving the use of today's antibiotics
- Promoting the development of new antibiotics and developing new diagnostic tests for resistant bacteria

Bacteria will inevitably find ways of resisting the antibiotics we develop, which is why aggressive action is needed now to keep new resistance from developing and to prevent the resistance that already exists from spreading.

Biggest Threats and Data

Antibiotic resistance is one of the biggest public-health challenges of our time. In 2013, the CDC published a comprehensive analysis outlining the top 18 antibiotic-resistant threats in the United States, titled Antibiotic Resistance Threats in the United States, 2013 (AR Threats Report). The report sounded the alarm to the danger of antibiotic resistance, stating that each year in the United States, at least 2 million people get an antibiotic-resistant infection, and at least 23,000 people die.

The report ranked the 18 threats (bacteria and fungi) into three categories based on the level of concern to human health—urgent, serious, and concerning—and identified:

- Minimum estimates of morbidity and mortality from antibiotic-resistant infections
- People at especially high risk
- Gaps in knowledge about antibiotic resistance
- Core actions to prevent infections caused by antibiotic-resistant bacteria, and slow spread of resistance
- What the CDC was doing at that time to combat the threat of antibiotic resistance

The data below is pulled from the 2013 Threats Report. The CDC is working toward releasing an updated AR threats report in Fall 2019.

Urgent Threats
Clostridioides difficile

C. difficile causes life-threatening diarrhea and colitis (an inflammation of the colon), mostly in people who have had both recent medical care and antibiotics

Carbapenem-Resistant Enterobacteriaceae

Some carbapenem-resistant Enterobacteriaceae (CRE), a family of germs, are resistant to nearly all antibiotics, including carbapenems, which are often considered the antibiotics of last resort.

Drug-Resistant Neisseria gonorrhoeae

N. gonorrhoeae causes the sexually transmitted disease gonorrhea and has progressively developed resistance to the antibiotic drugs prescribed to treat it.

Serious Threats
Multidrug-Resistant Acinetobacter

People with weakened immune systems, including hospitalized patients, are more at risk of getting an *Acinetobacter* infection, which is resistant to many commonly prescribed antibiotics.

Drug-Resistant Campylobacter

Campylobacter usually causes diarrhea, fever, and abdominal cramps, and can spread from animals to people through contaminated food, especially raw or undercooked chicken.

Fluconazole-Resistant Candida

Candida yeasts normally live on the skin and mucous membranes without causing infection; however, overgrowth of these microorganisms can cause symptoms to develop

Extended-Spectrum Beta-Lactamase-Producing Enterobacteriaceae

Extended-spectrum Beta-lactamase (ESBL)-producing Enterobacteriaceae are resistant to strong antibiotics, including extended-spectrum cephalosporins.

- ESBL is an enzyme that allows bacteria to become resistant to a wide variety of penicillin and cephalosporin drugs.

- Bacteria that contain this enzyme are known as ESBLs or ESBL-producing.

Vancomycin-Resistant Enterococcus

Vancomycin-resistant Enterococci (VRE) cause a range of illnesses, mostly among patients receiving healthcare.

Multidrug-Resistant Pseudomonas aeruginosa

Serious *Pseudomonas* infections usually occur in people with weakened immune systems, making it a common cause of healthcare-associated infections.

Drug-Resistant Nontyphoidal Salmonella

Salmonella spreads from animals to people mostly through food, and usually causes diarrhea, fever, and abdominal cramps.

Drug-Resistant Salmonella Serotype Typhi

Salmonella typhi causes a serious disease called typhoid fever, and is spread by contaminated food and water.

Drug-Resistant Shigella

Shigella spreads in feces through direct contact or through contaminated surfaces, food, or water, and most people infected with Shigella develop diarrhea, fever, and stomach cramps.

Methicillin-Resistant Staphylococcus aureus

Methicillin-resistant *Staphylococcus aureus* (MRSA) is *S. aureus* that has become resistant to certain antibiotics called "beta-lactams," including methicillin.

- Patients in healthcare settings frequently get severe or potentially life-threatening infections, and people can also get MRSA in their community.

Drug-Resistant Streptococcus pneumoniae

S. pneumoniae causes pneumococcal disease, which can range from ear and sinus infections to pneumonia and bloodstream infections.

Drug-Resistant Tuberculosis

Tuberculosis (TB) is caused by the bacteria M. tuberculosis and is among the most common infectious diseases and a frequent cause of death worldwide.

Concerning Threats
Vancomycin-Resistant Staphylococcus aureus

Vancomycin-resistant *Staphylococcus aureus* (VRSA) is *S. aureus* that has become resistant to the antibiotic vancomycin, the antibiotic most frequently used to treat serious *S. aureus* infections.

Erythromycin-Resistant Group A Streptococcus

Group A strep can cause many different infections that range from minor illnesses to very serious and deadly diseases, including strep throat, scarlet fever, and others.

Clindamycin-Resistant Group B Streptococcus

Group B strep can cause severe illness in people of all ages.

Part Six

Preventing
Infectious Diseases

Chapter 34

Transmission-Based Precautions

Transmission-based precautions are the second tier of basic infection control and are to be used in addition to standard precautions for patients who may be infected or colonized with certain infectious agents for which additional precautions are needed to prevent infection transmission.

Contact Precautions

- Ensure appropriate patient placement in a single patient space or room if available in acute-care hospitals. In long-term and other residential settings, make room placement decisions balancing risks to other patients. In ambulatory settings, place patients requiring contact precautions in an exam room or cubicle as soon as possible.

- Use personal protective equipment (PPE) appropriately, including gloves and gown. Wear a gown and gloves for all interactions that may involve contact with the patient or the patient's environment. Donning PPE upon room entry and properly discarding before exiting the patient room is done to contain pathogens.

This chapter includes text excerpted from "Transmission-Based Precautions," Centers for Disease Control and Prevention (CDC), January 7, 2016.

- Limit transport and movement of patients outside of the room to medically necessary purposes. When transport or movement is necessary, cover or contain the infected or colonized areas of the patient's body. Remove and dispose of contaminated PPE and perform hand hygiene prior to transporting patients on Contact Precautions. Don clean PPE to handle the patient at the transport location.

- Use disposable or dedicated patient-care equipment (e.g., blood pressure cuffs). If common use of equipment for multiple patients is unavoidable, clean and disinfect such equipment before use on another patient.

- Prioritize cleaning and disinfecting the rooms of patients on contact precautions, ensuring rooms are frequently cleaned and disinfected (e.g., at least daily or prior to use by another patient if an outpatient setting) and focusing on frequently touched surfaces and equipment in the immediate vicinity of the patient.

Droplet Precautions

- Source control: Put a mask on the patient.

- Ensure appropriate patient placement in a single room if possible. In acute-care hospitals, if single rooms are not available, utilize the recommendations for alternative patient placement considerations in the *Guideline for Isolation Precautions*. In long-term care and other residential settings, make decisions regarding patient placement on a case-by-case basis, considering infection risks to other patients in the room and available alternatives. In ambulatory settings, place patients who require droplet precautions in an exam room or cubicle as soon as possible and instruct patients to follow respiratory hygiene/cough etiquette recommendations.

- Use personal protective equipment (PPE) appropriately. Don a mask upon entry into the patient room or patient space.

- Limit transport and movement of patients outside of the room to medically necessary purposes. If transport or movement outside of the room is necessary, instruct patient to wear a mask and follow respiratory hygiene/cough etiquette.

428

Airborne Precautions

- Source control: Put a mask on the patient.

Ensure appropriate patient placement in an airborne-infection isolation room (AIIR) constructed according to the *Guideline for Isolation Precautions*. In settings where Airborne Precautions cannot be implemented due to limited resources, masking the patient and placing the patient in a private room with the door closed will reduce the likelihood of airborne transmission until the patient is either transferred to a facility with an AIIR or returned home.

- Restrict susceptible healthcare personnel from entering the rooms of patients known or suspected to have measles, chickenpox, disseminated zoster, or smallpox if other immune healthcare personnel are available.

- Use personal protective equipment (PPE) appropriately, including a fit-tested National Institute for Occupational Safety and Health (NIOSH)-approved N95 or higher-level respirator for healthcare personnel.

- Limit transport and movement of patients outside of the room to medically necessary purposes. If transport or movement outside an AIIR is necessary, instruct patients to wear a surgical mask, if possible, and observe respiratory hygiene/cough etiquette. Healthcare personnel transporting patients who are on Airborne Precautions do not need to wear a mask or respirator during transport if the patient is wearing a mask and infectious skin lesions are covered.

- Immunize susceptible persons as soon as possible following unprotected contact with vaccine-preventable infections (e.g., measles, varicella, or smallpox).

Chapter 35

Handwashing to Prevent Spread of Germs

Wash Your Hands Often to Stay Healthy

You can help yourself and your loved ones stay healthy by washing your hands often, especially during these key times when you are likely to get and spread germs:

- Before, during, and after preparing food
- Before eating food
- Before and after caring for someone at home who is sick with vomiting or diarrhea
- Before and after treating a cut or wound
- After using the toilet
- After changing diapers or cleaning up a child who has used the toilet
- After blowing your nose, coughing, or sneezing
- After touching an animal, animal feed, or animal waste
- After handling pet food or pet treats
- After touching garbage

This chapter includes text excerpted from "Wash Your Hands," Centers for Disease Control and Prevention (CDC), April 29, 2019.

Follow Five Steps to Wash Your Hands the Right Way

Washing your hands is easy, and it's one of the most effective ways to prevent the spread of germs. Clean hands can stop germs from spreading from one person to another and throughout an entire community—from your home and workplace to childcare facilities and hospitals.

Follow these five steps every time.

- Wet your hands with clean, running water (warm or cold), turn off the tap, and apply soap.

- Lather your hands by rubbing them together with the soap. Lather the backs of your hands, between your fingers, and under your nails.

- Scrub your hands for at least 20 seconds. Need a timer? Hum the "Happy Birthday" song from beginning to end twice.

- Rinse your hands well under clean, running water.

- Dry your hands using a clean towel or air dry them.

Use Hand Sanitizer Only When You Cannot Use Soap and Water

Washing your hands with soap and water is the best way to get rid of germs in most situations. If soap and water are not available, you can use an alcohol-based hand sanitizer that contains at least 60 percent alcohol. You can tell if the sanitizer contains at least 60 percent alcohol by looking at the product label.

Remember these key facts about alcohol-based hand sanitizers.

- Sanitizers can quickly reduce the number of germs on hands in some situations.

- Sanitizers do not get rid of all types of germs.

- Hand sanitizers may not be as effective when hands are visibly dirty or greasy.

- Hand sanitizers might not remove harmful chemicals such as pesticides and heavy metals from hands.

- Keep hand sanitizer out of the reach of young children and supervise their use. Swallowing alcohol-based hand sanitizers can cause alcohol poisoning if more than a couple of mouthfuls are swallowed.

How to Use Hand Sanitizer

- Apply the gel product to the palm of one hand (read the label to learn the correct amount).

- Rub your hands together.

- Rub the gel over all the surfaces of your hands and fingers until your hands are dry. This should take around 20 seconds.

Chapter 36

Eye Protection

The Centers for Disease Control and Prevention (CDC) recommends eye protection for a variety of potential exposure settings in which workers may be at risk of acquiring infectious diseases via ocular exposure. This document provides background information and specific details on eye protection that can be used to supplement eye protection recommendations provided in current CDC infection-control guidance documents. It is intended to familiarize workers with the various types of eye protection available, their characteristics, and their applicable use. Workers should understand that regular prescription eyeglasses and contact lenses are not considered eye protection.

Infectious diseases can be transmitted through various mechanisms, among which are infections that can be introduced through the mucous membranes of the eye (conjunctiva). These include viruses and bacteria that can cause conjunctivitis (e.g., adenovirus, herpes simplex, *Staphylococcus aureus*) and viruses that can cause systemic infections, including bloodborne viruses (e.g., hepatitis B and C viruses, human immunodeficiency virus), herpes viruses, and rhinoviruses. Infectious agents are introduced to the eye either directly (e.g., blood splashes, respiratory droplets generated during coughing or suctioning) or from touching the eyes with contaminated fingers or other objects.

This chapter includes text excerpted from "Eye Safety," Centers for Disease Control and Prevention (CDC), July 29, 2013. Reviewed May 2019.

Eye protection provides a barrier to infectious materials entering the eye and is often used in conjunction with other personal protective equipment (PPE) such as gloves, gowns, masks, or respirators.

What Types of Eye Protection Should Be Worn?

The eye protection chosen for specific work situations depends upon the circumstances of exposure, other PPE used, and personal vision needs. There is a wide variety in the types of protective eyewear, and appropriate selection should be based on a number of factors, the most important of which is the nature and extent of the hazard. Eye protection must be comfortable and allow for sufficient peripheral vision and must be adjustable to ensure a secure fit. It may be necessary to provide several different types, styles, and sizes. Selection of protective eyewear appropriate for a given task should be made from an evaluation of each activity, including regulatory requirements when applicable. These hazard assessments require a clear understanding of the work tasks, including knowledge of the potential routes of exposure and the opportunities for exposure in the task assessed (nature and extent of worker contact). Exposure incident reports should be reviewed to identify those incidents (whether or not infection occurred) that could have been prevented by the proper use of protective eyewear.

What Are Common Types of Eye Protection?
Goggles

Appropriately fitted, indirectly vented goggles* with a manufacturer's antifog coating provide the most reliable practical eye protection from splashes, sprays, and respiratory droplets. Newer styles of goggles may provide better indirect airflow properties to reduce fogging, as well as better peripheral vision and more size options for fitting goggles to different workers. Many styles of goggles fit adequately over prescription glasses with minimal gaps. However, to be efficacious, goggles must fit snugly, particularly from the corners of the eye across the brow. While highly effective as eye protection, goggles do not provide splash or spray protection to other parts of the face.

* *Directly-vented goggles may allow penetration by splashes or sprays; therefore, indirectly-vented or nonvented goggles are preferred for infection control.*

Face Shields

Face shields are commonly used as an infection control alternative to goggles.** As opposed to goggles, a face shield can also provide protection to other facial areas. To provide better face and eye protection from splashes and sprays, a face shield should have crown and chin protection and wrap around the face to the point of the ear, which reduces the likelihood that a splash could go around the edge of the shield and reach the eyes. Disposable face shields for medical personnel made of lightweight films that are attached to a surgical mask or fit loosely around the face should not be relied upon as optimal protection.

** *In a chemical exposure or industrial setting, face shields should be used in addition to goggles, not as a substitute for goggles (ANSI Z87.1-2003 Practice for occupational and educational eye and face protection).*

Safety Glasses

Safety glasses provide impact protection but do not provide the same level of splash or droplet protection as goggles and generally should not be used for infection-control purposes.

Full-Face Respirators

Full facepiece elastomeric respirators and powered air-purifying respirators (PAPRs) are designed and used for respiratory protection, but because of their design incidentally provide highly effective eye protection as well. Selection of this type of PPE should be based on an assessment of the respiratory hazard in an infection-control situation, but will also provide, as an additional benefit, optimal eye protection.

What Eye Protection Is Available for Prescription Lenses Users?

Many safety goggles or plano (nonprescription) safety glasses fit comfortably over street eyewear and can provide satisfactory protection without impairing the fit of the prescription eyewear. Prescription safety glasses with side protection are available, but do not protect against splashes or droplets as well as goggles. Special prescription inserts are available for goggles. When full facepiece elastomeric negative pressure (i.e., nonpowered) respirators or tight-fitting PAPRs are indicated for respiratory protection, these devices require appropriate prescription inserts to avoid compromising the seal around the face; PAPRs designed with loose-fitting facepieces or with hoods that completely cover the head and neck may be more accommodating to prescription lens wearers.

Contact lenses, by themselves, offer no infection-control protection. However, contact lenses may be worn with any of the recommended eye-protection devices, including full-face respirators. Contact lens users should rigorously adhere to handwashing guidelines when inserting, adjusting, or removing contact lenses.

What Combination of Eye Protection and Other Personal Protective Equipment Should Be Used?

Eye protection should be selected in the context of other PPE use requirements. Safety goggles may not fit properly when used with certain half-face respirators, and similarly, face shields may not fit properly over some respirators. Once PPE requirements have been established for a specific infection-control situation, the selected PPE should be pretested to assure suitable fit and protection when used as an ensemble. Elastomeric, full facepiece respirators and PAPRs have the advantage of incidentally providing optimal eye protection. In situations where all combinations of PPE may not be readily available to workers, judicious selection of complementary PPE is important to allow for appropriate protection.

How Should Potentially Contaminated Eye Protection Be Removed?

Eye protection should be removed by handling only the portion of this equipment that secures the device to the head (i.e., plastic temples, elasticized band, ties), as this is considered relatively "clean." The front and sides of the device (i.e., goggles, face shield) should not be touched, as these are the surfaces most likely to become contaminated by sprays, splashes, or droplets during patient care. Nondisposable eye protection should be placed in a designated receptacle for subsequent cleaning and disinfection. The sequence of PPE removal should follow a defined regimen that should be developed by infection-control staff and take into consideration the need to remove other PPE.

Is It Safe for Others to Reuse My Eye Protection?

The eyewear described above is generally not disposable and must be disinfected before reuse. Where possible, each individual worker should be assigned his or her own eye protection to insure appropriate fit and to minimize the potential of exposing the next wearer. A labeled container for used (potentially contaminated) eye protection should be available in the healthcare workers change-out/locker room. Eye protection deposited here can be collected, disinfected, washed, and then reused.

How Should Eye Protection Be Disinfected?

Healthcare setting-specific procedures for cleaning and disinfecting used patient-care equipment should be followed for reprocessing reusable eye-protection devices. Manufacturers may be consulted for their guidance and experience in disinfecting their respective products. Contaminated eye-protection devices should be reprocessed in an area where other soiled equipment is handled. Eye protection should be physically cleaned and disinfected with the designated hospital disinfectant, rinsed, and allowed to air dry. Gloves should be worn when cleaning and disinfecting these devices.

Chapter 37

Vaccination

Chapter Contents

Section 37.1

Facts about Infant, Childhood, Adolescent, and Adult Vaccinations

This section includes text excerpted from "Vaccines for Infants, Children, and Teens," Vaccines.gov, U.S. Department of Health and Human Services (HHS), December 15, 2017.

Vaccines for Infants, Children, and Teens

Vaccines help protect infants, children, and teens from serious diseases. Getting childhood vaccines means your child can develop immunity (protection) against diseases before they come into contact with them.

And did you know that getting your child vaccinated also protects others? Because of community immunity, vaccines help keep your child's younger siblings, older family members, and friends from getting sick, too.

In this section, you'll find vaccine information and schedules for:

- Infants and children from birth through age 6

- Preteens and teens ages 7 through 18

Why Do Vaccinations Start So Early?

Young children are at increased risk for infectious diseases because their immune systems have not yet built up the necessary defenses to fight serious infections and diseases. As a result, diseases such as whooping cough or pneumococcal disease can be very serious—and even deadly—for infants and young children. Vaccinations start early in life to protect children before they are exposed to these diseases.

Can Vaccines Overload My Child's Immune System?

No, vaccines do not overload the immune system. Your child's immune system successfully fights off thousands of germs every day. Even if your child gets several vaccines in a day, the vaccines make up only a tiny fraction of the germs their body fights off.

Why Does My Child Need More Than One Dose of a Vaccine?

Children—and adults, too—need more than one dose of some vaccines. That's because it can take more than one dose to build enough immunity against a disease. A vaccine's protection can also fade over time.

That's why every dose of a vaccine is important.

Do Some Vaccines Protect against More Than One Disease?

Yes. In many cases, your child can get combination vaccines—or vaccines that protect them from more than one disease. This means fewer vaccines for them and fewer trips to the doctor for you.

Can I Delay My Child's Vaccines or Spread Them out over a Longer Period of Time?

Experts do not recommend spreading out or delaying your child's vaccines. There is no benefit to spreading out vaccinations—and following the recommended schedule protects infants and children by providing immunity early in life. If your child misses vaccines or gets them late, they will be at risk for serious diseases that are preventable.

Can My Child Get Vaccinated If They Are Sick?

Probably, but ask your child's pediatrician first. Children can usually get vaccines when they have a mild illness such as cold, low fever, ear infection, or diarrhea (watery poop).

Vaccines for Adults

Every year, thousands of adults in the United States get sick and are hospitalized from vaccine-preventable diseases. Getting vaccinated will help you stay healthy, so you'll miss less work and also have more time for your family and friends.

And did you know that when you get vaccinated, you also help protect your family and your community? Because of community immunity, vaccines help keep diseases from spreading to people who may not be able to get certain vaccines, like newborn babies.

I Have Gotten All My Childhood Vaccines. Why Do I Need More?

Adults need vaccines for several reasons. For example:

- Some vaccines are recommended only for adults, who are more at risk for certain diseases—like shingles.

- Protection from childhood vaccines wears off over time so you need additional doses of certain vaccines to stay protected.

- You may not have gotten some of the newer vaccines that are now available.

- Some viruses, like the virus that causes the flu, can change over time.

- You may be at increased risk for diseases based on travel plans, your job, or health conditions.

How Do I Know Which Vaccinations I've Had and Which Ones I Need?

To find out which vaccinations you've had, you'll need to find your vaccination record. Your vaccination record is the history of all the vaccines you've had as a child and as an adult. To find your vaccination record:

- Ask your parents or caregivers if they have your vaccination record.

- Contact current or previous doctors and ask for your record.

- Contact your state health department—some states have registries (immunization information systems) that can provide information about your vaccination records.

- If you can't find your record, ask your doctor if you should get some vaccinations again.

Section 37.2

Vaccination for Your Children

This section includes text excerpted from "Vaccinate Your
Baby for Best Protection," Centers for Disease Control and
Prevention (CDC), April 29, 2019.

Immunization is one of the best ways parents can protect their
babies from 14 serious childhood diseases before the age of 2. Vaccinate your child according to the Centers for Disease Control and
Prevention's (CDC)-recommended immunization schedule for safe,
proven disease protection.

Diseases that vaccines prevent can be very serious—even deadly—
especially for infants and young children. Vaccines work with babies'
natural defenses to help them safely build immunity to these diseases.

Most parents today have never seen firsthand the devastating
consequences that vaccine-preventable diseases have on a family or
community. Some diseases that are prevented by vaccines, such as
pertussis (whooping cough) and chickenpox, remain common in the
United States.

Protect Your Child from Serious Diseases

Measles is an example of how serious vaccine-preventable diseases
can be. Cases and outbreaks still occur when the disease is brought
into the United States by unvaccinated travelers (Americans or foreign
visitors) who get infected when they are in other countries. Measles is
still a common disease in many parts of the world. The viral disease is
highly contagious and can spread easily when it reaches a community
where groups of people are unvaccinated. Measles can be serious and
can cause pneumonia, encephalitis (swelling of the brain), and even
death. Young children are at the highest risk for serious complications
from measles.

Another example is the whooping cough. The United States has
experienced an increase in whooping-cough cases and outbreaks
reported over the last few decades. Whooping cough can be deadly,
especially for young babies who are too young to get their own vaccines.
Since 2010, there have been tens of thousands of whooping cough cases
reported each year nationwide, with a peak of more than 48,000 cases
reported in 2012.

The Diseases Vaccines Prevent

- Diphtheria

- Haemophilus influenzae type B (Hib)

- Hepatitis A

- Hepatitis B

- Influenza (flu)

- Measles

- Mumps

- Pertussis

- Pneumococcal disease

- Polio

- Rubella (German measles)

- Tetanus (lockjaw)

- Rotavirus

- Varicella (chickenpox)

Stay Current with Your Child's Vaccines

It is very important to stay up-to-date on your baby's vaccinations. It can take weeks for a vaccine to help your baby make protective disease-fighting antibodies, and some vaccines require multiple doses to provide best protection. If you wait until you think your child could be exposed to a serious illness—such as when your child starts attending childcare or during a disease outbreak—there may not be enough time for the vaccine to work.

Fortunately, most parents choose to vaccinate their children. However, some children have not received all of their vaccines, so they are not fully protected. It is important that children receive all doses of the vaccines according to the recommended immunization schedule. Not receiving all doses of a vaccine leaves a child vulnerable to catching serious diseases.

That's why it is important to make sure that your child is up to date on all vaccinations. Ask your child's doctor if your child is due for any vaccinations. You can also review the CDC's parent-friendly immunization schedule for infants and children (from birth through six years) at www.cdc.gov/vaccines/schedules/parents-adults/index. html.

Paying for Vaccinations

Most health insurance plans cover the cost of vaccinations, but you should check with your insurance provider before going to the doctor. If you do not have health insurance or your insurance policy does not cover all recommended childhood vaccines, your child may be eligible for vaccines through the Vaccines for Children (VFC) program. Ask if your child's doctor is a VFC program provider.

Section 37.3

FAQs about Vaccinations

This section includes text excerpted from "Common Immunization Questions," Centers for Disease Control and Prevention (CDC), July 12, 2018.

What Are the Possible Side Effects from Vaccines?

Any vaccine can cause side effects. For the most part these are minor (for example, a sore arm or low-grade fever) and go away within a few days. Listed below are vaccines licensed in the United States and side effects that have been associated with each of them. This information is copied directly from the CDC's Vaccine Information Statements, which in turn are derived from the Advisory Committee on Immunization Practices (ACIP) recommendations for each vaccine.

Remember, vaccines are continually monitored for safety, and like any medication, vaccines can cause side effects. However, a decision not to immunize children also involves risk and could put the children and others who come into contact with them at risk of contracting a potentially deadly disease.

What Are the Differences between Active and Passive Immunity?

Immunity Types

Immunity to a disease is achieved through the presence of antibodies to that disease in a person's system. Antibodies are proteins produced by the body to neutralize or destroy toxins or disease-carrying organisms. Antibodies are disease specific. For example, a measles antibody will protect a person who is exposed to measles disease, but will have no effect on exposure to mumps.

There are two types of immunity: active and passive.

Active Immunity

Active immunity results when exposure to a disease organism triggers the immune system to produce antibodies to that disease. Exposure to the disease organism can occur through infection with the actual disease (resulting in natural immunity) or introduction of a killed or weakened form of the disease organism through vaccination (vaccine-induced immunity). Either way, if an immune person comes into contact with that disease in the future, their immune system will recognize it and immediately produce the antibodies needed to fight it.

Active immunity is long-lasting, and sometimes lifelong.

Passive Immunity

Passive immunity is provided when a person is given antibodies to a disease rather than producing them through her or his own immune system.

A newborn baby acquires passive immunity from its mother through the placenta. A person can also get passive immunity through antibody-containing blood products such as immune globulin, which may be given when immediate protection from a specific disease is needed. This is the major advantage to passive immunity; protection is immediate, whereas active immunity takes time (usually several weeks) to develop.

However, passive immunity lasts only for a few weeks or months. Only active immunity is long lasting.

What Are the Risks of Not Vaccinating?

As a parent, you want to protect your little ones from harm. Before you decide to vaccinate, you may wish to know more about:

- How vaccines work

- How vaccines work with your baby's immune system

- Vaccine side effects/risks

- Vaccine ingredients

- Vaccine safety

Visit the CDC's Parents' Guide to Immunizations on their website to find the information you need to make the vaccine decision. If you have more questions, talk with your child's doctor or explore the site further.

How Vaccines Prevent Diseases

The diseases vaccines prevent can be dangerous, or even deadly. Vaccines reduce your child's risk of infection by working with their body's natural defenses to help them safely develop immunity to disease.

When germs such as bacteria or viruses invade the body, they attack and multiply. This invasion is called an "infection," and the infection is what causes illness. The immune system then has to fight the infection. Once it fights off the infection, the body has a supply of cells that help recognize and fight that disease in the future. These supplies of cells are called "antibodies."

Vaccines help develop immunity by imitating an infection, but this "imitation" infection does not cause illness. Instead it causes the immune system to develop the same response as it does to a real infection so the body can recognize and fight the vaccine-preventable disease in the future. Sometimes, after getting a vaccine, imitation infection can cause minor symptoms, such as fever. Such minor symptoms are normal and should be expected as the body builds immunity.

As children get older, they require additional doses of some vaccines for best protection. Older kids also need protection against additional diseases they may encounter.

What Diseases Do Vaccines Prevent?
Recommended Vaccines by Disease

Vaccines are available for these 18 dangerous or deadly diseases. Over the years, these vaccines have prevented countless cases of disease and saved millions of lives. Infants, children, adolescents, teens, and adults need different vaccinations, depending on their age, location, job, lifestyle, travel schedule, health conditions, or previous vaccinations.

- Chickenpox (varicella)
- Diphtheria
- Flu (influenza)
- Hepatitis A
- Hepatitis B
- Hib (Haemophilus influenzae type b)
- HPV (human papillomavirus)
- Measles
- Meningococcal
- Mumps
- Pneumococcal
- Polio (poliomyelitis)
- Rotavirus
- Rubella (German measles)
- Shingles (Herpes zoster)
- Tetanus (lockjaw)
- Whooping cough (pertussis)

Vaccines Recommended for Travel and Some Specific Groups

People in certain research jobs and travel situations may be exposed to dangerous or deadly diseases that are no longer common in the United States. Because of the increased risk of disease exposure in these instances, the nonroutine vaccines listed below. These are considered nonroutine vaccines because they are not part of the recommended immunization schedules for children, adolescents, and adults.

- Adenovirus
- Anthrax
- Cholera
- Japanese encephalitis (JE)

- Rabies
- Smallpox
- Tuberculosis
- Typhoid fever
- Yellow fever

What Do You Need to Know about Immunizations?

1. **Why your child should be vaccinated**

   Immunizations protect children from dangerous childhood diseases. Any of these diseases can cause serious complications and can even kill.

2. **Diseases that childhood vaccines prevent**

   - Diphtheria
   - Haemophilus influenzae type b (Hib disease—a major cause of bacterial meningitis)
   - Hepatitis A
   - Hepatitis B
   - Human papillomavirus (HPV—a major cause of cervical and other cancers)
   - Influenza
   - Measles
   - Meningococcal
   - Mumps
   - Pertussis
   - Pneumococcal (causes bacterial meningitis and blood infections)
   - Polio
   - Rotavirus
   - Rubella
   - Tetanus
   - Varicella

3. **The number of doses your child needs**

   The following vaccinations are recommended by age two and can be given over five visits to a doctor or clinic:

   - 4 doses of diphtheria, tetanus, and pertussis vaccine (DTaP)
   - 3 to 4 doses of Hib vaccine (depending on the brand used)
   - 4 doses of pneumococcal vaccine
   - 3 doses of polio vaccine
   - 2 doses of hepatitis A vaccine
   - 3 doses of hepatitis B vaccine
   - 1 dose of measles, mumps, and rubella vaccine (MMR)
   - 2 to 3 doses of rotavirus vaccine (depending on the brand used)
   - 1 dose of varicella vaccine
   - 1 or 2 annual doses of influenza vaccine (the number of doses depends on influenza vaccine history)

4. **Like any medicine, vaccines can cause minor side effects**

   Side effects can occur with any medicine, including vaccines. Depending on the vaccine, these can include a slight fever, rash, or soreness at the site of injection. Slight discomfort is normal and should not be a cause for alarm. Your healthcare provider can give you additional information.

5. **It is extremely rare, but vaccines can cause serious reactions—weigh the risks!**

   Serious reactions to vaccines are extremely rare. The risk of serious complications from a disease that could have been prevented by vaccination is far greater than the risk of a serious reaction to a vaccine.

6. **What to do if your child has a serious reaction**

   If you think your child is experiencing a persistent or severe reaction, call your doctor or get the child to a doctor right away. Write down what happened and the date and time it happened. Ask your doctor, nurse, or health department to file a VAERS (Vaccine Adverse Event Reporting System) report or go to (vaers.hhs.gov) to file this form yourself electronically.

7. **Why you should not wait to vaccinate**

   Children under five are especially susceptible to disease because their immune systems have not built up the necessary defenses to fight infection. By immunizing on time (by age two), you can protect your child from disease and also protect others at school or daycare.

8. **Be sure to track your shots via a health record**

   A vaccination health record helps you and your healthcare provider keep your child's vaccinations on schedule. If you move or change providers, having an accurate record might prevent your child from having to repeat vaccinations she or he has already had. A shot record should be started when your child receives the first vaccination and updated with each vaccination visit.

9. **Some children are eligible for free vaccinations**

   The federal program Vaccines for Children provides free vaccines to eligible children, including those without health-insurance coverage, those enrolled in Medicaid, American Indians and Alaskan Natives, and those whose health insurance does not cover vaccines.

10. **More information is available**

    - General immunization questions can be answered by the CDC Contact Center at 800-CDC-INFO (800-232-4636) English and Español Contact CDC-INFO at (www.cdc.gov/cdc-info/index.html)

    - Questions about vaccines and vaccine-preventable diseases frequently asked by people calling the TTY Service Hotline at 888-232-6348 (TTY hotline)

What Are the Common Questions Parents Ask about Infant Immunizations?
Are Vaccines Safe?

Yes. Vaccines are very safe. The United States' long-standing vaccine safety system ensures that vaccines are as safe as possible. Currently, the United States has the safest vaccine supply in its history. Millions of children safely receive vaccines each year. The most common side effects, such as pain or swelling at the injection site, are typically very mild.

What Are the Side Effects of the Vaccines? How Do I Treat Them?

Vaccines, like any medication, may cause some side effects. Most of these side effects, such as soreness where the shot was given, fussiness, or a low-grade fever, are very minors. These side effects typically only last a couple of days and are treatable. For example, you can apply a cool, wet washcloth on the sore area to ease discomfort.

Serious reactions are very rare. However, if your child experiences any reactions that concern you, call the doctor's office.

What Are the Risks and Benefits of Vaccines?

Vaccines can prevent infectious diseases that once killed or harmed many infants, children, and adults. Without vaccines, your child is at risk for getting seriously ill and suffering pain, disability, and even death from diseases such as measles and whooping cough. The main risks associated with getting vaccines are side effects, which are almost always mild (redness and swelling at the injection site) and go away within a few days. Serious side effects after vaccination, such as a severe allergic reaction, are very rare and doctors and clinic staff are trained to deal with them. The disease-prevention benefits of getting vaccines are much greater than the possible side effects for almost all children. The only exceptions to this are cases in which a child has a serious chronic medical condition, such as cancer or a disease that weakens the immune system, or has had a severe allergic reaction to a previous vaccine dose.

Is There a Link between Vaccines and Autism?

No. Scientific studies and reviews continue to show no relationship between vaccines and autism.

Some people have suggested that thimerosal (a compound that contains mercury) in vaccines given to infants and young children might be a cause of autism. Others have suggested that the MMR (measles-mumps-rubella) vaccine may be linked to autism. However, numerous scientists and researchers have studied and continue to study the MMR vaccine and thimerosal, and they reach the same conclusion: There is no link between the MMR vaccine or thimerosal and autism.

Can Vaccines Overload My Baby's Immune System?

Vaccines do not overload the immune system. Every day, a healthy baby's immune system successfully fights off thousands of germs.

Antigens are parts of the germs that cause the body's immune system to go to work to build antibodies, which fight off diseases.

The antigens in vaccines come from the germs themselves, but the germs are weakened or killed so they cannot cause serious illness. Even if babies receive several vaccinations in one day, vaccines contain only a tiny fraction of the antigens they encounter every day in their environment. Vaccines give your child the antibodies they need to fight off serious vaccine-preventable diseases.

Why Are So Many Doses Needed for Each Vaccine?

Getting every recommended dose of each vaccine provides your child with the best protection possible. Depending on the vaccine, your child will need more than one dose to build high enough immunity to prevent disease or to boost immunity that fades over time. Your child may also receive more than one dose to make sure they are protected if they did not get immunity from a first dose, or to protect them against germs that change over time, such as flu. Every dose is important because each protects against infectious diseases that can be especially serious for infants and very young children.

Why Do Vaccines Start So Early?

The recommended schedule protects infants and children by providing immunity early in life, before they come into contact with life-threatening diseases. Children receive immunization early because they are susceptible to diseases at a young age. The consequences of these diseases can be very serious, even life-threatening, for infants and young children.

What about Delaying Some Vaccines or Following a Nonstandard Schedule?

Children do not receive any known benefits from following schedules that delay vaccines. Infants and young children who follow immunization schedules that spread out or leave out shots are at risk of developing diseases during the time you delay their shots. Some vaccine-preventable diseases remain common in the United States and children may be exposed to these diseases during the time they are not protected by vaccines, placing them at risk for a serious case of the disease that might cause hospitalization or death.

Have Not We Gotten Rid of Most of These Diseases in This Country?

Some vaccine-preventable diseases, such as pertussis (whooping cough) and chickenpox, remain common in the United States. On the other hand, other diseases that vaccines prevent are no longer common in this country because of vaccines. However, if we stopped vaccinating, the few cases we have in the United States could very quickly become tens or hundreds of thousands of cases. Even though many serious vaccine-preventable diseases are uncommon in the United States, some are common in other parts of the world. Even if your family does not travel internationally, you could come into contact with international travelers anywhere in your community. Children who do not receive all vaccinations and are exposed to a disease can become seriously sick and spread it through a community.

What Are Combination Vaccines? Why Are They Used?

Combination vaccines protect your child against more than one disease with a single shot. They reduce the number of shots and office visits your child needs, which not only saves you time and money, but also is easier on your child.

Some common combination vaccines are Pediarix®, which combines DTap, Hep B, and IPV (polio), and ProQuad®, which combines MMR and varicella (chickenpox).

Cannot I Just Wait until My Child Goes to School to Catch up on Immunizations?

Before entering school, young children can be exposed to vaccine-preventable diseases from parents and other adults, siblings, on a plane, at daycare, or even at the grocery store. Children under age five are especially susceptible to diseases because their immune systems have not built up the necessary defenses to fight infection. Do not wait to protect your children and risk their getting these diseases when they need protection now.

Why Does My Child Need a Chickenpox Shot? Is Not It a Mild Disease?

Your child needs a chickenpox vaccine because chickenpox can actually be a serious disease. In many cases, children experience a mild case of chickenpox, but other children may have blisters that become infected. Others may develop pneumonia. There is no way to tell in advance how severe your child's symptoms will be.

Before vaccine was available, about 50 children died every year from chickenpox, and about 1 in 500 children who got chickenpox was hospitalized.

My Child Is Sick Right Now. Is It Okay to Still Get Shots?

Talk with your child's doctor, but children can usually get vaccinated even if they have a mild illness such as a cold, earache, mild fever, or diarrhea. If the doctor says it is okay, your child can still get vaccinated.

What Are the Ingredients in Vaccines and What Do They Do?

Vaccines contain ingredients that cause the body to develop immunity. Vaccines also contain very small amounts of other ingredients. All ingredients play necessary roles either in making the vaccine or in ensuring that the final product is safe and effective.

Do Not Infants Have Natural Immunity? Is Not Natural Immunity Better Than the Kind from Vaccines?

Fetuses may get some temporary immunity (protection) from their mothers during the last few weeks of pregnancy, but only for diseases to which their mother is immune. Breastfeeding may also protect your baby temporarily from minor infections such as colds. These antibodies do not last long, leaving your baby vulnerable to disease.

Natural immunity occurs when your child is exposed to a disease and becomes infected. It is true that natural immunity usually results in better immunity than vaccination, but the risks are much greater. A natural chickenpox infection may result in pneumonia, whereas the vaccine might only cause a sore arm for a couple of days.

Cannot I Just Wait to Vaccinate If My Baby Is Not Exposed to Disease at Daycare?

No, even young children who are cared for at home can be exposed to vaccine-preventable diseases, so it is important for them to get all their vaccines at the recommended ages. Children can catch these illnesses from any number of people or places, including from parents, siblings, visitors to the home, on playgrounds, or even at the grocery store. Regardless of whether or not your baby is cared for outside the home, your child comes in contact with people throughout the day—some of whom may be sick but not know it yet.

Some people who have a vaccine-preventable disease may not have symptoms or the symptoms may be mild, and they can end up spreading disease to babies or young children. Remember, many of these diseases can be especially dangerous to young children, so it is safest to vaccinate your children at the recommended ages to protect them, whether or not they are in daycare.

Do I Have to Vaccinate My Baby on Schedule If I Am Breastfeeding?

Yes, even breastfed babies need to be protected with vaccines at the recommended ages. The immune system is not fully developed at birth, which puts newborns at greater risk for infections.

Breast milk provides important protection from some infections as your baby's immune system is developing. For example, babies who are breastfed have a lower risk of ear infections, respiratory-tract infections, and diarrhea. However, breast milk does not protect children against all diseases. Even in breastfed infants, vaccines are the most effective way to prevent many diseases. Babies needs the long-term protection that can only come from making sure that they receive all vaccines according to the CDC's recommended schedule.

What Is Wrong with Delaying Some of My Baby's Vaccines If I Am Planning to Get Them All Eventually?

Young children have the highest risk of having a serious case of disease that could cause hospitalization or death. Delaying or spreading out vaccine doses leaves your child unprotected during the time when they need vaccine protection the most. For example, diseases such as Hib or pneumococcus almost always occur in the first two years of a baby's life. And some diseases, such as hepatitis B and whooping cough (pertussis), are more serious when babies get them at a younger age. Vaccinating your child according to the CDC's recommended immunization schedule offers protection at a young age.

I Got the Whooping Cough and Flu Vaccines during My Pregnancy. Why Does My Baby Need These Vaccines Too?

The protection (antibodies) you passed to your fetus before birth will offer some early protection against whooping cough and flu. However, these antibodies will only give your baby short-term protection. It is very important for your baby to get vaccines on time and start building protection against these serious diseases.

Who Is Eligible for Free Vaccines?

The Vaccines for Children (VFC) program offers vaccines at no cost for eligible children through VFC-enrolled doctors. Find out if your child qualifies below and at www.cdc.gov/vaccines/programs/vfc/parents/qa-detailed.html. Vaccinating on time means healthier children, families, and communities.

Which Children Are Eligible?

Children through 18 years of age who meet at least one of the following criteria are eligible to receive VFC vaccines:

- **Medicaid eligible:** A child who is eligible for the Medicaid program (For the purposes of the VFC program, the terms "Medicaid-eligible" and "Medicaid-enrolled" are equivalent and refer to children who have health insurance covered by a state Medicaid program.)

- **Uninsured:** A child who has no health-insurance coverage

- **American Indian or Alaska Native:** A child who is defined as an American Indian or Alaska Native by the Indian Health Care Improvement Act (25 U.S.C. 1603)

Children whose health insurance covers the cost of vaccinations are not eligible for VFC vaccines, even when a claim for the cost of the vaccine and its administration would be denied for payment by the insurance carrier because the plan's deductible had not been met.

What Is a Federally Qualified Health Center?

A Federally Qualified Health Center (FQHC) is a health center that is designated by the Bureau of Primary Health Care (BPHC) of the Health Resources and Services Administration (HRSA) to provide healthcare to a medically underserved population. FQHCs include community and migrant health centers, special health facilities such as those for the homeless and persons with acquired immunodeficiency syndrome (AIDS) that receive grants under the Public Health Service (PHS) Act, and "lookalikes" that meet the qualifications but do not actually receive grant funds. They also include health centers within public housing and Indian health centers.

What Is an Rural Health Clinic?

An rural health clinic (RHC) is a clinic located in a Health Professional Shortage Area (HPSA), Medically Underserved Area (MUA), or a governor-designated shortage area. RHCs are required to be staffed by physician assistants, nurse practitioners, or certified nurse midwives at least half of the time that the clinic is open.

Where Can I Get Vaccines?

VFC vaccines can be administered by any enrolled VFC program provider (a private doctor, private clinic, hospitals, public health clinic, community health clinic, schools, etc.).

Most pediatricians (doctors who specialize in the treatment of children) in the United States and its territories are now VFC-enrolled providers. Additionally, many family-practice providers are enrolled, as well as general practitioners, and many other subspecialty healthcare providers. In some states, schools are enrolled. Altogether, there are over 44,000 providers enrolled in the VFC program nationwide.

Your state or territory health department is responsible for managing the VFC program where you reside. Each state or territory has a VFC program coordinator who is responsible for enrolling providers and monitoring the provider's participation in the program.

What Is the Cost?

If your child meets one of the VFC eligibility criteria listed above, the vaccine must always be provided free of charge.

"Free of charge" means just that. The vaccines have already been paid for with federal tax dollars. This means that no one can charge a fee for the vaccine itself.

However, each state immunization provider has been granted (by law) the ability to charge what is called an "administrative fee." An administrative fee is similar to a patient's health insurance copayment in that it helps providers offset their costs of doing business.

The amount of the administrative fee differs from state to state, based on a regional scale determined by the Centers for Medicare and Medicaid Services (CMS).

These regional administrative charges are maximum fees that providers may ask patients to pay. This means that if a state's administrative fee is $15.00, a provider may charge a patient any amount up to, but not exceeding, that $15.00 charge for each vaccine administered. There is no lower limit, so providers have the option to charge what they feel is fair, including no charge at all.

What Vaccines Are Provided? What Diseases Are Prevented?

Many single and combination vaccines licensed in the United States protect children against 16 preventable diseases. The vaccines available through the VFC are determined by the Advisory Committee on Immunization Practices (ACIP). The CDC, as the administrator of the VFC, purchases and distributes the vaccines. The VFC covers any vaccines included in the immunization schedules:

- Parent version of recommended immunizations for children from birth through 6 years old (www.cdc.gov/vaccines/parents/downloads/parent-ver-sch-0-6yrs.pdf)

- Parent version of recommended immunizations for children 7 through 18 years old (www.cdc.gov/vaccines/schedules/downloads/teen/parent-version-schedule-7-18yrs.pdf)

Diseases that are preventable by recommended childhood vaccines recommended by the ACIP include the following. Each disease is briefly described on the second page of the above-linked documents.

- Diphtheria

- Haemophilus influenzae type b (Hib)

- Hepatitis A

- Hepatitis B

- Human papillomavirus (HPV)

- Influenza (flu)

- Measles

- Meningococcal

- Mumps

- Pertussis

- Pneumococcal

- Polio

- Rotavirus

- Rubella

- Tetanus

- Varicella

Should I Believe Information I Read on the Web?

Before considering vaccine information found on the Internet, check that the information comes from a credible source and is updated on a regular basis.

The CDC's vaccines and immunization web content is researched, written, and approved by subject-matter experts, including physicians, researchers, epidemiologists, and analysts. Content is based on peer-reviewed science. CDC leadership makes the final decision on the words, images, and links to best serve the information needs of the public as well as healthcare providers, public-health professionals, partners, educators, and researchers. Science and public-health data are frequently updated. Most pages are reviewed yearly.

The CDC's National Center for Immunization and Respiratory Diseases (NCIRD) is a member of the World Health Organization's (WHO) Vaccine Safety Net and follows web content and credibility criteria defined by the Global Advisory Committee on Vaccine Safety (GACVS).

The CDC's vaccines safety site is one of the WHO's twenty English language—certified websites.

As you surf for vaccine information, consider guidance from these sources:

- The Immunization Action Coalition suggests questions you should ask.

- The National Network for Immunization Information (NNii) suggests questions to ask when evaluating information.

- The University of California San Francisco's Evaluating Health Information lists "red flags" every consumer needs to know.

- The Medical Library Association translates medical jargon ("medspeak") into language everyone can understand.

While it' is a useful tool for researching health-related issues, the Internet does not replace a discussion with a healthcare professional.

Why Immunize

Why do we immunize our children? Sometimes we are confused by the messages in the media. First we are assured that, thanks to vaccines, some diseases are almost gone from the United States. But we are also warned to immunize our children, ourselves as adults, and the elderly.

Diseases Are Becoming Rare Due to Vaccinations

It is true, some diseases (such as polio and diphtheria) are becoming very rare in the United States. Of course, they are becoming rare largely because we have been vaccinating against them. But it is still reasonable to ask whether it is really worthwhile to keep vaccinating.

It is much like bailing out a boat with a slow leak. When we started bailing, the boat was filled with water. But we have been bailing fast and hard, and now it is almost dry. We could say, "Good. The boat is dry now, so we can throw away the bucket and relax." But the leak has not stopped. Before long we would notice a little water seeping in, and soon it might be back up to the same level as when we started.

Keep Immunizing until Disease Is Eliminated

Unless we can "stop the leak" (eliminate the disease), it is important to keep immunizing. Even if there are only a few cases of disease today, if we take away the protection given by vaccinations, more and more people will become infected and will spread the disease to others. Soon we will undo the progress we have made over the years.

Japan Reduced Pertussis Vaccinations, and an Epidemic Occurred

In 1974, Japan had a successful pertussis (whooping cough) vaccination program, with nearly 80 percent of Japanese children vaccinated. That year only 393 cases of pertussis were reported in the entire country and there were no deaths from pertussis. But then rumors began to

463

spread that the pertussis vaccination was no longer needed and that the vaccine was not safe, and by 1976 only 10 percent of infants were getting vaccinated. In 1979 Japan suffered a major pertussis epidemic, with more than 13,000 cases of whooping cough and 41 deaths. In 1981 the government began vaccinating with the acellular pertussis vaccine and the number of pertussis cases dropped again.

What If We Stopped Vaccinating

So what would happen if we stopped vaccinating here? Diseases that are almost unknown would stage a comeback. Before long we would see epidemics of diseases that are nearly under control today. More children would get sick and more would die.

We Vaccinate to Protect Our Future

We do not vaccinate just to protect our children. We also vaccinate to protect our grandchildren and their grandchildren. With one disease, smallpox, we "stopped the leak" in the boat by eradicating the disease. Our children do not have to get smallpox shots anymore because the disease no longer exists. Smallpox is now only a memory, and if we keep vaccinating against other diseases, the same will someday be true for them too. Vaccinations are one of the best ways to put an end to the serious effects of certain diseases.

What about the Safety of Vaccines

The United States has the safest, most effective vaccine supply in its history. The vaccine safety system ensures that vaccines are as safe as possible.

Scientists ensure the safety of vaccines by conducting different types of studies:

- Clinical trials are studies conducted before a vaccine is made available. These studies are carried out by vaccine manufacturers and help the U.S. Food and Drug Administration (FDA) make decisions about whether a vaccine is safe, effective, and ready to be licensed for use.

- Postlicensure studies are conducted after a vaccine is approved by the FDA and made available to the public. These studies continue to monitor vaccine safety and often include groups that are often underrepresented in clinical trials. These studies can look for rare adverse events.

What Ingredients and Additives Are Found in Vaccines?

Chemicals commonly used in the production of vaccines include a suspending fluid (sterile water, saline, or fluids containing protein); preservatives and stabilizers (for example, albumin, phenols, and glycine); and adjuvants or enhancers that help improve the vaccine's effectiveness. Vaccines also may contain very small amounts of the culture material used to grow the virus or bacteria used in the vaccine, such as chicken-egg protein.

What You Should Know

- Millions of doses of vaccines are administered to children in this country each year. Ensuring that those vaccines are potent, sterile, and safe requires the addition of minute amounts of chemical additives.

- Chemicals are added to vaccines to inactivate a virus or bacteria and stabilize the vaccine, helping to preserve the vaccine and prevent it from losing its potency over time.

- The amount of chemical additives found in vaccines is very small.

- All routinely recommended pediatric vaccines manufactured for the U.S. market are available in formulations that contain no thimerosal or only trace amounts.

How Do Vaccines Prevent Disease?

It is always better to prevent a disease than to treat it after it occurs.

Diseases that used to be common in this country and around the world—including polio, measles, diphtheria, pertussis (whooping cough), rubella (German measles), mumps, tetanus, rotavirus, and Haemophilus influenzae type b (Hib)—can now be prevented by vaccination. Thanks to a vaccine, one of the most terrible diseases in history—smallpox—no longer exists outside the laboratory. Over the years vaccines have prevented countless cases of disease and saved millions of lives.

Immunity Protects Us from Disease

Immunity is the body's way of preventing disease. Children are born with an immune system composed of cells, glands, organs, and fluids located throughout the body. The immune system recognizes germs that enter the body as "foreign invaders" (called "antigens") and produces proteins called "antibodies" to fight them.

The first time a child is infected with a specific antigen (say, the measles virus), the immune system produces antibodies designed to fight it. This takes time. Usually, the immune system can't work fast enough to prevent the antigen from causing disease, so the child still gets sick. However, the immune system "remembers" that antigen. If it ever enters the body again, even after many years, the immune system can produce antibodies fast enough to keep it from causing disease a second time. This protection is called "immunity."

It would be nice if there were a way to give children immunity to a disease without their having to get sick first.

Vaccines contain the same antigens (or parts of antigens) that cause diseases. For example, the measles vaccine contains the measles virus. But the antigens in the vaccines are either killed or weakened to the point that they do not cause disease. However, they are strong enough to make the immune system produce antibodies that lead to immunity. In other words, a vaccine is a safer substitute for a child's first exposure to a disease. The child gets protection without having to get sick. Through vaccination, children can develop immunity without suffering from the actual diseases that vaccines prevent.

Section 37.4

Types of Vaccines and Vaccine Strategies

This section includes text excerpted from "Vaccine Types," National Institute of Allergy and Infectious Diseases (NIAID), April 3, 2012. Reviewed May 2019.

Scientists take many approaches to design vaccines against a microbe. These choices are typically based on fundamental information about the microbe, such as how it infects cells and how the immune system responds to it, as well as practical considerations, such as regions of the world where the vaccine would be used. The following are some of the options that researchers might pursue:

- Live, attenuated vaccines

- Inactivated vaccines

- Subunit vaccines

- Toxoid vaccines

- Conjugate vaccines

- DNA vaccines

- Recombinant vector vaccines

Live, Attenuated Vaccines

Live, attenuated vaccines contain a version of the living microbe that has been weakened in the lab so it can't cause disease. Because a live, attenuated vaccine is the closest thing to a natural infection, these vaccines are good "teachers" of the immune system: They elicit strong cellular and antibody responses and often confer lifelong immunity with only one or two doses.

Despite the advantages of live, attenuated vaccines, there are some downsides. It is the nature of living things to change, or mutate, and the organisms used in live, attenuated vaccines are no different. The remote possibility exists that an attenuated microbe in the vaccine could revert to a virulent form and cause disease. Also, not everyone can safely receive live, attenuated vaccines. For their own protection, people who have damaged or weakened immune systems—because they've undergone chemotherapy or have HIV, for example—cannot be given live vaccines.

Another limitation is that live, attenuated vaccines usually need to be refrigerated to stay potent. If the vaccine needs to be shipped overseas and stored by healthcare workers in developing countries that lack widespread refrigeration, a live vaccine may not be the best choice.

Live, attenuated vaccines are relatively easy to create for certain viruses. Vaccines against measles, mumps, and chickenpox, for example, are made by this method. Viruses are simple microbes containing a small number of genes, and scientists can, therefore, more readily control their characteristics. Viruses often are attenuated through a method of growing generations of them in cells in which they do not reproduce very well. This hostile environment takes the fight out of viruses: As they evolve to adapt to the new environment, they become weaker with respect to their natural host, human beings.

467

Live, attenuated vaccines are more difficult to create for bacteria. Bacteria have thousands of genes and thus are much harder to control. Scientists working on a live vaccine for a bacterium, however, might be able to use recombinant DNA technology to remove several key genes. This approach has been used to create a vaccine against the bacterium that causes cholera, *Vibrio cholerae*, although the live cholera vaccine has not been licensed in the United States.

Inactivated Vaccines

Scientists produce inactivated vaccines by killing the disease-causing microbe with chemicals, heat, or radiation. Such vaccines are more stable and safer than live vaccines: The dead microbes can't mutate back to their disease-causing state. Inactivated vaccines usually do not require refrigeration, and they can be easily stored and transported in a freeze-dried form, which makes them accessible to people in developing countries.

Most inactivated vaccines, however, stimulate a weaker immune system response than do live vaccines. So it would likely take several additional doses, or booster shots, to maintain a person's immunity. This could be a drawback in areas where people do not have regular access to healthcare and cannot get booster shots on time.

Subunit Vaccines

Instead of the entire microbe, subunit vaccines include only the antigens that best stimulate the immune system. In some cases, these vaccines use epitopes—the very specific parts of the antigen that antibodies or T cells recognize and bind to. Because subunit vaccines contain only the essential antigens and not all the other molecules that make up the microbe, the chances of adverse reactions to the vaccine are lower.

Subunit vaccines can contain anywhere from 1 to 20 or more antigens. Of course, identifying which antigens best stimulate the immune system is a tricky and time-consuming process. Once scientists do that, however, they can make subunit vaccines in one of two ways:

- They can grow the microbe in the laboratory and then use chemicals to break it apart and gather the important antigens.

- They can manufacture the antigen molecules from the microbe using recombinant DNA technology. Vaccines produced this way are called "recombinant subunit vaccines."

A recombinant subunit vaccine has been made for the hepatitis B virus. Scientists inserted hepatitis B genes that code for important antigens into common baker's yeast. The yeast then produced the antigens, which the scientists collected and purified for use in the vaccine. Research is continuing on a recombinant subunit vaccine against hepatitis C virus.

Toxoid Vaccines

For bacteria that secrete toxins, or harmful chemicals, a toxoid vaccine might be the answer. These vaccines are used when a bacterial toxin is the main cause of illness. Scientists have found that they can inactivate toxins by treating them with formalin, a solution of formaldehyde and sterilized water. Such "detoxified" toxins, called "toxoids," are safe for use in vaccines.

When the immune system receives a vaccine containing a harmless toxoid, it learns how to fight off the natural toxin. The immune system produces antibodies that lock onto and block the toxin. Vaccines against diphtheria and tetanus are examples of toxoid vaccines.

Conjugate Vaccines

If a bacterium possesses an outer coating of sugar molecules called "polysaccharides," as many harmful bacteria do, researchers may try making a conjugate vaccine for it. Polysaccharide coatings disguise a bacterium's antigens so that the immature immune systems of infants and younger children cannot recognize or respond to them. Conjugate vaccines, a special type of subunit vaccine, get around this problem.

When making a conjugate vaccine, scientists link antigens or toxoids from a microbe that an infant's immune system can recognize to the polysaccharides. The linkage helps the immature immune system react to polysaccharide coatings and defend against the disease-causing bacterium.

The vaccine that protects against Haemophilus influenzae type B (Hib) is a conjugate vaccine.

Deoxyribonucleic Acid Vaccines

Once the genes from a microbe have been analyzed, scientists could attempt to create a DNA vaccine against it.

Still in the experimental stages, these vaccines show great promise, and several types are being tested in humans. DNA vaccines take immunization to a new technological level. These vaccines dispense with both the whole organism and its parts and get right down to the essentials: The microbe's genetic material. In particular, DNA vaccines use the genes that code for those all-important antigens.

Researchers have found that when the genes for a microbe's antigens are introduced into the body, some cells will take up that DNA. The DNA then instructs those cells to make the antigen molecules. The cells secrete the antigens and display them on their surfaces. In other words, the body's own cells become vaccine-making factories, creating the antigens necessary to stimulate the immune system.

A DNA vaccine against a microbe would evoke a strong antibody response to the free-floating antigen secreted by cells, and the vaccine also would stimulate a strong cellular response against the microbial antigens displayed on cell surfaces. The DNA vaccine could not cause the disease because it would not contain the microbe, just copies of a few of its genes. In addition, DNA vaccines are relatively easy and inexpensive to design and produce.

So-called naked DNA vaccines consist of DNA that is administered directly into the body. These vaccines can be administered with a needle and syringe or with a needleless device that uses high-pressure gas to shoot microscopic gold particles coated with DNA directly into cells. Sometimes, the DNA is mixed with molecules that facilitate its uptake by the body's cells. Naked DNA vaccines being tested in humans include those against the viruses that cause influenza and herpes.

Recombinant Vector Vaccines

Recombinant vector vaccines are experimental vaccines similar to DNA vaccines, but they use an attenuated virus or bacterium to introduce microbial DNA to cells of the body. "Vector" refers to the virus or bacterium used as the carrier.

In nature, viruses latch on to cells and inject their genetic material into them. In the lab, scientists have taken advantage of this process. They have figured out how to take the roomy genomes of certain harmless or attenuated viruses and insert portions of the genetic material from other microbes into them. The carrier viruses then ferry that microbial DNA to cells. Recombinant vector vaccines closely mimic a natural infection, and therefore, do a good job of stimulating the immune system.

Attenuated bacteria also can be used as vectors. In this case, the inserted genetic material causes the bacteria to display the antigens of other microbes on its surface. In effect, the harmless bacterium mimics a harmful microbe, provoking an immune response.

Researchers are working on both bacterial and viral-based recombinant vector vaccines for HIV, rabies, and measles.

Section 37.5

Recommended Vaccines by Age

This section includes text excerpted from "Recommended Vaccines by Age," Centers for Disease Control and Prevention (CDC), November 22, 2016.

Vaccination is one of the best ways parents can protect infants, children, and teens from 16 potentially harmful diseases that can be very serious, may require hospitalization, or even be deadly.

And immunizations are not just for children. Protection from some childhood vaccines can wear off over time. Adults may also be at risk for vaccine-preventable disease due to age, job, lifestyle, travel, or health conditions.

Review the sections below to learn what other vaccines you and your family may need. Check with your family's healthcare professionals to make sure everyone is up to date on recommended vaccines.

Birth

Before leaving the hospital or birthing center, your baby receives the first of three doses of the vaccine that protects against hepatitis B. Hepatitis B virus can cause chronic swelling of the liver and possible lifelong complications. It is important to protect infants and young children from hepatitis B because they are more likely than adults to develop incurable chronic (long-term) infection that can result in liver damage and liver cancer.

1 to 2 Months

Protect your baby by providing immunity early in life. Starting at one to two months of age, your baby receives the following vaccines to develop immunity from potentially harmful diseases:

- Hepatitis B (second dose)
- Diphtheria, tetanus, and whooping cough (pertussis) (DTaP)
- Haemophilus influenzae type b (Hib)
- Polio (IPV)
- Pneumococcal (PCV)
- Rotavirus (RV)

4 Months

Protect your baby by providing immunity early in life. Stay on track with the recommended vaccine schedule. At four months of age, your baby receives the following vaccines to develop immunity from potentially harmful diseases:

- Diphtheria, tetanus, and whooping cough (pertussis) (DTaP)
- Haemophilus influenzae type b (Hib)
- Polio (IPV)
- Pneumococcal (PCV)
- Rotavirus (RV)
- Hepatitis B (HepB)

6 Months

Protect your baby by providing immunity early in life. Stay on track with the recommended vaccine schedule. At six months of age, your baby receives the following vaccines to develop immunity from potentially harmful diseases:

- Diphtheria, tetanus, and whooping cough (pertussis) (DTaP)
- Haemophilus influenzae type b (Hib)
- Polio (IPV)

- Pneumococcal (PCV)

- Rotavirus (RV)

- Influenza (flu)

7 to 11 Months

There are usually no vaccinations scheduled between 7 and 11 months of age. However, if your baby has missed an earlier vaccination, now is a good time to "catch up."

Babies 6 months and older should receive a flu vaccination every flu season.

1 to 2 Years

By following the recommended schedule and fully immunizing your child by two years of age, your child should be protected against 14 vaccine-preventable diseases. Between one to two years of age, your child receives the following vaccines to continue developing immunity from potentially harmful diseases:

- Chickenpox (Varicella)

- Diphtheria, tetanus, and whooping cough (pertussis) (DTaP)

- Haemophilus influenzae type b (Hib)

- Measles, mumps, rubella (MMR)

- Polio (IPV) (between 6 through 18 months)

- Pneumococcal (PCV)

- Hepatitis A (HepA)

- Hepatitis B (HepB)

Additionally, children should receive a flu vaccination every flu season.

2 to 3 Years

Between two and three years of age, your child should visit the doctor once a year for checkups.

Additionally, children should receive a flu vaccination every flu season.

4 to 6 Years

Between four through six years of age, your child should visit the doctor once a year for checkups. During this time, your child receives the following vaccines:

- Diphtheria, tetanus, and whooping cough (pertussis) (DTaP)
- Polio (IPV)
- Measles, mumps, and rubella (MMR)
- Chickenpox (varicella)
- Influenza (flu) every year

7 to 10 Years

Between 7 and 10 years of age, your child should visit the doctor once a year for checkups.

Additionally, children should receive a flu vaccination every flu season.

11 to 12 Years

There are four vaccines recommended for preteens—these vaccines help protect your children, their friends, and their family members.

- Meningococcal conjugate vaccine
- HPV vaccine
- Tdap
- Flu vaccine every flu season

13 to 18 Years

Between 13 through 18 years old, your child should visit the doctor once each year for checkups. This can be a great time to get any vaccines your teen may have missed or may need if traveling outside the United States.

Additional, everyone six months and older should receive a flu vaccination every flu season.

19 to 26 Years

In addition to a seasonal flu (influenza) vaccine and Td or Tdap vaccine (tetanus, diphtheria, and pertussis), you should also get an

HPV vaccine, which protects against the human papillomaviruses that causes most cervical cancers, anal cancer, and genital warts. It is recommended for women up to age 26 years, men up to age 21 years, and men ages 22 to 26 who have sex with men.

Some vaccines may be recommended for adults because of particular job- or school-related requirements, health conditions, lifestyle, or other factors. Some states require students entering colleges and universities to be vaccinated against certain diseases such as meningitis due to increased risk among college students living in residential housing.

27 to 60 Years

All adults need a seasonal flu (influenza) vaccine every year. A flu vaccine is especially important for people with chronic health conditions, pregnant women, and older adults.

Every adult should get the Tdap vaccine once if they did not receive it as an adolescent to protect against pertussis (whooping cough), and then a Td (tetanus, diphtheria) booster shot every 10 years. In addition, women should get the Tdap vaccine each time they are pregnant, preferably at 27 through 36 weeks.

Healthy adults aged 50 years and older should get a zoster vaccine to prevent shingles and the complications from the disease.

Some vaccines may be recommended for adults because of particular job- or school-related requirements, health conditions, lifestyle, or other factors.

60 Years or Older

In addition to a seasonal flu (influenza) vaccine and Td or Tdap vaccine (tetanus, diphtheria, and pertussis), people 65 years and older should also get:

- Pneumococcal vaccines, which protect against pneumococcal disease, including infections in the lungs and bloodstream (recommended for all adults over 65 years old, and for adults younger than 65 years who have certain chronic-health conditions)

- Zoster vaccine, which protects against shingles (recommended for adults 50 years or older)

Section 37.6

Potential Problems with Vaccinations

This section contains text excerpted from the following
sources: Text under the heading "Adverse Event" is excerpted from
"Adverse Event," Centers for Disease Control and Prevention (CDC),
August 28, 2015. Reviewed May 2019; Text under the heading
"Vaccine Side Effects" is excerpted from "Vaccine Side Effects,"
Vaccines.gov, U.S. Department of Health and Human
Services (HHS), December 2017.

Adverse Event

An "adverse event" is any health problem that happens after receiving a shot or other vaccine. An adverse event might be truly caused by a vaccine, or it might be pure coincidence.

Types of adverse events include:

- True reactions to the vaccine

These include both common, known side effects and serious reactions, such as allergic reactions.
Side effect caused by a vaccine.

- A side effect is any health problem shown by studies to be caused by a vaccine. As with any medication, vaccines can cause side effects. Usually, vaccine side effects are minor (for example, a sore arm where a shot was given or a low-grade fever after a vaccine) and go away on their own within a few days.

- Unrelated health problems

These are experiences that would have occurred even if the person had not been vaccinated. They happen after vaccination but are not caused by the vaccine.

- Health problems that cannot be related directly to the vaccine

The cause of these events is unknown, and there is not enough evidence to say whether they are caused by a vaccine.

One of the main jobs of the CDC's Immunization Safety Office is doing research to find out if adverse events that are reported by doctors, vaccine manufacturers, and the public are truly caused by a vaccine.

Vaccine Side Effects

Most people do not have any serious side effects from vaccines. The most common side effects—like soreness where the shot was given—are usually mild and go away quickly on their own.

What Are Common Side Effects of Vaccines?

The most common side effects after vaccination are mild. They include:

- Pain, swelling, or redness where the shot was given
- Mild fever
- Chills
- Feeling tired
- Headache
- Muscle and joint aches

Most common side effects are a sign that your body is starting to build immunity (protection) against a disease.

What about Serious Side Effects

Serious side effects from vaccines are extremely rare. For example, if one million doses of a vaccine are given, one to two people may have a severe allergic reaction.

Keep in mind that getting vaccinated is much safer than getting the diseases vaccines prevent.

What If I Feel Sick after Getting Vaccinated

Talk with your doctor if you are concerned about your health after getting vaccinated. You or your doctor can choose to report the side effect to the Vaccine Adverse Event Reporting System (VAERS).

In the very rare event that a vaccine causes a serious problem, the National Vaccine Injury Compensation Program (VICP) may offer financial help to individuals who file a petition.

Section 37.7

Vaccine Adverse Event Reporting Systems

This section includes text excerpted from "Vaccine Adverse Event
Reporting System (VAERS)," Centers for Disease Control and
Prevention (CDC), August 28, 2015. Reviewed May 2019.

The Vaccine Adverse Event Reporting System (VAERS) is a national
vaccine safety surveillance program run by the Centers for Disease
Control and Prevention (CDC) and the U.S. Food and Drug Administration (FDA). VAERS serves as an early warning system to detect
possible safety issues with U.S. vaccines by collecting information
about adverse events (possible side effects or health problems) that
occur after vaccination.

VAERS was created in 1990 in response to the National Childhood Vaccine Injury Act (NCVIA). If any health problem happens
after vaccination, anyone—doctors, nurses, vaccine manufacturers, and any member of the general public—can submit a report to
VAERS.

How the Vaccine Adverse Event Reporting System Is Used

VAERS is used to detect possible safety problems—called "signals"—that may be related to vaccination. If a vaccine safety signal is
identified through VAERS, scientists may conduct further studies to
find out if the signal represents an actual risk.

The main goals of VAERS are to:

- Detect new, unusual, or rare adverse events that happen after
  vaccination

- Monitor increases in known side effects, such as arm soreness
  where a shot was given

- Identify potential patient risk factors for particular types of
  health problems related to vaccines

- Assess the safety of newly licensed vaccines

- Watch for unexpected or unusual patterns in adverse event
  reports

- Serve as a monitoring system in public-health emergencies

How to Report Adverse Events to the Vaccine Adverse Event Reporting System

There are two ways to submit a report to VAERS:

- Report online
- Complete a VAERS form online at: vaers.hhs.gov/External

What to Report to the Vaccine Adverse Event Reporting System

Anyone who gives or receives a licensed vaccine in the United States is encouraged to report any significant health problem that occurs after vaccination. An adverse event can be reported even if it is uncertain or unlikely that the vaccine caused it. Reporting to VAERS helps scientists at the CDC and FDA better understand the safety of vaccines.

The Reportable Events Table (RET) lists conditions that are believed to be caused by vaccines. It is used by the National Vaccine Injury Compensation Program, which is operated by the United States. Health Resources and Services Administration (HRSA). Healthcare providers are required by law to report any conditions on the RET to VAERS and are strongly encouraged to report clinically significant or unexpected events following vaccination.

What Happens after a Vaccine Adverse Event Reporting System Report is Submitted

Each VAERS report is assigned a VAERS identification number. This number can be used to provide additional information to VAERS if necessary. The CDC or FDA scientists follow up on selected cases of serious adverse events immediately by obtaining medical records to better understand the event. Then, letters are sent one year after vaccination to check the recovery status of the patient for all serious reports that listed recovery status as "not recovered" on the initial report.

The Vaccine Injury Compensation Program (VICP), administered by HRSA, compensates people whose injuries may have been caused by certain vaccines. The VICP is separate from VAERS, and reporting an event to VAERS does not file a claim for compensation to the VICP.

479

What We Can Learn from Vaccine Adverse Event Reporting System Data

Approximately 30,000 VAERS reports are filed each year. About 85 to 90 percent of the reports describe mild side effects such as fever, arm soreness, and crying or mild irritability. The remaining reports are classified as serious, which means that the adverse event resulted in permanent disability, hospitalization, life-threatening illness, or death. While these problems happen after vaccination, they are rarely caused by the vaccine.

The VAERS form collects information about:

- The type of vaccine received

- The timing of the vaccination

- The onset of the adverse event

- Current illnesses or medication

- Past history of adverse events following vaccination

- Demographic information

The FDA and CDC use VAERS data to monitor vaccine safety and conduct research studies.

Strengths and Limitations of Vaccine Adverse Event Reporting System Data

When evaluating VAERS data, it is important to understand the strengths and limitations. VAERS data contain both coincidental events and those truly caused by vaccines.

Table 37.1. Strengths and Limitations of Vaccine Adverse Event Reporting System

Strengths	Limitations
VAERS collects national data from all U.S. states and territories.	It is generally not possible to find out from VAERS data if a vaccine caused the adverse event.
VAERS accepts reports from anyone.	Reports submitted to VAERS often lack details and sometimes contain errors.
The VAERS form collects information about the vaccine, the person vaccinated, and the adverse event.	Serious adverse events are more likely to be reported than mild side effects.

Table 37.1. Continued

Strengths	Limitations
Data are publicly available.	Rate of reports may increase in response to media attention and increased public awareness.
VAERS can be used as an early warning system to identify rare adverse events.	It is not possible to use VAERS data to calculate how often an adverse event occurs in a population.
It is possible to follow-up with patients to obtain health records, when necessary.	

Section 37.8

Vaccine Records

This section includes text excerpted from "Keeping
Your Vaccine Records Up to Date," Centers for Disease
Control and Prevention (CDC), May 2, 2016.

Your vaccination record (sometimes called your "immunization record") provides a history of all the vaccines you received as a child and adult. This record may be required for certain jobs, travel abroad, or school registration.

How to Locate Your Vaccination Records

Unfortunately, there is no national organization that maintains vaccination records. The CDC does not have this information. The records that exist are the ones you or your parents were given when the vaccines were administered and the ones in the medical record of the doctor or clinic or health department where the vaccines were given.

If you need official copies of vaccination records, or if you need to update your personal records, there are several places you can look:

- Ask your parents or other caregivers if they have records of your childhood immunizations.

- Try looking through baby books or other saved documents from your childhood.

- Check with your high school and/or college health services for dates of any immunizations. Keep in mind that generally records are kept only for one to two years after students leave the system.

- Check with previous employers (including the military) that may have required immunizations.

- Check with your doctor or public-health clinic. Keep in mind that vaccination records are maintained at doctor's office for a limited number of years.

- Contact your state's health department. Some states have registries (Immunization Information Systems) that include adult vaccines.

What to Do If You Cannot Find Your Records

If you cannot find your personal records or records from the doctor, you may need to get some of the vaccines again. While this is not ideal, it is safe to repeat vaccines. The doctor can also sometimes do blood tests to see if you are immune to certain vaccine-preventable diseases.

Tools to Record Your Vaccinations

Today we move, travel, and change healthcare providers more than we did in previous generations. Finding old immunization information can be difficult and time consuming. Therefore, it is critical that you keep an accurate and up-to-date record of the vaccinations you have received. Keeping an immunization record and storing it with other important documents (or in a safe place) will save you time and unnecessary hassle.

Ask your doctor, pharmacist, or other vaccine providers for an immunization record form or download and use this form (www.immunize.org/catg.d/p2023.pdf). Bring this record with you to health visits, and ask your vaccine provider to sign and date the form for each vaccine you receive. That way, you can be sure that the immunization information is current and correct.

If your vaccine provider participates in an immunization registry, ask that your vaccines be documented there as well.

Chapter 38

Healthcare-Associated Infections

Chapter Contents

Section 38.1

Understanding
Healthcare-Associated Infections

This section includes text excerpted from
"Healthcare-Associated Infections," Office of Disease
Prevention and Health Promotion (ODPHP), U.S. Department of
Health and Human Services (HHS), May 7, 2019.

Healthcare-associated infections (HAIs) are infections people get while they are receiving healthcare for another condition. HAIs can happen in any healthcare facility, including hospitals, ambulatory surgical centers, end-stage renal disease facilities, and long-term care facilities. HAIs can be caused by bacteria, fungi, viruses, or other, less common pathogens.

HAIs are a significant cause of illness and death—and they can have devastating emotional, financial, and medical consequences. At any given time, about 1 in 25 inpatients have an infection related to hospital care. These infections lead to the loss of tens of thousands of lives and cost the U.S. healthcare system billions of dollars each year.

These factors raise the risk of HAIs:

- Catheters (bloodstream, endotracheal, and urinary)

- Surgery

- Injections

- Healthcare settings that are not properly cleaned and disinfected

- Communicable diseases passing between patients and healthcare workers

- Overuse or improper use of antibiotics

Common HAIs patients get in hospitals include:

- Central-line associated bloodstream infections (CLABSI)

- *Clostridium difficile* infections

- Pneumonia

- Methicillin-resistant *Staphylococcus aureus* (MRSA) infections

- Surgical site infections (SSI)

- Urinary tract infections (UTI)

484

Catheter-associated urinary tract infections (CAUTI) are some of the most common HAIs.

Healthcare-Associated Infections and Antibiotic Resistance

As healthcare quality activities progress, it is important to recognize how HAIs, antibiotic use, and antibiotic resistance are related. Prevention of HAIs leads to fewer illnesses requiring antibiotic treatment—and proper use of antibiotics slows the development and spread of antibiotic-resistant organisms that can be difficult to treat.

Since the 1940s, antibiotics have greatly reduced illness and death—but using them also creates selective pressure that can lead to resistance. Widespread and indiscriminate use of antibiotics has accelerated the development of antibiotic-resistant organisms, making many antibiotics less effective.

Using antibiotics judiciously is essential if we are to slow the development of resistance and extend the useful lifetime of our most urgently needed antibiotics.

Antibiotic Stewardship

Antibiotic stewardship is among the most effective approaches to improving antibiotic use. Antibiotic stewardship can:

- Optimize clinical outcomes
- Minimize unintended consequences
- Improve patient safety
- Improve cost effectiveness
- Reduce inappropriate antibiotic use

Antibiotic stewardship is important across the spectrum of healthcare.

Section 38.2

Diseases and Organisms in Healthcare Settings

This section includes text excerpted from
"Healthcare-Associated Infections," Centers for
Disease Control and Prevention (CDC), January 2, 2019.

Acinetobacter

Acinetobacter is a group of bacteria commonly found in soil and water. Outbreaks of *Acinetobacter* infections typically occur in intensive care units and healthcare settings housing very ill patients. While there are many types or "species" of *Acinetobacter* and all can cause human disease, *Acinetobacter baumannii* accounts for about 80 percent of reported infections. *Acinetobacter* infections rarely occur outside of healthcare settings.

Burkholderia cepacia

Burkholderia cepacia (also called "*B. cepacia*") is the name for a group or "complex" of bacteria that can be found in soil and water. *Burkholderia cepacia* bacteria are often resistant to common antibiotics. *Burkholderia cepacia* poses little medical risk to healthy people; however, it is a known cause of infections in hospitalized patients. People with certain health conditions, such as weakened immune systems or chronic lung diseases (particularly cystic fibrosis), may be more susceptible to infections with *Burkholderia cepacia*.

Candida auris

Healthcare facilities in several countries have reported that a type of yeast called "*Candida auris*" has been causing severe illness in hospitalized patients. In some patients, this yeast can enter the bloodstream and spread throughout the body, causing serious invasive infections. This yeast often does not respond to commonly used antifungal drugs, making infections difficult to treat. Patients who have been hospitalized in a healthcare facility a long time, have a central venous catheter or other lines or tubes entering their body, or have previously received antibiotics or antifungal medications appear to be at highest risk of infection with this yeast.

Clostridioides difficile

Clostridioides difficile (formerly known as *"Clostridium difficile"* and often called *"C. difficile"* or *"C. diff"*) is a bacterium (germ) that causes diarrhea and an inflammation of the colon called "colitis."

Diarrhea and fever are the most common symptoms of *C. diff* infection. Overuse of antibiotics is the most important risk for getting *C. diff*.

Clostridium sordellii

Clostridium sordellii is a rare bacterium that causes pneumonia, endocarditis, arthritis, peritonitis, and myonecrosis. *Clostridium sordellii* bacteremia (when bacteria is present in the bloodstream) and sepsis (when bacteremia or another infection triggers a serious body-wide response) occur rarely. Most cases of sepsis from *Clostridium sordellii* occur in patients with other health conditions. Severe toxic shock syndrome among previously healthy persons has been described in a small number of *Clostridium sordellii* cases, most often associated with gynecologic infections in women and infection of the umbilical stump in newborns.

Enterobacteriaceae (Carbapenem Resistance)

Carbapenem-resistant Enterobacteriaceae (CRE) are a family of germs that are difficult to treat because they have high levels of resistance to antibiotics. Klebsiella species and *Escherichia coli* (*E. coli*) are examples of Enterobacteriaceae, a normal part of the human gut bacteria, that can become carbapenem resistant.

In healthcare settings, CRE infections most commonly occur among patients who are receiving treatment for other conditions. Patients whose care requires devices such as ventilators (breathing machines), urinary (bladder) catheters, or intravenous (vein) catheters, and patients who are taking long courses of certain antibiotics are most at risk for CRE infections.

Gram-Negative Bacteria

Gram-negative bacteria cause infections such as pneumonia, bloodstream infections, wound or surgical site infections, and meningitis in healthcare settings. Gram-negative bacteria are resistant to multiple drugs and are increasingly resistant to most available antibiotics. Gram-negative infections include those caused by *Klebsiella, Acineto-bacter, Pseudomonas aeruginosa,* and *E. coli,* as well as many other less common bacteria.

Hepatitis

The word "hepatitis" means inflammation of the liver and also refers to a group of viral infections that affect the liver. The most common types are hepatitis A, hepatitis B, and hepatitis C.

The delivery of healthcare has the potential to transmit hepatitis to both healthcare workers and patients. Outbreaks have occurred in outpatient settings, hemodialysis units, long-term care facilities, and hospitals, primarily as a result of unsafe injection practices; reuse of needles, fingerstick devices and syringes, and other lapses in infection control.

Human Immunodeficiency Virus

Human immunodeficiency virus (HIV) is the virus that can lead to acquired immune deficiency syndrome (AIDS). HIV destroys blood cells called CD4+ T cells, which are crucial to helping the body fight disease. This results in a weakened immune system, making persons with HIV or AIDS at risk for many different types of infections. Transmission of HIV to patients in healthcare settings is rare. Most exposures do not result in infection.

Influenza

Influenza is an infection that is transmitted in households and community settings. Each year, 5 to 20 percent of U.S. residents acquire an influenza virus infection, and many will seek medical care in ambulatory healthcare settings (e.g., pediatricians' offices, urgent-care clinics). In addition, more than 200,000 persons, on average, are hospitalized each year for influenza (flu).

Healthcare-associated influenza infections can occur in any healthcare setting and are most common when influenza is also circulating in the community. Therefore, influenza prevention measures should be implemented in all healthcare settings. Supplemental measures may need to be implemented during influenza season if outbreaks of healthcare-associated influenza occur within certain facilities, such as long-term care facilities and hospitals.

Klebsiella

Klebsiella is a type of Gram-negative bacteria that can cause health-care-associated infections including pneumonia, bloodstream infections, wound or surgical site infections, and meningitis. Increasingly, *Klebsiella* bacteria have developed antimicrobial resistance, most recently to the class of antibiotics known as "carbapenems." *Klebsiella* bacteria are normally found in the human intestines (where they do not cause disease). They are also found in human stool (feces). In healthcare settings, *Klebsiella* infections commonly occur among sick patients who are receiving treatment for other conditions. Patients who have devices such as ventilators (breathing machines) or intravenous (vein) catheters, and patients who are taking long courses of certain antibiotics are most at risk for *Klebsiella* infections. Healthy people usually do not get *Klebsiella* infections.

Methicillin-Resistant Staphylococcus aureus

Methicillin-resistant *Staphylococcus aureus* (MRSA) is a type of staph bacteria that is resistant to certain antibiotics called beta-lactams. These antibiotics include methicillin and other more common antibiotics such as oxacillin, penicillin, and amoxicillin. In the community, most MRSA infections are skin infections. More severe or potentially life-threatening MRSA infections occur most frequently among patients in healthcare settings.

Mycobacterium abscessus

Mycobacterium abscessus is a bacterium distantly related to the ones that cause tuberculosis and leprosy. It is found in water, soil, and dust. It has been known to contaminate medications and products, including medical devices. Healthcare-associated *Mycobacterium abscessus* can cause a variety of infections that require medical attention. Infections due to this bacterium are usually of the skin and the soft tissues under the skin. It can also cause lung infections in persons with various chronic lung diseases.

Norovirus

Noroviruses are a group of viruses that cause gastroenteritis in people. Gastroenteritis is an inflammation of the lining of the stomach and intestines, causing an acute onset of severe vomiting and diarrhea. Norovirus illness is usually brief in people who are otherwise healthy.

489

Young children, the elderly, and people with other medical illnesses are most at risk for more severe or prolonged infection. Like all viral infections, noroviruses are not affected by treatment with antibiotics.

Pseudomonas aeruginosa

Pseudomonas infection is caused by strains of bacteria found widely in the environment; the most common type causing infections in humans is called *"Pseudomonas aeruginosa."* Serious *Pseudomonas* infections usually occur in people in the hospital and/or with weakened immune systems.

Staphylococcus aureus

Staphylococcus aureus (staph), is a bacterium commonly found on the skin and in the nose of about 30 percent of individuals. Most of the time, staph does not cause any harm. These infections can look like pimples, boils, or other skin conditions and most are able to be treated.

Tuberculosis

Tuberculosis (TB) is caused by a bacterium called "Mycobacterium tuberculosis." Transmission of Mycobacterium tuberculosis is a recognized risk to patients and healthcare personnel in healthcare facilities. Transmission is most likely to occur from patients who have unrecognized pulmonary tuberculosis or tuberculosis related to their larynx, are not on effective antituberculosis therapy, and have not been placed in tuberculosis isolation. Transmission of *Mycobacterium* tuberculosis in healthcare settings has been associated with close contact with persons who have infectious tuberculosis, particularly during the performance of cough-inducing procedures such as bronchoscopy and sputum induction. Mycobacterium tuberculosis is spread through the air and can travel long distances. Cases of multidrug-resistant tuberculosis (MDR-TB, which includes extensively drug-resistant tuberculosis (XDR-TB)), have been recognized and are more difficult to treat.

Vancomycin-Intermediate Staphylococcus aureus and *Vancomycin-Resistant* Staphylococcus aureus

Vancomycin-intermediate *Staphylococcus aureus* (also called "S. aureus") and vancomycin-resistant *Staphylococcus aureus* are specific staph bacteria that have developed resistance to the antimicrobial agent vancomycin. Persons who develop this type of staph infection may have underlying health conditions (such as diabetes and kidney disease), devices going into their bodies (such as catheters), previous infections with methicillin-resistant *Staphylococcus aureus*, and recent exposure to vancomycin and other antimicrobial agents.

Vancomycin-Resistant Enterococci

Vancomycin-resistant enterococci are specific types of antimicrobial-resistant bacteria that are resistant to vancomycin, the drug often used to treat infections caused by enterococci. Enterococci are bacteria that are normally present in the human intestines and in the female genital tract and are often found in the environment. These bacteria can sometimes cause infections. Most vancomycin-resistant enterococci infections occur in hospitals.

Section 38.3

Preventing Healthcare-Associated Infections

This section contains text excerpted from the following sources: Text in this section begins with excerpts from "Healthcare-Associated Infections," Agency for Healthcare Research and Quality (AHRQ), U.S. Department of Health and Human Services (HHS), January 2019; Text beginning with the heading "Action Plan Development" is excerpted from "National Action Plan to Prevent Healthcare-Associated Infections: Road Map to Elimination," Office of Disease Prevention and Health Promotion (ODPHP), U.S. Department of Health and Human Services (HHS), May 7, 2019.

A cornerstone of healthcare-associated infection (HAI) prevention is appropriate to hand hygiene. Although the effectiveness of simple handwashing in preventing infection transmission has been known for decades, until recently hand hygiene rates among all clinicians were low. Strategies to improve hand hygiene that rely on traditional educational approaches as well as enhanced monitoring of hand hygiene, feedback on hand hygiene practice in a facility, and sociocultural approaches have resulted in improved hand hygiene at many hospitals and other healthcare facilities. What's more, strong evidence links higher hand hygiene rates to lower overall HAI rates.

The Centers for Disease Control and Prevention (CDC) offers evidence-based guidelines that detail methods to prevent specific HAIs in the inpatient and outpatient setting. The challenge has been making it easy for clinicians and healthcare executives to establish and adopt the recommended methods as standard practice in healthcare-delivery organizations. Organizations that successfully overcome this obstacle represent some of the major successes of the patient safety movement. For example, the development and implementation of the AHRQ-supported Comprehensive Unit-based Safety Program (CUSP) has brought about significant advances in HAI prevention. CUSP combines improvement in safety culture, teamwork, and communications with a checklist that incorporates a manageable set of evidence-based measures to prevent a particular HAI. The implementation of CUSP to prevent central line-associated bloodstream infection (CLABSI) has resulted in dramatic nationwide reductions in these serious infections, thanks in part to Agency for Healthcare Research and Quality (AHRQ)-funded research and dissemination programs that fostered the use of CUSP in intensive care units across the country. Conceptually similar approaches have also been successful in reducing rates of SSIs, and AHRQ is currently funding a large nationwide effort to promote the use of CUSP to reduce rates of catheter-associated UTI (CAUTI). A combination of improvement in organizational culture and use of the checklist has powered the reductions in CLABSI. In-depth analysis of the project has identified other important components of the program, such as rigorous data measurement and feedback and reframing of CLABSI as a social problem in a clinical environment.

The increasing threat posed by infections such as *C. difficile* is also stimulating efforts to address this issue. Strategies to prevent *C. difficile* infections primarily involve limiting antibiotic use (a major cause of these infections), particularly through antibiotic stewardship programs, preventing patient-to-patient transmission of the bacteria through isolation procedures and hand hygiene, and increased and improved cleaning of the environment of care, including patient rooms. Toolkits to help hospitals establish antibiotic stewardship programs targeting *C. difficile* have been developed and disseminated. Prevention of transmission of antibiotic-resistant bacteria follows similar principles.

Action Plan Development

In recognition of healthcare-associated infections (HAIs) as an important public-health and patient-safety issue, the U.S. Department of Health and Human Services (HHS) convened the Federal Steering Committee for the Prevention of Healthcare-Associated Infections (originally called the "HHS Steering Committee," but this name was changed to reflect the addition of agencies outside of HHS). The Steering Committee's charge is to coordinate and maximize the efficiency of prevention efforts across the federal government. Members of the Steering Committee include clinicians, scientists, and public-health leaders representing:

- Administration for Community Living (ACL)
- Agency for Healthcare Research and Quality (AHRQ)
- Centers for Disease Control and Prevention (CDC)
- Centers for Medicare & Medicaid Services (CMS)
- U.S. Food and Drug Administration (FDA)
- Health Resources and Services Administration (HRSA)
- Indian Health Service (IHS)
- National Institutes of Health (NIH)
- Office of the Secretary (OS)
  - National Vaccine Program Office (NVPO)
  - Office of Disease Prevention and Health Promotion (ODPHP)
- Office of the Assistant Secretary for Planning and Evaluation (ASPE)
- Office of the Assistant Secretary for Public Affairs (ASPA)
- Office of the National Coordinator for Health Information Technology (ONC)
- U.S. Department of Defense (DoD)
- U.S. Department of Labor (DOL)
- U.S. Department of Veterans Affairs (VA)

The Steering Committee marshaled the extensive and diverse resources of the Department, formed public and private partnerships, and initiated discussions that identified new approaches to

493

HAI prevention and collaborations. Along with scientists and program officials across HHS, the Steering Committee released the National Action Plan to Prevent Healthcare-Associated Infections: Road Map to Elimination (HAI Action Plan). The HAI Action Plan provides a road map for preventing HAIs in acute-care hospitals, ambulatory surgical centers, end-stage renal disease facilities, and long-term care facilities, and for implementing antibiotic stewardship efforts as a means of HAI prevention. The HAI Action Plan also includes a chapter on increasing influenza coverage of healthcare personnel.

Phases one, two, and three of the HAI Action Plan led to meaningfully enhanced coordination of federal efforts to address HAIs by establishing a structure to regularly share best practices, resources, and lessons learned among federal partners. Phase four, which was finalized in February 2018, reviews current federal antibiotic stewardship efforts across various healthcare settings, highlights the importance of antibiotic stewardship to prevent resistance in HAIs, and showcases the coordination between various health agencies.

Phase One: Acute-Care Hospitals

Phase one of the HAI Action Plan addresses the most common infections in inpatient acute-care settings and outlines a:

- Prioritized research agenda

- Integrated information systems strategy

- Policy options for linking payment incentives or disincentives to quality of care

outlines a plan to enhance regulatory oversight of hospitals, and a national messaging and communications plan to raise awareness of HAIs among the general public, and prevention strategies among healthcare workers.

Phase Two: Ambulatory Surgical Centers, End-Stage Renal Disease Facilities, and Increasing Influenza Vaccination among Healthcare Personnel

The healthcare and public-health communities are increasingly challenged to identify, respond to, and prevent HAIs across the continuum of settings where healthcare is delivered. The public-health model's population-based perspective can increasingly be deployed to enhance the prevention of HAIs, particularly given the shifts in healthcare delivery from acute-care settings to ambulatory and long-term care settings. The Steering Committee clearly articulated the need to:

- Maintain the HAI Action Plan as a "living document"
- Develop successor plans in collaboration with public and private stakeholders incorporate
  - Advances in science and technology
  - Shifts in the ways healthcare is delivered
  - Hanges in healthcare-system processes and cultural norms and other factors

Phase Three: Long-Term Care Facilities

The 2009 publication of the original HAI Action Plan, which focused on the acute-care setting, increased awareness of the need for strategies to address HAIs in long-term care facilities. A growing number of individuals are receiving care in long-term care settings such as skilled nursing facilities and nursing homes. The population in these facilities is requiring more complex medical care as a result of increased transitions between healthcare settings. These trends can create an increased risk for HAIs, which can worsen health status and increase healthcare costs. The Steering Committee chose to address HAIs in long-term care facilities for Phase Three.

Phase Four: Antibiotic Stewardship

Phase Four showcases the essential coordination and collaboration among federal partners engaged in HAI prevention and antibiotic stewardship. It highlights the work of the Federal Steering Committee for the Prevention of Healthcare-Associated Infections (FSC) to leverage existing relationships—including with the Presidential Advisory Council on Combatting Antibiotic Resistance (PACCARB). These partners are working collaboratively to realize a goal of the CARB Action Plan to slow the emergence of resistant bacteria through antibiotic stewardship programs in healthcare settings.

Evaluation of the Healthcare-Associated Infections Action Plan

The Office of Disease Prevention and Health Promotion (ODPHP), Division of Healthcare Quality, the Agency for Healthcare Research and Quality (AHRQ), and the CDC contracted with Insight Policy Research, IMPAQ International (IMPAQ) and the Research ANd Development (RAND) Corporation to produce iterative and comprehensive evaluations of HHS programs related to the National Action Plan to Prevent Healthcare-Associated Infections.

The Longitudinal Program Evaluation of the Healthcare-Associated Infections HHS Action Plan-Year 1 Report (September 2011), the first report of the evaluation, examined initial progress toward achieving action plan targets. The evaluation found that measurable progress has been made in reducing HAIs and specifically aimed to:

- Record current and future design, content, and progress of the HAI action plan

- Provide feedback on how to strengthen monitoring capabilities

- Offer insights to identify prospective high-yield opportunities to reduce HAIs

In addition to the successes noted to date, the evaluation also identified several areas for improved coordination and outreach.

State Healthcare-Associated Infection Prevention Plans

The 2009 Omnibus Law required states receiving Preventive Health and Health Services (PHHS) block-brant funds to certify that they will submit a plan to prevent HAIs to the Secretary of Health and Human Services by January 2010. HHS received plans from all 50 states, the District of Columbia (DC), and Puerto Rico.

The HHS Report to Congress on Healthcare-Associated Infections: FY 2010 State Action Plans addresses the adequacy of State Healthcare-Associated Infection (HAI) Action Plans for achieving state and national goals for reducing HAIs. It responds to the joint explanatory statement to accompany H.R. 1105, the Omnibus Appropriations Law, 2009 (Public Law 111-8):

...Each State plan shall be consistent with the Department of Health and Human Services' national action plan for reducing healthcare-associated infections and include measurable 5-year goals and interim milestones for reducing such infections: Provided further, That the Secretary shall conduct a review of the State plans submitted pursuant to the preceding proviso and report to the Committees on Appropriations of the House of Representatives and the Senate...

Section 38.4

Workplace Safety: Healthcare Workers

This section includes text excerpted from "Healthcare," Occupational
Safety and Health Administration (OSHA), January 13, 2017.

What Is Healthcare?

Healthcare is involved, directly or indirectly, with the provision of
health services to individuals. These services can occur in a variety
of work settings, including hospitals, clinics, dental offices, outpatient surgery centers, birthing centers, emergency medical care, home
healthcare, and nursing homes.

What Types of Hazards Do Workers Face?

Healthcare workers face a number of serious safety and health
hazards. They include bloodborne pathogens and biological hazards,
potential chemical and drug exposures, waste anesthetic gas exposures, respiratory hazards, ergonomic hazards from lifting and repetitive tasks, laser hazards, workplace violence, hazards associated with
laboratories, and radioactive material and X-ray hazards. Some of the
potential chemical exposures include formaldehyde, used for preservation of specimens for pathology; ethylene oxide, glutaraldehyde, and
peracetic acid used for sterilization; and numerous other chemicals
used in healthcare laboratories.

How Many Workers Get Sick or Injured?

More workers are injured in the healthcare and social-assistance
industry sector than any other. This industry has one of the highest
rates of work-related injuries and illnesses. In 2010, the healthcare
and social-assistance industry reported more injury and illness cases
than any other private industry sector—653,900 cases. That is 152,000
more cases than the next industry sector: manufacturing. In 2010,
the incidence rate for work-related nonfatal injuries and illnesses
in healthcare and social assistance was 139.9; the incidence rate for
nonfatal injury and illnesses in all private industry was 107.7.

Nursing aides, orderlies, and attendants had the highest rates
of musculoskeletal disorders (MSDs) of all occupations in 2010. The
incidence rate of work-related musculoskeletal disorders for these

occupations was 249 per 10,000 workers. This compares to the average rate for all workers in 2010 of 34.

Other than Doctors and Nurses, What Workers Are Exposed?

In addition to the medical staff, large healthcare facilities employ a wide variety of trades that have health and safety hazards associated with them. These include mechanical maintenance, medical equipment maintenance, housekeeping, food service, building and grounds maintenance, laundry, and administrative staff.

Infectious Diseases

Healthcare workers (HCWs) are occupationally exposed to a variety of infectious diseases during the performance of their duties. The delivery of healthcare services requires a broad range of workers, such as physicians, nurses, technicians, clinical laboratory workers, first responders, building maintenance, security and administrative personnel, social workers, food service, housekeeping, and mortuary personnel. Moreover, these workers can be found in a variety of workplace settings, including hospitals, nursing care facilities, outpatient clinics (e.g., medical and dental offices, and occupational-health clinics), ambulatory care centers, and emergency response settings. The diversity among HCWs and their workplaces makes occupational exposure to infectious diseases especially challenging. For example, not all workers in the same healthcare facility, not all individuals with the same job title, and not all healthcare facilities will be at equal risk of occupational exposure to infectious agents.

The primary routes of infectious disease transmission in the U.S. healthcare settings are contact, droplet, and airborne. Contact transmission can be subdivided into direct and indirect contact. Direct contact transmission involves the transfer of infectious agents to a susceptible individual through physical contact with an infected individual (e.g., direct skin-to-skin contact). Indirect contact transmission occurs when infectious agents are transferred to a susceptible individual when the individual makes physical contact with contaminated items and surfaces (e.g., door knobs, patient-care instruments or equipment, bed rails, and examination table). Two examples of contact transmissible infectious agents include Methicillin-resistant *Staphylococcus aureus* (MRSA) and Vancomycin-resistant Enterococcus (VRE).

Droplets containing infectious agents are generated when an infected person coughs, sneezes, or talks, or during certain medical procedures, such as suctioning or endotracheal intubation. Transmission occurs when droplets generated in this way come into direct contact with the mucosal surfaces of the eyes, nose, or mouth of a susceptible individual. Droplets are too large to be airborne for long periods of time, and droplet transmission does not occur through the air over long distances. Two examples of droplet transmissible infectious agents are the influenza virus which causes the seasonal flu and Bordetella pertussis which causes pertussis (i.e., whooping cough).

Airborne transmission occurs through very small particles or droplet nuclei that contain infectious agents and can remain suspended in air for extended periods of time. When they are inhaled by a susceptible individual, they enter the respiratory tract and can cause infection. Since air currents can disperse these particles or droplet nuclei over long distances, the airborne transmission does not require face-to-face contact with an infected individual. Airborne transmission only occurs with infectious agents that are capable of surviving and retaining infectivity for relatively long periods of time in airborne particles or droplet nuclei. Only a limited number of diseases are transmissible via the airborne route. Two examples of agents that can be spread through the airborne route include Mycobacterium tuberculosis, which causes tuberculosis (TB), and the measles virus (Measles morbillivirus), which causes measles (sometimes called "rubeola," among other names).

Several Occupational Safety and Health Administration (OSHA) standards and directives are directly applicable to protecting workers against the transmission of infectious agents. These include OSHA's Bloodborne Pathogens standard (29 CFR 1910.1030), which provides protection of workers from exposures to blood and body fluids that may contain bloodborne infectious agents; OSHA's Personal Protective Equipment standard (29 CFR 1910.132) and Respiratory Protection standard (29 CFR 1910.134), which provide protection for workers when exposed to contact, droplet, and airborne transmissible infectious agents; and OSHA's TB compliance directive, which protects workers against exposure to TB through enforcement of existing applicable OSHA standards and the General Duty Clause of the OSHA.

Section 38.5

Veterinary Healthcare Workers

This section includes text excerpted from "Veterinary Safety and Health," Centers for Disease Control and Prevention (CDC), April 27, 2018.

Veterinary medicine and animal care workers provide medical, surgical, preventive health, or animal care services for a variety of animal species in many different workplace settings. These workers are exposed to biological, chemical, physical, and psychological hazards depending on their workplace setting, species of animals worked with, and type of tasks performed.

In the United States, there are more than 455,000 veterinary medicine and animal care workers, including 79,600 veterinarians, 102,000 veterinary technologists and technicians, 83,800 veterinary assistants and laboratory animal caretakers, and 190,520 nonfarm animal caretakers [BLS 2017a-d].

The National Institute for Occupational Safety and Health (NIOSH) National Occupational Research Agenda (NORA), Healthcare and Social Assistance Sector Program is working with industry, labor, other stakeholders, and academics to identify and address the priority workplace safety and health hazards of these workers.

Hazard Prevention and Infection Control
Recommendations for Employers

Employers have the responsibility to provide a safe workplace. Effective safety and health programs (also known as injury and illness prevention programs) have been shown to reduce workplace injuries and illnesses and associated costs. Employers should develop a comprehensive written safety and health program that addresses key elements:

- Management leadership
- Worker participation
- Hazard identification and assessment
- Hazard prevention and control
- Education and training
- Program evaluation and improvement

- Communication and coordination for host employers, contractors, and staffing agencies

Employers of veterinary medicine and animal care workers should:

- Develop and implement a comprehensive written workplace-specific safety and health program
- Review and update the written safety and health program periodically
- Document and maintain staff records of training, immunizations, and work-related injuries and illnesses
- Comply with federal and state occupational hazard laws
- Comply with relevant federal, state, and local laws such as proper veterinary waste management and disposal
- Inform all workers and volunteers about potential workplace hazards
- Promote safe work habits including best infection control practices
- Have a medical surveillance system in place to record and report workplace-related injuries and illnesses
- Ensure that equipment is maintained and operated safely

Prevention through Design

One of the best ways to prevent and control workplace injuries, illnesses, and fatalities is to "design out," or minimize, hazards and risks early in the design process. Prevention through design efforts in veterinary facilities and processes can protect workers and animals and be cost-effective.

- Consider safety in the design and construction of animal handling, restraint, housing, and other veterinary facilities
- Consider safety in the design of processes such as animal restraint and anesthetic gas control systems

Hierarchy of Controls

The hierarchy of controls listed below should be followed to most effectively protect veterinary medicine and animal care workers from workplace hazards. Different categories of methods for controlling hazards are listed in general order of effectiveness. However, an individual preventive intervention may be more or less important than suggested by its' general category. Some examples are provided. Often a combination of engineering and administrative controls and personal protective equipment (PPE) are needed to adequately protect workers from workplace hazards. PPE should be used only when other controls cannot effectively reduce hazardous exposures.

- **Elimination:** Remove the hazard from the workplace

  - e.g., do not admit animals for which the facility is not properly equipped

- **Substitution:** Switch to the use of a less risky hazard

  - e.g., switch to the use of safer chemicals

- **Engineering controls:** Prevent exposure to a hazard or place a barrier between the hazard and the worker

  - e.g., install an effective waste anesthetic gas scavenging system

- **Administrative controls:** Implement changes in work practices and management policies

  - e.g., require rabies preexposure vaccination for workers at risk

- **Personal protective equipment (PPE):** Use gloves, safety eyewear, masks, hearing protection, respirators, or other protective equipment

  - e.g., require the use of hearing protection in an animal shelter with barking dogs

Worker Training

Veterinary medicine and animal care workers should be trained about hazards before they begin work. Refresher training should be conducted at regular intervals as required or as needed. Training should include information about the following:

- Potential workplace hazards

- Occupational risks for pregnant and immunocompromised workers

- Effective use of controls for reducing workplace exposures
- Veterinary standard precautions including infection control practices
- Safe handling, restraint, and care of animals
- Preventing needlestick, scalpel, and sharps injury
- Proper care and use of PPE
- Prompt reporting of work-related injuries and illnesses
- Emergency and evacuation procedures

Chapter 39

Quarantine and Isolation to Control the Spread of Infectious Diseases

Isolation and Quarantine

Isolation and quarantine help protect the public by preventing exposure to people who have or may have a contagious disease.

- Isolation separates sick people with a contagious disease from people who are not sick.

- Quarantine separates and restricts the movement of people who were exposed to a contagious disease to see if they become sick.

In addition to serving as medical functions, isolation and quarantine also are "police power" functions, derived from the right of the state to take action affecting individuals for the benefit of society.

This chapter contains text excerpted from the following sources: Text beginning with the heading "Isolation and Quarantine" is excerpted from "Legal Authorities for Isolation and Quarantine," Centers for Disease Control and Prevention (CDC), October 8, 2014. Reviewed May 2019; Text beginning with the heading "A Comprehensive Quarantine System" is excerpted from "Quarantine Stations," Centers for Disease Control and Prevention (CDC), September 29, 2017.

Federal Law

The federal government derives its authority for isolation and quarantine from the Commerce Clause of the U.S. Constitution.

Under section 361 of the Public Health Service Act (42 U.S. Code § 264), the U.S. Secretary of Health and Human Services (HHS) is authorized to take measures to prevent the entry and spread of communicable diseases from foreign countries into the United States and between states.

The authority for carrying out these functions on a daily basis has been delegated to the Centers for Disease Control and Prevention (CDC).

Centers for Disease Control and Prevention's Role

Under 42 Code of Federal Regulations parts 70 and 71, the CDC is authorized to detain, medically examine, and release persons arriving into the United States and traveling between states who are suspected of carrying these communicable diseases.

As part of its federal authority, the CDC routinely monitors persons arriving at U.S. land-border crossings and passengers and crew arriving at U.S. ports of entry for signs or symptoms of communicable diseases.

When alerted about an ill passenger or crew member by the pilot of a plane or captain of a ship, the CDC may detain passengers and crew as necessary to investigate whether the cause of the illness on board is a communicable disease.

State, Local, and Tribal Law

States have police power functions to protect the health, safety, and welfare of persons within their borders. To control the spread of disease within their borders, states have laws to enforce the use of isolation and quarantine.

These laws can vary from state to state and can be specific or broad. In some states, local health authorities implement state law. In most states, breaking a quarantine order is a criminal misdemeanor.

Tribes also have police power authority to take actions that promote the health, safety, and welfare of their own tribal members. Tribal health authorities may enforce their own isolation and quarantine laws within tribal lands, if such laws exist.

Who Is in Charge?
The Federal Government

- Acts to prevent the entry of communicable diseases into the United States. Quarantine and isolation may be used at U.S. ports of entry.

- Is authorized to take measures to prevent the spread of communicable diseases between states

- May accept state and local assistance in enforcing federal quarantine

- May assist state and local authorities in preventing the spread of communicable diseases

State, Local, and Tribal Authorities

- Enforce isolation and quarantine within their borders

It is possible for federal, state, local, and tribal health authorities to have and use all at the same time separate but coexisting legal quarantine power in certain events. In the event of a conflict, federal law is supreme.

Enforcement

If a quarantinable disease is suspected or identified, the CDC may issue a federal isolation or quarantine order.

Public-health authorities at the federal, state, local, and tribal levels may sometimes seek help from police or other law-enforcement officers to enforce a public-health order.

U.S. Customs and Border Protection and U.S. Coast Guard officers are authorized to help enforce federal quarantine orders.

Breaking a federal quarantine order is punishable by fines and imprisonment.

Federal law allows the conditional release of persons from quarantine if they comply with medical monitoring and surveillance.

Federal Quarantine Rarely Used

Large-scale isolation and quarantine were last enforced during influenza ("Spanish Flu") pandemic in 1918–1919. In recent history, only a few public-health events have prompted federal isolation or quarantine orders.

A Comprehensive Quarantine System

The U.S. quarantine stations are part of a comprehensive quarantine system that serves to limit the introduction of infectious diseases into the United States and to prevent their spread.

The U.S. quarantine stations are located at 20 ports of entry and land-border crossings where international travelers arrive. They are staffed with quarantine medical and public-health officers from the CDC. These health officers decide whether ill persons can enter the United States and what measures should be taken to prevent the spread of infectious diseases.

Quarantine officers are responsible for varied activities, such as responding to reports of illnesses, screening cargo, inspecting animals and animal products, and monitoring the health of and collecting any medical information of new immigrants, refugees, asylees, and parolees.

Contacting U.S. Quarantine Stations

Quarantine stations are charged with the responsibility of enforcing foreign quarantine regulations at all ports of entry within their assigned area of jurisdiction.

All telephone numbers operate with 24-hour access, unless an alternate number is provided.

Shipping note: For shipping to quarantine stations using a delivery service other than FedEx (such as UPS, DHL, or freight), confirm the correct shipping address prior to sending.

Time zones: All hours of operation are based on the local time of the station's geographical location.

Chapter 40

National Notifiable Diseases Surveillance System

To protect Americans from serious disease, the National Notifiable Diseases Surveillance System (NNDSS) helps public-health departments monitor, control, and prevent about 120 diseases. These diseases are important to monitor nationwide and include infectious diseases such as Zika, foodborne outbreaks such as *E. coli*, and noninfectious conditions such as lead poisoning. About 3,000 public-health departments gather and use data on these diseases to protect their local communities. Through NNDSS, the Centers for Disease Control and Prevention (CDC) receives and uses these data to keep people healthy and defend the United States from health threats.

The National Notifiable Diseases Surveillance System is a multi-faceted program that includes the surveillance system for collection, analysis, and sharing of health data. It also includes policies, laws, electronic messaging standards, people, partners, information systems, processes, and resources at the local, state, territorial, and national levels.

This chapter includes text excerpted from "National Notifiable Diseases Surveillance System (NNDSS)," Centers for Disease Control and Prevention (CDC), March 13, 2019.

Supporting Public Health Surveillance in Jurisdictions and at the Centers for Disease Control and Prevention

Notifiable disease surveillance begins at the level of local, state, and territorial public-health departments (also known as jurisdictions). Jurisdictional laws and regulations mandate the reporting of cases of specified infectious and noninfectious conditions to health departments. The health departments work with healthcare providers, laboratories, hospitals, and other partners to obtain the information needed to monitor, control, and prevent the occurrence and spread of these health conditions.

The CDC Division of Health Informatics and Surveillance (DHIS) supports NNDSS by receiving, securing, processing, and providing nationally notifiable infectious diseases data to disease-specific CDC programs. DHIS also supports local, state, and territorial public-health departments by helping them collect, manage, and submit case notification data to the CDC for NNDSS. DHIS provides this support through funding, health information exchange standards and frameworks, electronic health information systems, and technical support through the NNDSS website, tools, and training. DHIS and the CDC programs publish statistical data based on NNDSS to support recognition of outbreaks, monitor shifts in disease patterns, and evaluate disease control activities.

These programs collaborate with the Council of State and Territorial Epidemiologists (CSTE) to determine which conditions reported to local, state, and territorial public-health departments are nationally notifiable. The CDC programs, in collaboration with subject-matter experts in CSTE and in health departments, determine what data elements are included in national notifications. Health departments participating in NNDSS voluntarily submit case notification data to DHIS and also submit some data directly to CDC programs.

National Notifiable Diseases Surveillance System Modernization Initiative

With the evolution of technology and data and exchange standards, the CDC is strengthening and modernizing the infrastructure supporting NNDSS. As part of the CDC Surveillance Strategy, the NNDSS Modernization Initiative (NMI) is enhancing the system's ability to provide more comprehensive, timely, and higher quality data than ever before for public health decision making.

Part Seven

Additional Help and Information

Chapter 41

Glossary of Terms Related to Infectious Diseases

active immunity: The production of antibodies against a specific disease by the immune system. Active immunity can be acquired in two ways, either by contracting the disease or through vaccination. Active immunity is usually permanent, meaning an individual is protected from the disease for the duration of their lives.

addiction: A chronic, relapsing disease characterized by compulsive drug seeking and use despite serious adverse consequences, and by long-lasting changes in the brain.

adjuvant: A substance that is added to a vaccine to increase and improve the body's immune response to the vaccine antigen(s). Antigens are the components of the flu vaccine that prompt your body to have an immune response. Vaccine adjuvants can allow flu vaccines to be produced using less antigen. Therefore, use of adjuvants can allow vaccine manufacturers to produce more doses of vaccine with less antigen.

air changes: Ratio of the volume of air flowing through a space in a certain period of time (air flow rate) to the volume of that space (room volume); usually expressed as the number of room air changes per hour (ACH).

This glossary contains terms excerpted from documents produced by several sources deemed reliable.

airborne transmission: Occurs by dissemination of either airborne droplet nuclei (small-particle residue [5 μm or smaller] of evaporated droplets containing microorganisms that remain suspended in the air for long periods of time) or dust particles containing the infectious agent. Microorganisms carried in this manner can be dispersed widely by air currents and may become inhaled by a susceptible host in the same room or over a longer distance from the source patient, depending on environmental factors.

allergy: A condition in which the body has an exaggerated response to a substance (e.g., food or drug). Also known as hypersensitivity.

alcohol: A chemical substance found in drinks such as beer, wine, and liquor. It is also found in some medicines, mouthwashes, household products, and essential oils (scented liquid taken from certain plants). It is made by a chemical process called "fermentation" that uses sugars and yeast.

anesthetic: A drug that causes insensitivity to pain and is used for surgeries and other medical procedures.

anthrax: An acute infectious disease caused by the spore-forming bacterium *Bacillus anthracis*. Anthrax most commonly occurs in hoofed mammals and can also infect humans.

antibiotic: A drug that kills or stops the growth of bacteria. Antibiotics are a type of antimicrobial. Penicillin and ciprofloxacin are examples of antibiotics.

antibody: A protein made by plasma cells (a type of white blood cell) in response to an antigen (a substance that causes the body to make a specific immune response). Each antibody can bind to only one specific antigen.

antigen: Any substance that causes the body to make an immune response against that substance. Antigens include toxins, chemicals, bacteria, viruses, or other substances that come from outside the body.

antimicrobial: A substance, such as an antibiotic, that kills or stops the growth of microbes, including bacteria, fungi, or viruses. Antimicrobials are grouped according to the microbes they act against (antibiotics, antifungals, and antivirals). Also referred to as drugs.

anxiety: Feelings of fear, dread, and uneasiness that may occur as a reaction to stress. A person with anxiety may sweat, feel restless, and tense, and have a rapid heartbeat.

514

arthritis: A term used to describe more than 100 rheumatic diseases and conditions that affect joints, the tissues which surround the joint and other connective tissue.

assessment: The process of gathering evidence and documentation of a student's learning.

asthma: A chronic disease in which the bronchial airways in the lungs become narrowed and swollen, making it difficult to breathe.

asymptomatic infection: The presence of an infection without symptoms. Also known as inapparent or subclinical infection.

bacteria: Single-celled organisms that live in and around us with a distinct structure from other microbes. Bacteria can be helpful, but can also cause illnesses such as strep throat, ear infections, and pneumonia.

bias: Flaws in the collection, analysis or interpretation of research data that lead to incorrect conclusions.

bladder: The organ in the human body that stores urine. It is found in the lower part of the abdomen.

blood: A tissue with red blood cells (RBCs), white blood cells (WBCs), platelets, and other substances suspended in fluid called plasma. Blood takes oxygen and nutrients to the tissues, and carries away wastes.

bone: A living, growing tissue made mostly of collagen.

bronchoscopy: Procedure for visually examining the respiratory tract and/or obtaining specimens for diagnostic purposes; requires inserting an instrument (bronchoscope) through a patient's mouth or nose into the trachea.

calcium: A mineral that is an essential nutrient for bone health. It is also needed for the heart, muscles, and nerves to function properly and for blood to clot.

calorie: A unit of energy in food. Carbohydrates, fats, protein, and alcohol in the foods and drinks we eat provide food energy or "calories."

cancer: A term for diseases in which abnormal cells in the body divide without control. Cancer cells can invade nearby tissues and can spread to other parts of the body through the blood and lymphatic system, which is a network of tissues that clears infections and keeps body fluids in balance.

central nervous system (CNS): Comprised of the nerves in the brain and spinal cord. These nerves are used to send electrical impulses throughout the body, resulting in voluntary and reflexive movement. Information about the environment is received by the senses and sent to the central nervous system, which causes the body to respond appropriately.

chemotherapy: Treatment with anticancer drugs.

chronic disease: A disease that has one or more of the following characteristics: is permanent; leaves residual disability; is caused by nonreversible pathological alteration; requires special training of the patient for rehabilitation; or may be expected to require a long period of supervision, observation, or care.

clinical trial: A research study in which one or more human subjects are prospectively assigned to one or more interventions (which may include placebo or other control) to evaluate the effects of those interventions on health-related biomedical or behavioral outcomes.

coronavirus: One of a group of viruses that have a halo or crown-like (corona) appearance when viewed under a microscope. These viruses are a common cause of mild to moderate upper-respiratory illness in humans and are associated with respiratory, gastrointestinal, liver, and neurologic disease in animals.

corticosteroids: Steroid-type hormones that have antitumor activity in lymphomas and lymphoid leukemias. In addition, corticosteroids may be used for hormone replacement and for the management of some of the complications of cancer and its treatment.

Creutzfeldt-Jakob disease (CJD): A degenerative neurological disorder of humans thought to be transmitted by abnormal isoforms of neural proteins called prions. CJD is one of a group of related diseases known as transmissible spongiform encephalopathies (TSEs).

culture: A test to see whether there are tuberculosis (TB) bacteria in your phlegm or other body fluids. This test can take 2 to 4 weeks in most laboratories.

deoxyribonucleic acid (DNA): The double-helix molecule that provides the basis of genetic heredity, about two nanometers in diameter but often several millimeters in length.

diabetes: A condition in which blood glucose (blood sugar) levels are above or below normal.

diet: What a person eats and drinks. Any type of eating plan.

disinfection: The destruction of pathogenic and other kinds of microorganisms by physical or chemical means. Disinfection is less lethal than sterilization, because it destroys most recognized pathogenic microorganisms, but not necessarily all microbial forms, such as bacterial spores. Disinfection does not ensure the margin of safety associated with sterilization processes.

droplet transmission: Occurs when droplets containing infectious agents are propelled a short distance through the air (e.g., by coughing, sneezing, or talking) and deposited in the eyes, nose, or mouth of a susceptible person.

encephalopathy: A general term describing brain dysfunction. Examples include encephalitis, meningitis, seizures, and head trauma.

enzyme: A protein that speeds up chemical reactions in the body.

ergonomics: It is the science of designing the job and the workplace to suit the capabilities of the workers. Simply stated, ergonomics means "fitting the task to the worker." The aim of ergonomics is the evaluation and design of facilities, workstations, jobs, training methods, and equipment to match the capabilities of users and workers, and thereby reduce stress and eliminate injuries and disorders associated with the overuse of muscles, bad posture, and repeated tasks.

exercise: A type of physical activity that involves planned, structured, and repetitive bodily movement done to maintain or improve one or more components of physical fitness.

exposure: Contact with infectious agents (bacteria or viruses) in a manner that promotes transmission and increases the likelihood of disease.

extensively drug-resistant TB (XDR TB): A rare type of TB disease that is resistant to nearly all medicines used to treat TB.

fetus: A developing unborn offspring in the uterus (womb). This stage of pregnancy begins eight weeks after conception and lasts until birth.

fracture: Broken bone. People with osteoporosis, osteogenesis imperfecta, and Paget disease are at greater risk for bone fracture.

genes: Genes, which are made up of DNA, are the basic units that define the characteristics of every organism. Genes carry information that determine traits, such as eye color in humans and resistance to antibiotics in bacteria.

genetics: The study of particular genes, deoxyribonucleic acid (DNA), and heredity.

genome: An organism's complete set of genes that carry the genetic instructions for building and maintaining that organism.

hand hygiene: A general term that applies to any one of the following: 1. handwashing with plan (nonantimicrobial) soap and water, 2. antiseptic handwash (soap containing antiseptic agents and water), 3. antiseptic hand rub (waterless antiseptic product, most often alcohol-based, rubbed on surfaces of hands), or 4. surgical hand antisepsis.

healthcare worker: Any employee in a healthcare facility who has close contact with patients, patient-care areas, or patient-care items; also referred to as "healthcare personnel."

hepatitis A: A minor viral disease, that usually does not persist in the blood; transmitted through ingestion of contaminated food or water.

hepatitis C: A liver disease caused by the hepatitis C virus (HCV), which is found in the blood of persons who have the disease. HCV is spread by contact with the blood of an infected person.

hepatitis D: A defective virus that needs the hepatitis B virus to exist. Hepatitis D virus (HDV) is found in the blood of persons infected with the virus.

hormone: Substance produced by one tissue and conveyed by the bloodstream to another to affect a function of the body, such as growth or metabolism.

human immunodeficiency virus (HIV): A virus that infects and destroys the body's immune cells and causes a disease called acquired immunodeficiency syndrome (AIDS).

hypertension: Also called high blood pressure, it is having blood pressure greater than 140 over 90 mmHg (millimeters of mercury). Long-term high blood pressure can damage blood vessels and organs, including the heart, kidneys, eyes, and brain.

immune system: A complex system of cellular and molecular components having the primary function of distinguishing self from not self and defense against foreign organisms or substances.

immunity: Protection against a disease. Immunity is indicated by the presence of antibodies in the blood and can usually be determined with a laboratory test.

immunization: The process by which a person becomes immune, or protected, against a disease. This term is often used interchangeably with vaccination or inoculation. However, the term "vaccination" is defined as the injection of a killed or weakened infectious organism in order to prevent the disease. Thus, vaccination, by inoculation with a vaccine, does not always result in immunity.

inflammation: Redness, swelling, heat, and pain resulting from injury to tissue (parts of the body underneath the skin). Also known as swelling.

influenza: A highly contagious viral infection characterized by sudden onset of fever, severe aches and pains, and inflammation of the mucous membrane.

jaundice: Yellowing of the skin and eyes. This condition is often a symptom of hepatitis infection.

larynx: The area of the throat containing the vocal cords and used for breathing, swallowing, and talking. Also called voice box.

lesion: An area of abnormal tissue. A lesion may be benign (not cancer) or malignant (cancer).

magnetic resonance imaging (MRI): A noninvasive procedure that uses magnetic fields and radio waves to produce three-dimensional computerized images of areas inside the body.

meningitis: Inflammation of the meninges, the membranes that envelop the brain and the spinal cord; may cause hearing loss or deafness.

metabolism: The chemical changes that take place in a cell or an organism. These changes make energy and the materials cells and organisms need to grow, reproduce, and stay healthy. Metabolism also helps get rid of toxic substances.

microbes: Living organisms, like bacteria, fungi, or viruses, which can cause infections or disease. Also referred to as germs.

mutation: A change in a DNA sequence that can result from DNA copying mistakes made during cell division, exposure to ionizing radiation, exposure to chemical mutagens, or infection by viruses.

Mycobacterium tuberculosis: Bacteria that cause latent TB infection and TB disease.

nutrition: The taking in and use of food and other nourishing material by the body. Nutrition is a three-part process. First, food or drink is consumed. Second, the body breaks down the food or drink into nutrients.

obesity: Excess body fat. Because body fat is usually not measured directly, a ratio of body weight to height is often used instead.

organ: A part of the body that performs a specific function. For example, the heart is an organ.

organism: Any living thing, including humans, animals, plants, and microbes.

over-the-counter (OTC): Medicine that can be bought without a prescription (doctor's order). Examples include analgesics (pain relievers), such as aspirin and acetaminophen. Also called nonprescription.

overweight: An excessive amount of body weight that includes muscle, bone, fat, and water. A person who has a body mass index (BMI) of 25 to 29.9 is considered overweight.

papillomavirus: Group of viruses that can cause noncancerous wart-like tumors to grow on the surface of skin and internal organs, such as the respiratory tract; can be life-threatening.

perception (hearing): Process of knowing or being aware of information through the ear.

personal protective equipment (PPE): A specialized clothing or equipment worn by an employee for protection against a hazard (e.g., gloves, masks, protective eyewear, gowns). General work clothes (e.g., uniforms, pants, shirts or blouses) not intended to function as protection against a hazard are not considered to be personal protective equipment.

physical activity: Any bodily movement that is produced by the contraction of skeletal muscle and that substantially increases energy expenditure.

precaution: A condition in a recipient which may result in a life-threatening problem if the vaccine is given, or a condition which could compromise the ability of the vaccine to produce immunity.

pregnancy: The condition between conception (fertilization of an egg by a sperm) and birth, during which the fertilized egg develops in the uterus. In humans, pregnancy lasts about 288 days.

prevalence: The number of disease cases (new and existing) within a population over a given time period.

preventions: Actions that reduce exposure or other risks, keep people from getting sick, or keep disease from getting worse.

prognosis: The likely outcome or course of a disease; the chance of recovery or recurrence.

protein: A molecule made up of amino acids. Proteins are needed for the body to function properly. They are the basis of body structures, such as skin and hair, and of other substances such as enzymes, cytokines, and antibodies.

quarantine: The isolation of a person or animal who has a disease (or is suspected of having a disease) in order to prevent further spread of the disease.

radiation: Energy moving in the form of particles or waves. Familiar radiations are heat, light, radio, and microwaves.

resistance gene: A gene that gives microbes the ability to resist the effects of one or more drugs. The gene may be naturally present in the microbe, or it may be transferred from other microbes.

resistance pattern: A description of the antibiotic resistance testing results for an isolate.

resistance profile: A description of the resistance patterns for all isolates in an investigation. A resistance profile differs from a resistance pattern, which refers to the characteristics of a single isolate.

resistant isolate: An isolate that is resistant to one or more antibiotics.

rheumatoid arthritis (RA): An inflammatory disease that causes pain, swelling, stiffness, and loss of function in the joints. It occurs when the immune system, which normally defends the body from invading organisms, attacks the membrane lining the joints. Studies have found an increased risk of bone loss and fracture in individuals with RA.

rubella (German measles): Viral infection that is milder than normal measles but as damaging to the fetus when it occurs early in pregnancy.

seizure: The sudden onset of a jerking or staring spell. Many seizures following a vaccination are caused by fever. Seizures are also known as convulsions.

severe combined immunodeficiency (SCID): Included in a group of rare, life-threatening disorders caused by at least 15 different single gene defects that result in profound deficiencies in T- and B- lympho-cyte function.

smallpox: An acute, highly infectious, often fatal disease caused by a poxvirus and characterized by high fever and aches with subsequent widespread eruption of pimples that blister, produce pus, and form pockmarks. Also called variola.

smear: A test to see whether there are TB bacteria in your phlegm. To do this test, lab workers smear the phlegm on a glass slide, stain the slide with a special stain, and look for any TB bacteria on the slide. This test usually takes 1 day to get the results.

smell: To perceive odor or scent through stimuli affecting the olfactory nerves.

sodium: A mineral and an essential nutrient needed by the human body in relatively small amounts (provided that substantial sweating does not occur).

specimen: A sample collected for laboratory testing. During out-break investigations, samples may be collected from the blood, stool, or another location of a human or animal, and from food and the environment.

sputum: Phlegm coughed up from deep inside the lungs. Sputum is examined for TB bacteria using a smear; part of the sputum can also be used to do a culture.

steroid: Any of a group of lipids (fats) that have a certain chemical structure. Steroids occur naturally in plants and animals or they may be made in the laboratory.

stroke: Also known as a cerebrovascular accident (CVA); caused by a lack of blood to the brain, resulting in the sudden loss of speech, lan-guage, or the ability to move a body part, and, if severe enough, death.

tobacco: A plant with leaves that have high levels of the addictive chemical nicotine. After harvesting, tobacco leaves are cured, aged, and processed in various ways. The resulting products may be smoked (in cigarettes, cigars, and pipes), applied to the gums (as dipping and chewing tobacco), or inhaled (as snuff).

typhoid fever: Typhoid fever is a life-threatening illness caused by the bacterium *Salmonella typhi*. Persons with typhoid fever carry the bacteria in their bloodstream and intestinal tract.

urinary tract infection (UTI): An infection anywhere in the urinary tract, or organs that collect and store urine and release it from your body (the kidneys, ureters, bladder, and urethra).

vaccine: A product that produces immunity, therefore, protecting the body from the disease. Vaccines are administered through needle injections, by mouth and by aerosol.

virus: A small organism that can infect a person and cause illness or disease.

vitamin D: A nutrient that the body needs to absorb calcium.

whole genome sequencing: A technology that determines the genetic code (genome) of an organism (for example, people, bacteria, and viruses).

X-ray: A type of high-energy radiation. In low doses, X-rays are used to diagnose diseases by making pictures of the inside of the body.

Chapter 42

Directory of Resources Providing Information about Infectious Diseases

Government Organizations

Agency for Healthcare Research and Quality (AHRQ)
Office of Communications and
Knowledge Transfer (OCKT)
5600 Fishers Ln.
Seventh Fl.
Rockville, MD 20857
Phone: 301-427-1104
Website: www.ahrq.gov

AIDSinfo
P.O. Box 4780
Rockville, MD 20849-6303
Toll-Free: 800-HIV-0440
(800-448-0440)
Toll-Free TTY: 888-480-3739
Fax: 301-315-2818
Website: www.aidsinfo.nih.gov
E-mail: ContactUs@aidsinfo.nih.
gov

CDC Division of STD Prevention (DSTDP)
Centers for Disease Control and
Prevention (CDC)
1600 Clifton Rd.
Atlanta, GA 30329
Toll-Free: 800-CDC-INFO
(800-232-4636)
Toll-Free TTY: 888-232-6348
Website: www.cdc.gov/std/dstdp/
default.htm

Resources in this chapter were compiled from several sources deemed reliable;
all contact information was verified and updated in May 2019.

CDC Division of Viral Hepatitis (DVH)
Centers for Disease Control and Prevention (CDC)
1600 Clifton Rd. N.E.
MS G-37
Atlanta, GA 30329-4018
Toll-Free: 800-CDC-INFO
(800-232-4636)
Toll-Free TTY: 888-232-6348
Website: www.cdc.gov/hepatitis

CDC National Prevention Information Network (NPIN)
P.O. Box 6003
Rockville, MD 20849
Toll-Free: 800-CDC-INFO
(800-232-4636)
Toll-Free TTY: 888-232-6348
Website: www.npin.cdc.gov
E-mail: NPIN-Info@cdc.gov

CDC Vaccines and Immunizations
1600 Clifton Rd.
Atlanta, GA 30333
Toll-Free: 800-CDC-INFO
(800-232-4636)
Toll-Free TTY: 888-232-6348
Website: www.cdc.gov/vaccines

Centers for Disease Control and Prevention (CDC)
1600 Clifton Rd.
Atlanta, GA 30329-4027
Toll-Free: 800-CDC-INFO
(800-232-4636)
Toll-Free TTY: 888-232-6348
Website: www.cdc.gov

Eunice Kennedy Shriver
National Institute of Child Health and Human Development (NICHD)
NICHD Information Resource Center (IRC)
P.O. Box 3006
Rockville, MD 20847
Toll-Free: 800-370-2943
Toll-Free TTY: 888-320-6942
Toll-Free Fax: 866-760-5947
Website: www.nichd.nih.gov
E-mail: NICHDInformation
ResourceCenter@mail.nih.gov

FDA MedWatch
5600 Fishers Ln.
Rockville, MD 20857
Toll-Free: 800-332-1088
Toll-Free Fax: 800-332-0178
Website: www.fda.gov/Safety/
MedWatch/default.htm
E-mail: webmail@oc.fda.gov

Federal Trade Commission (FTC)
Consumer Response Center (CRC)
600 Pennsylvania Ave. N.W.
Washington, DC 20580
Toll-Free: 877-FTC-HELP
(877-382-4357)
Toll-Free TDD/TTY:
866-653-4261
Website: www.ftc.gov
E-mail: antitrust@ftc.gov

Genetic and Rare Diseases Information Center (GARD)
P.O. Box 8126
Gaithersburg, MD 20898-8126
Toll-Free: 888-205-2311
Phone: 301-251-4925
Toll-Free TTY: 888-205-3223
Fax: 301-251-4911
Website: www.rarediseases.info.nih.gov

Genetics Home Reference (GHR)
8600 Rockville Pike
Bethesda, MD 20894
Website: www.ghr.nlm.nih.gov

GlobalChange.gov
1800 G St. N.W.
Ste. 9100
Washington, DC 20006
Phone: 202-223-6262
Fax: 202-223-3065
Website: www.globalchange.gov

Health Resources and Services Administration (HRSA)
Information Center
P.O. Box 2910
Merrifield, VA 22116
Toll-Free: 888-275-4772
Toll-Free TTY: 877-489-4772
Fax: 703-821-2098
Website: www.hrsa.gov
E-mail: ask@hrsa.gov

Healthfinder®
National Health Information Center (NHIC)
P.O. Box 1133
Washington, DC 20013
Fax: 301-984-4256
Website: www.healthfinder.gov

HealthyPeople.gov
Office of Disease Prevention and Health Promotion (ODPHP)
1101 Wootton Pkwy LL-100
Rockville, MD 20852
Website: www.healthypeople.gov
E-mail: healthypeople@hhs.gov

MedlinePlus
National Library of Medicine (NLM)
8600 Rockville Pike
Bethesda, MD 20894
Toll-Free: 888-346-3656
Website: www.medlineplus.gov

National Cancer Institute (NCI)
Public Inquiries Office
6116 Executive Blvd.
Rm. 3036A
Bethesda, MD 20892
Toll-Free: 800-4-CANCER (800-422-6237)
Toll-Free TTY: 800-332-8615
Website: www.cancer.gov
E-mail: cancergovstaff@mail.nih.gov

National Center for Biotechnology Information (NCBI)
8600 Rockville Pike
Bethesda, MD 20894
Website: www.ncbi.nlm.nih.gov
E-mail: info@ncbi.nlm.nih.gov

National Center for Complementary and Integrative Health (NCCIH)
NCCIH Clearinghouse
9000 Rockville Pike
Bethesda, MD 20892
Toll-Free: 888-644-6226
Toll-Free TTY: 866-464-3615
Website: www.nccih.nih.gov
E-mail: info@nccih.nih.gov

National Diabetes Information Clearinghouse (NDIC)
1 Information Way
Bethesda, MD 20892-3560
Toll-Free: 800-860-8747
Phone: 301-654-3327
Fax: 703-738-4929
Website: diabetes.niddk.nih.gov
E-mail: healthinfo@niddk.nih.gov

National Health Information Center (NHIC)
P.O. Box 1133
Washington, DC 20013
Toll-Free: 800-336-4797
Phone: 301-565-4167
Fax: 301-984-4256
Website: www.health.gov/NHIC
E-mail: nhic@hhs.gov

National Heart, Lung, and Blood Institute (NHLBI)
P.O. Box 30105
Bethesda, MD 20824
Phone: 301-592-8573
TTY: 240-629-3255
Fax: 240-629-3246
Website: www.nhlbi.nih.gov
E-mail: nhlbiinfo@nhlbi.nih.gov

National Human Genome Research Institute (NHGRI)
National Institutes of Health (NIH)
31 Center Dr., MSC 2152
Bldg. 31, Rm 4B09
Bethesda, MD 20892-2152
Phone: 301-402-0911
Fax: 301-402-2218
Website: www.genome.gov

National Institute of Allergy and Infectious Diseases (NIAID)
Office of Communications and Government Relations (OCGR)
5601 Fishers Ln., MSC 9806
Bethesda, MD 20892-9806
Toll-Free: 866-284-4107
Phone: 301-496-5717
Toll-Free TDD: 800-877-8339
Fax: 301-402-3573
Website: www.niaid.nih.gov
E-mail: ocpostoffice@niaid.nih.gov

National Institute of Diabetes and Digestive and Kidney Diseases (NIDDK)
Office of Communications and
Public Liaison (OCPL)
Bldg. 31 Rm. 9A06
31 Center Dr. MSC 2560
Bethesda, MD 20892
Toll-Free: 800-891-5390
Phone: 301-496-3583
Website: www2.niddk.nih.gov
E-mail: healthinfo@niddk.nih.gov

National Institute of Environmental Health Sciences (NIEHS)
MD K3-16
P.O. Box 12233
Research Triangle Park, NC 27709
Phone: 919-541-3345
Fax: 919-541-4395
Website: www.niehs.nih.gov

National Institute of General Medical Sciences (NIGMS)
Office of Communications and
Public Liaison (OCPL)
45 Center Dr., MSC 6200
Bethesda, MD 20892-6200
Phone: 301-496-7301
Website: www.nigms.nih.gov
E-mail: info@nigms.nih.gov

National Institute of Neurological Disorders and Stroke (NINDS)
NIH Neurological Institute
P.O. Box 5801
Bethesda, MD 20824
Toll-Free: 800-352-9424
Website: www.ninds.nih.gov

National Institute on Aging (NIA)
Bldg. 31 Rm. 5C27
31 Center Dr. MSC 2292
Bethesda, MD 20892
Toll-Free: 800-222-2225
Phone: 301-496-1752
Toll-Free TTY: 800-222-4225
Fax: 301-496-1072
Website: www.nia.nih.gov
E-mail: niaic@nia.nih.gov

National Institutes of Health (NIH)
9000 Rockville Pike
Bethesda, MD 20892
Phone: 301-496-4000
TTY: 301-402-9612
Website: www.nih.gov

National Vaccine Injury Compensation Program (VICP)
Parklawn Bldg. Rm. 8A-35
5600 Fishers Ln.
Rockville, MD 20857
Toll-Free: 800-338-2382
Website: www.hrsa.gov/
vaccinecompensation
E-mail: healthit@hrsa.gov

National Women's Health Information Center (NWHIC)
200 Independence Ave. S.W.
Washington, DC 20201
Toll-Free: 800-994-9662
Toll-Free TDD: 888-220-5446
Website: www.womenshealth.gov
E-mail: womenshealth@hhs.gov

Occupational Safety and Health Administration (OSHA)
U.S. Department of Labor (DOL)
200 Constitution Ave. N.W.
Rm. N3626
Washington, DC 20210
Toll-Free: 800-321-OSHA
(800-321-6742)
Website: www.osha.gov

Office of Dietary Supplements (ODS)
6100 Executive Blvd.
Rm. 3B01 MSC 7517
Bethesda, MD 20892
Phone: 301-435-2920
Fax: 301-480-1845
Website: dietary-supplements.
info.nih.gov
E-mail: ods@nih.gov

Public Health Emergency (PHE)
Office of the Assistant Secretary
for Preparedness and Response
(ASPR)
200 Independence Ave. S.W.
Rm. 638G
Washington, DC 20201
Website: www.phe.gov

U.S. Department of Agriculture (USDA)
1400 Independence Ave. S.W.
Washington, DC 20250
Phone: 202-720-2791
Website: www.usda.gov

U.S. Department of Health and Human Services (HHS)
200 Independence Ave. S.W.
Washington, DC 20201
Toll-Free: 877-696-6775
Website: www.hhs.gov

U.S. Environmental Protection Agency (EPA)
1200 Pennsylvania Ave. N.W.
Washington, DC 20460
Phone: 202-272-0167
TTY: 202-272-0165
Website: www.epa.gov
E-mail: r8eisc@epa.gov

U.S. Food and Drug Administration (FDA)
10903 New Hampshire Ave.
Silver Spring, MD 20993-0002
Toll-Free: 888-INFO-FDA
(888-463-6332)
Phone: 301-796-8240
Website: www.fda.gov
E-mail: druginfo@fda.hhs.gov

U.S. National Library of Medicine (NLM)
8600 Rockville Pike
Bethesda, MD 20894
Toll-Free: 888-346-3656
Phone: 301-594-5983
Website: www.nlm.nih.gov

Vaccine Adverse Event Reporting System (VAERS)
P.O. Box 1100
Rockville, MD 20849-1100
Toll-Free: 800-822-7967
Toll-Free Fax: 877-721-0366
Website: vaers.hhs.gov

Private Organizations

American Academy of Allergy, Asthma, and Immunology (AAAAI)
555 E. Wells St.
Ste. 1100
Milwaukee, WI 53202
Phone: 414-272-6071
Website: www.aaaai.org
E-mail: Info@aaaai.org

American Academy of Family Physicians (AAFP)
P.O. Box 11210
Shawnee Mission, KS 66207
Toll-Free: 800-274-2237
Phone: 913-906-6000
Website: www.aafp.org
E-mail: aafp@aafp.org

American Association of Blood Banks (AABB)
8101 Glenbrook Rd.
Bethesda, MD 20814
Phone: 301-907-6977
Fax: 301-907-6895
Website: www.aabb.org
E-mail: aabb@aabb.org

American Cancer Society (ACS)
250 Williams St. N.W.
Atlanta, GA 30303
Toll-Free: 800-227-2345
Toll-Free TTY: 866-228-4327
Website: www.cancer.org

American Liver Foundation (AAFP)
75 Maiden Ln.
Ste. 603
New York, NY 10038
Toll-Free: 800-GO-LIVER (800-465-4837) / 888-4HEP-USA (888-443-7872)
Phone: 212-668-1000
Fax: 212-483-8179
Website: www.liverfoundation.org
E-mail: support@liverfoundation.org

American Lung Association (ALA)
1301 Pennsylvania Ave. N.W.
Ste. 800
Washington, DC 20004
Toll-Free: 800-586-4872 (for location of nearest ALA group);
800-548-8252 (to speak with a lung health professional)
Phone: 212-315-8700
Website: www.lungusa.org
E-mail: info@lung.org

American Medical Association (AMA)
515 N. State St.
Chicago, IL 60610
Toll-Free: 800-621-8335
Phone: 312-464-5000
Fax: 312-464-5600
Website: www.ama-assn.org
E-mail: profilescs@ama-assn.org

American Social Health Association (ASHA)
P.O. Box 13827
Research Triangle Park, NC 27709
Toll-Free: 800-656-4673
Phone: 919-361-8400
Fax: 919-361-8425
Website: www.ashastd.org
E-mail: info@ashasexualhealth.org

Hepatitis Foundation International (HFI)
8121 Georgia Ave.
Silver Spring, MD 20910
Toll-Free: 800-891-0707
Phone: 301-565-9410
Website: www.hepatitisfoundation.org
E-mail: Info@hepatitisfoundation.org

Immunization Safety Review Committee (ISR)
Institute of Medicine (IOM)
500 Fifth St. N.W.
Washington, DC 20001
Phone: 202-334-2352
Fax: 202-334-1412
Website: www.iom.edu/imsafety
E-mail: iowww@nas.edu

National Foundation for Infectious Diseases (NFID)
Institute of Medicine (IOM)
Bethesda, MD 20814
Phone: 301-656-0003
Fax: 301-907-0878
Website: www.nfid.org
E-mail: idcourse@nfid.org

National Network for Immunization Information (NNii)
301 University Blvd.
Galveston, TX 77555
Phone: 409-772-0199
Fax: 409-772-5208
Website: www.immunizationinfo.org
E-mail: nnii@i4ph.org

National Patient Advocate Foundation (NPAF)
725 15th St. N.W
10th Fl.
Washington, DC 20005
Phone: 202-347-8009
Fax: 202-347-5579
Website: www.npaf.org
E-mail: caitlin.donovan@npaf.org

The Nemours Foundation
Center for Children's Health Media
1600 Rockland Rd.
Wilmington, DE 19803
Phone: 302-651-4000
Website: www.kidshealth.org or www.teenshealth.org
E-mail: info@kidshealth.org

World Health Organization (WHO)
Ave. Appia 20
1202 Geneva
Switzerland
Phone: 41-22-7912111
Website: www.who.int

Index

Index

Page numbers followed by 'n' indicate a footnote. Page numbers in *italics* indicate a table or illustration.

537